Pharmaceutical Homicide

A Forensic Approach to Patent Safety

David B. Brushwood, RPh, JD, FAPhA

innovativeink
PUBLISHING

innovativeink PUBLISHING

www.innovativeinkpublishing.com
Send all inquiries to:
4050 Westmark Drive
Dubuque, IA 52004-1840

Print ISBN: 979-8-7657-9696-2
eBook ISBN: 979-8-7657-9697-9

Published in the United States of America

Dedication

This book is dedicated to my wife Chris, whose curiosity about the subject of pharmaceutical homicide led to my professional investigations and to the development of this project with her constant support.

Acknowledgments

The author wishes to thank the following colleagues for their assistance in reviewing an early version of this manuscript: David M. Angaran, MS, FCCP, FASHP; William E. Fassett, PhD, RPh, FAPhA; Randy C. Hatton, PharmD, FCCP; Larry Lopez, PharmD, FCCP, BCPS. All errors and omissions remaining in the manuscript are the responsibility of the auth r.

Pharmaceutical Homicide: A Forensic Approach to Patient Safety

Table of Contents

Foreword

Clinton, Indiana, in the mid-1990s, was what many people would refer to as a "typical small Midwest town," with tree-lined streets, well-equipped schools, pleasant parks, and many other community resources that are characteristic of comfortable Midwestern living. It was a pleasant place in which to grow up, to work, to raise a family, and to retire. The Clinton Downtown Historic District had many banks and offices and restaurants and retail stores. Vermilion County Hospital (VCH) provided a broad range of healthcare services for the approximately 10,000 people who lived in Clinton and in the surrounding communities. What the area residents did not know, until several years later, was that the hospital employed a serial killer, a nurse, who was murdering patients using medications that had been acquired through the hospital's pharmacy department.

Orville Lynn Majors was a native of the State of Indiana who graduated from a practical nursing school program in 1989 and began working at VCH in 1993.[1] Almost immediately, the death rate at the hospital increased dramatically. It took two years for the hospital to recognize that the spike in patient deaths was happening during Majors' shifts. An internal investigation disclosed that family members of deceased patients remembered seeing Majors "inject something" into their relatives immediately prior to the death of their loved ones. Several of Majors' nursing colleagues indicated that they felt uncomfortable while working with Majors because of his unprofessional approach to patient care. One of Majors' roommates reported that he had seen Majors bring home vials of potassium chloride and epinephrine.

In March 1995, a formal law enforcement investigation was initiated into the series of suspicious patient deaths at the hospital. The investigation revealed that Majors had been on duty in the patient care area during the sudden and unexpected deaths of seven patients and that no one else had been present during all seven incidents. Investigators concluded that Majors killed these patients by injecting them with potassium chloride and/or with epinephrine. There were approximately 150 patients whose deaths occurred while under Majors' care. For the sake of efficiency, and to avoid confusing the jury, the state prosecutor charged Majors with only seven counts of murder. The jury found Majors guilty of murdering six of these seven patients. The trial court sentenced him to 360 years in prison. This sentence was affirmed on appeal. Majors died in prison in 2017.

One might be tempted to ask: Why weren't Majors' murderous ways discovered sooner? How many lives could have been saved if an earlier investigation had associated Majors' nursing shifts with an unexpected increase in patient deaths during those shifts? How much easier might it have been to identify Majors as a serial killer if an early analysis of the spike in unexpected patient deaths had incorporated the first-hand observations of patients' family members, along with the unease of his fellow nurses, and the testimony of the roommate?

Perhaps the delay in recognizing Majors as a murderer occurred because it seems so bizarrely implausible that any licensed healthcare professional would intentionally use medicines to kill patients. That kind of investigative delay is understandable given the public trust that is extended to healthcare professionals, but it is unacceptable from the perspective of what is known today about pharmaceutical homicide. Delay can be deadly.

One key purpose of this book is to openly address the reality that pharmaceutical homicide occurs in healthcare settings. It may be possible, through greater awareness of the problem, to find early solutions that save lives. As has been said many times, "Justice delayed is justice denied." Many of the perpetrators who commit pharmaceutical homicides think that they have committed "the perfect crime." They think that since pharmaceuticals are so commonly found in American society, they will be overlooked as a murder weapon. Perpetrators of pharmaceutical homicide may be right. They may actually be able to accomplish the perfect crime, until an alert pharmacist or nurse or other healthcare professional notices something that just doesn't seem right, and an investigation is initiated. From a patient safety perspective, the sooner these concerns are raised and investigated, the better.

Anyone who has access to potentially lethal medications has the means to commit murder. This includes the patients for whom potentially lethal medications have been prescribed and to whom they have been dispensed. For example, Myrle Miller of Mifflinburg Pennsylvania was convicted in July 2023 of murdering her 77-year-old husband by administering to him an overdose of her prescribed verapamil. Miller had emptied her husband's bank accounts, and she was designated as beneficiary on several of his life insurance policies. A representative from the local area agency on aging alerted law enforcement to Miller's suspicious activities related to her husband's finances. Based on this tip, an investigation was conducted to determine whether the husband had died for a reason other than natural causes. It was due to this alert notification from the agency on aging that the otherwise unnoticed drug overdose came to the attention of law enforcement. Miller will spend the rest of her life in prison. This tragic case raises questions about how Miller knew that an overdose of her calcium channel blocker could be fatal and how she knew that this type of overdose is difficult to diagnose and manage. Did she read online about this drug's toxic effects? Did a pharmacist inadvertently "teach" her how to murder her husband by counseling her that an overdose of verapamil should be avoided to prevent death of the person taking the drug? With these questions in mind, it is important to consider what steps can be taken by pharmacists, other health professionals, and patients themselves, to prevent the intentional use of medications as murder weapons once they leave a pharmacy.

It takes time to bring a pharmaceutical murderer to justice. Sometimes, it takes a long time. Respiratory therapist Jennifer Hall was suspected of murdering nine of her patients with succinylcholine in 2002.[3] Hall was employed by Hedrick Medical Center in Chillicothe, Missouri. Families of the patients who unexpectedly died while under Hall's care urged the local police chief and prosecutor to investigate and bring murder charges if the evidence warranted prosecution. But Hall had previously been acquitted of charges that she had set fire to a hospital in Harrisonville, Missouri, and law enforcement authorities were wary of once again devoting substantial resources to a complex criminal prosecution without hard proof of guilt. For twenty years the case languished until a new chief of police and a new prosecutor were persuaded by the local coroner to take a closer look at the evidence. Since there is no statute of limitations for murder, the new prosecutor chose to file murder charges against Hall, and in August 2023 Hall was convicted of two counts of involuntary manslaughter. Forensic evidence was key to the successful prosecution, as there was no direct evidence of guilt. Hall has been sentenced to 18 years in prison. The outcome of this case suggests that it may be appropriate to consider other cold cases of suspected pharmaceutical homicide, and to give them a second look with a fresh set of eyes, using updated tools for forensic analysis.

This book describes how medicines that have been placed under the control of pharmacists, and which are intended for use in therapy for patients who need them, are sometimes used instead by criminals to kill people. A surprisingly large number of healthcare professionals have intentionally killed patients within healthcare settings. Healthcare professionals have also stolen pharmaceuticals from healthcare settings and used them to kill relatives, friends, and acquaintances outside a healthcare setting. Patients who have acquired medications from a pharmacy as authorized for them by a prescriber have used these medications as murder weapons. Pharmacies have dispensed defective drugs that have killed patients. This book focuses on identifying the zone of risk for innocent victims who could be intentionally harmed by medications that are weaponized in the commission of a crime. The book also investigates the development and adoption of best practices to protect patients and others from the harm that can be caused by otherwise beneficial medications if these medications are used criminally as murder weapons.

The dictionary definition of "forensics" is "the application of scientific methods and techniques to the investigation of crimes." Most pharmacy laws are not associated with the field of forensics, because they do not relate to the commission of crimes. The focus of forensic pharmacy, as a subset of the larger field of pharmacy law, is specifically on the patterns through which crimes are committed with pharmaceuticals, and the strategies that can be utilized to prevent crimes using pharmaceuticals.

This *Pharmaceutical Homicide* book begins with materials that describe the elements of a crime and the role of pharmacists in the detection and prevention of crimes. The book then describes how pharmaceuticals have been used by notorious criminals in the commission of serial murders. The book also describes the hazards that pharmaceuticals present to certain vulnerable persons who may find themselves in harm's way due to their proximity to a pharmaceutical murderer.

The final sections of the book focus on the pharmaceuticals themselves and on the criminality that may be associated with the production and distribution of defective and/or inherently lethal pharmaceuticals. The book ends with a discussion of the potential exposure to civil liability for malpractice and government prosecution of a negligent healthcare professional following a victim's death due to the lethal effects of medications.

Please note that there is intentional overlap and repetition between the materials in some of the chapters. This has been done to contextualize the materials in each chapter, without requiring cross-references to other chapters. Although the book is organized as a cohesive whole, the chapters in the book have been designed to stand alone with sufficient background information to promote a clear understanding of the basic principles of patient safety and pharmacy regulation.

This book is intended primarily for practicing pharmacists and for student pharmacists. Pharmacists have the responsibility to control access to all medications that can be used in the commission of pharmaceutical homicide.

Pharmacists are the last link in a long chain of drug discovery, experimentation, approval, development, formulation, distribution, and selection. Pharmacists are strategically positioned as a "last best chance" or the "safety-net" to protect patients from harm due to the diversion of pharmaceuticals from therapeutic use to criminal use.

Practitioners and students in fields such as medicine, nursing, respiratory therapy, patient safety, healthcare administration, law, criminal justice, regulatory compliance, and journalism will also find the information in this book to be of significant interest and value.

The goal of this book is to promote successful patient safety activities in healthcare generally and in pharmacy practice specifically. Pharmaceutical homicide occurs in both the inpatient and outpatient settings. The challenges and recommendations discussed in this book are significant for both institutional pharmacy practice and for community pharmacy practice. Pharmacists must have assistance from others to effectively address the problem of pharmaceutical homicide. Readers of this book who work collaboratively with pharmacists will quickly see a role for themselves in sharing responsibility for preventing murder with medications. All readers of this book are cordially invited to consider a contribution that they might make to patient safety activities that are directed toward preventing pharmaceutical homicide. It will require a unified and substantial effort to raise awareness of this problem and to implement effective solutions.

References

1. Majors v. State, 773 N.E.2d 231 (ind. 2002).

2. Strawser J. Convicted killer Myrle Miller seeking new trial, to overturn conviction. The Daily Item. (March 19, 2024). **https://www.dailyitem.com/news/convicted-killer-myrle-miller-seeking-new-trial-to-overturn-conviction/article_005c4ad2-e623-11ee-8443-d7cd4e65f3e5.html**

3. Yeatman D. Missouri respiratory therapist Jennifer Hall is sentenced to 18 years in prison for causing deaths of at least two patients, aged 75 and 37. The Daily Mail (August 21, 2023). **https://www.dailymail.co.uk/news/article-12429309/Missouri-respiratory-therapist-Jennifer-Hall-sentenced-18-years-prison-causing-deaths-two-patients-aged-75-37.html**

Chapter 1

Patient Safety and Healthcare Killings

Pharmaceuticals are among the most dangerous consumer products in American commerce. When used appropriately, pharmaceuticals can prevent or cure disease. When used inappropriately, pharmaceuticals can be deadly. In the absence of intense and comprehensive oversight by government agencies, healthcare institutions, and healthcare professionals, the misuse of pharmaceuticals would cause significant harm to the public. An unregulated market in pharmaceuticals cannot protect people from the hazards of medication use. These hazards are an example of the market failure that economists and regulatory scholars generally refer to as "information asymmetry." According to regulatory theory, a market failure can serve as justification for government regulation.

Market Failure of Pharmaceuticals

Information asymmetry occurs when two parties to a transaction are not equally informed as to the nature of the potential benefits and detriments of a product or a service that is the subject of the transaction between the parties. For example, the technical complexity of a product such as a cellphone or a computer may lead to some purchasers becoming "dazed, dazzled, and confused" by the intricate attributes of the product, so that they purchase the product without a complete understanding of what is being purchased. The sellers of the product usually know much more about their product than do the purchasers of the product. This knowledge imbalance is a type of information asymmetry.

A profession that is dedicated to proficiency in the field "information technology" has evolved to provide expertise for those who need guidance in the use of computer systems and other technological products. By following the advice of experts who understand the complexities of IT, users who lack that technical understanding can acquire a product that is appropriate for them, and they can use the product in a manner that is of most benefit to them.

Fortunately, most commercial products are not subject to the market failure of information asymmetry. For example, a kitchen knife is often considered to be a "pre-experience good" because the value of a kitchen knife (or virtually any other kitchen utensil) can be discerned prior to its purchase by anyone based on mere visualization and manipulation of the product using common knowledge rather than technical expertise. The same can generally be said of furniture, hand tools, office supplies, and other retail products for which size and shape and utility are obvious to any person prior to purchasing the product. There is no information asymmetry. There is no market failure with these pre-experience goods.

Consistent with this approach, there is another category of goods and services that can be classified as "experience goods" because their value can easily be known, although only through an actual circumstance of using the good or service and not by examination prior to their use or acquisition. A haircut or a restaurant meal falls into this category. It is difficult to know the value of these items until they are experienced, but once that experience occurs, it is relatively easy to separate good quality from poor quality. General knowledge allows one to recognize a bad haircut or a bad restaurant meal after it has been experienced, although it is difficult to evaluate this sort of product until it has been experienced. Again, no technical expertise is required. There is no market failure with experience goods.

Medications are very different. Regulatory theory classifies medications as "post-experience goods," because it is often impossible to know the value of medications until long after they have been used, perhaps even months if not years after their use. In an open market, where any uninformed user would be able to purchase any pharmaceutical product for any reason or for no reason at all, the market would fail to efficiently provide an acceptable therapeutic return on investment. There would be therapeutic failures and toxicities that cause harm to the uninformed product user. The safety and efficacy aspects of a pharmaceutical product are invisible to those who lack formal training in pharmacotherapy. Uninformed choices can lead to inappropriate actions that produce harmful results for untrained product users. This is information asymmetry. It is a market failure. The market failure justifies government regulation.

A government solution to a market failure of information asymmetry, as it relates to pharmaceuticals, is to require that medications be provided to users only under the supervision of a person who is educated and experienced in the safe and effective use of the product. The government requires formal education and training of this person and licenses this person. The government then assigns to this person the responsibility for assuring safe and effective product use, based on this professional person's specialized technical expertise. Educated and trained professionals who prescribe, dispense, and administer pharmaceuticals can apply knowledge and skill that will convert a post-experience good into a pre-experience good, by anticipating in advance the effects that the product is likely to deliver in the future, thereby enhancing the beneficial aspects of those effects and minimizing the detrimental effects.

Malevolent Use of Professional Expertise

It is quite clear that the rationale for government regulation is for the professional knowledge and skill of dedicated licensed caregivers to be used in promoting beneficial outcomes from medication use. The unfortunate reality is that a small number of criminally motivated professionals may instead use their pharmaceutical expertise to cause harm. An article by Johnstone, Katz, and Stanley reports four tragic examples of pharmaceutical homicide that were committed by skillful and knowledgeable healthcare professionals.[1] These three anesthesiologists also describe how they personally assisted in the successful prosecution of the murderers.

The four homicides described in the article are significantly different, yet they share the common element that the murder weapon was a medication that had been removed from a healthcare setting with criminal intent:

- A nurse was convicted of murdering her husband with rocuronium. The nurse set fire to the house that she shared with her husband, with her husband's body inside. The husband's body was badly burned, but rocuronium levels were detected in the husband's blood and liver samples. A charred needle cap similar to those used at the hospital where the nurse worked was found in the burned house. Expert testimony described the effects of rocuronium and the availability of rocuronium in the hospital where the nurse had been employed.
- An anesthesiologist's wife died unexpectedly from what was initially thought to be natural causes. The wife's father suspected foul play and an investigation was begun. An investigator discovered that the anesthesiologist had previously been acquitted of murdering the husband of a woman with whom he was having an affair. Both women's bodies were exhumed, and evidence of an injection of succinylcholine in the buttocks of both victims was discovered. Expert testimony described the effects of injected succinylcholine. The anesthesiologist was convicted of both murders.
- A pharmacist stole fentanyl patches along with injectable fentanyl from the crime laboratory where she worked. Her husband died from a fentanyl overdose administered by the pharmacist through fentanyl-laced soup and through the application of patches. Evidence showed the husband had discovered the pharmacist's addiction to

methamphetamine that the she obtained from her workplace. The husband had threatened to reveal this information to the pharmacist's employer. The pharmacist was convicted and sentenced to life in prison. Expert testimony was used to establish the lethal dose of fentanyl.

- A small-town physician was convicted of murdering a former patient who was described as "mentally challenged." The bizarre facts showed that the physician had administered fentanyl and midazolam to the victim for no medical purpose. The physician had then practiced intubation and cardiopulmonary resuscitation on the victim as a means to hone the physician's skills with these procedures. The victim had supposedly given his consent, and the entire proceedings were videotaped for later educational purposes. Expert testimony established that the drug doses were lethal and that the drugs caused the victim's death.

In reporting these criminal actions, the authors emphasize how important it is for pharmaceutical expertise to be used in the investigation and prosecution of crimes. The safety of future patients is enhanced when criminally motivated healthcare professionals are disabused of the notion that they can get away with murder by malevolently applying their expertise with medications. Pharmaceuticals are not the perfect weapons for committing perfect crimes, as long as forensic principles are applied by benevolent healthcare professionals in collaboration with law enforcement authorities.

System of Regulatory Oversight for Pharmaceuticals

Pharmaceutical regulation is designed to promote patient safety in the use of medications. Drugs are the most commonly chosen therapeutic agents in healthcare. All drugs have risks. The purpose of the drug regulatory system is to minimize unintended adverse patient outcomes and also to protect people from intentional criminality in medication use. The focus of pharmaceutical regulation is on drug safety, which is a key element of patient safety.

Before a new drug can be marketed, the drug must undergo extensive clinical trials to demonstrate through substantial evidence that the drug will safely produce beneficial therapeutic effects when used as directed. Pharmaceutical labeling is carefully crafted to provide truthful and non-misleading information that promotes patient safety. Special packaging may be developed to facilitate safe medication use. Regulatory safeguards are in place to minimize product adulteration and/or counterfeiting. Pharmaceuticals that are in violation of government regulations can be seized, their further distribution can be enjoined, and the distributor can be criminally prosecuted.

Most new drugs are classified as prescription-only, because the effects of the drugs in a large number of users are not yet known. A systematic program of post-marketing surveillance is conducted by the government to determine whether there may be unexpected adverse drug effects in a large population of users. Serious but infrequent adverse effects may not be detected in pre-marketing clinical trials that have been conducted with a relatively small number of subjects.

State-licensed prescribers utilize a methodic approach to diagnosis and treatment that results in an order for medication that meets a specific patient's needs. Pharmacists evaluate prescriptions to assure that potential problems such as drug–drug interactions are resolved before a patient receives a medication and that the right patient receives the right medication with the right directions at the right time.

The complex system of drug development, distribution, and therapeutic use is premised on the assumption that all involved parties are well intentioned. Patient safety considerations are built on a foundation of both professional responsibility and a firm commitment to the public good. Yet this is not a consistently valid assumption. An article by Menshawey and Menshawey evaluates the motives of healthcare murderers, and the authors conclude that "There needs to be serious consideration of the intentional harm of a patient as part of training healthcare workers in patient safety."[2] The authors contend that reliance on law enforcement to effectively detect and prevent pharmaceutical homicide is a mistaken approach.

Menshawey and Menshawey describe the many challenges faced by prosecutors in proving, beyond a reasonable doubt, that a pharmaceutical homicide has been committed and that the alleged perpetrator committed the crime. Given the significant barriers to a successful investigation and prosecution, law enforcement cannot be relied on to protect a community from pharmaceutical homicide. The authors challenge healthcare institutions and healthcare professionals to incorporate pharmaceutical homicide into existing patient safety programs to promote the best interests of the community being served.

The many layers of established regulatory oversight within the healthcare system can promote patient safety by reducing the risk of unsafe medication use, but regulatory oversight cannot remove all risks. This is why institutional patient safety activities are often referred to as "risk management" rather than as "risk elimination." The frequency of medication use, the ubiquitousness of medications in the healthcare system, and the unavoidability of risks, all of these continually challenge pharmaceutical regulators to develop new strategies that promote patient safety. The intent of pharmaceutical regulation is to promote reasonable and measured risks, where the likelihood of benefit outweighs the likelihood of harm. Medication use safety is a critical component of patient safety. Safe drugs can be used safely, but safe drugs can also be used unsafely, and the goal of patient safety activities is to assure the safe use of safe drugs.

Patient Safety Orphan

Current patient safety activities do not address all risks of medication use. Two scholars who have spent their careers studying pharmaceutical homicide have expressed concern that what they call "health care serial murder" (HCSM) is a "patient safety orphan."[3] They use the phrase "orphan" to emphasize that HCSM receives little attention when issues of patient safety are formally addressed. Kenneth Kizer and Beatrice Yorker contend that the complexity of the issues related to HCSM have led to low prioritization of system changes that would prevent intentional killings by healthcare professionals in healthcare settings. They speculate that the incidence of HCSM may be much larger than has been reported, because the accumulation and aggregation of data on HCSM is not conducted through any recognized program. They suggest that it may be misleading and counterproductive to view HCSM as a horrifying yet insignificant outlier in the grand scheme of medication adverse events.

Kizer and Yorker contend that HCSM should be incorporated into patient safety programs because HCSM has many of the same characteristics as other patient safety challenges. An approach that incorporates HCSM into patient safety programs could indirectly facilitate the prevention of inadvertent errors while the purposeful consideration of HCSM would also directly addresses the prevention of intentional harm. There are similarities between harms caused by inadvertence and harms caused by intentionality. The investigations of both intentional and unintentional harms are hampered by a disinclination by healthcare professionals to share information about potentially problematic healthcare colleagues. This understandable reticence to "rat out" a teammate can lead to delayed recognition of obvious problems, to inadequate examination of adverse events, and to a failure to investigate the cause of unexpected and unexplained fatalities.

A Perfect Place for Homicide

One of the most chilling explanations of why and how pharmaceutical homicide occurs is told by Bruce Sackman, who spent his career as a Special Agent in Charge with the Department of Veterans Affairs Office of Inspector General. Sackman describes hospitals as the "perfect hunting ground" for serial killers.[4] Sackman explains that patients have no choice but to place their implicit trust in healthcare professionals. Sometimes, that trust is betrayed by healthcare murderers. Furthermore, hospitals are an environment in which death is common and is usually attributed to an underlying medical condition rather than to criminal activity.

Hospitals are also an environment with systems and responsibilities that are confusing to law enforcement officers. Healthcare professionals use technical medical language, and detectives find themselves on very uncomfortable territory when they investigate alleged criminality in a hospital setting. Specialized healthcare practices and procedures are difficult to interpret, and patient privacy is zealously guarded. After a patient dies, there is understandable financial pressure to thoroughly clean the hospital room to make it available for the next patient who is waiting for care. Evidence of a crime may be discarded before law enforcement has the opportunity to investigate the potential crime scene.

Murderers who work in hospitals often volunteer for unpopular night shifts when there is little supervision. There is no need to bring a murder weapon into the hospital because lethal pharmaceuticals are readily available. The evidence of an attack on a patient is difficult to discover because it may be only a tiny pinprick on the victim's skin or an indiscernible puncture of a patient's existing intravenous line.

Nurse Mary Sullivan reported an ominous quote from Special Agent Sackman at a "Forensics in Healthcare Conference" in Omaha, during his presentation titled, "Red Flags of Healthcare Serial Killers."[5] At the conference, Sackman reportedly said: "If I were inclined to want to kill a lot of people over a long time period and not get caught, I'd search for a place where I could do this without much difficulty. It would have to be somewhere that death is a common occurrence with a wide choice of prey who wouldn't give me much resistance; a place I could work alone and where privacy with a victim is actually encouraged; a place I wouldn't have a supervisor looking over my shoulder, especially if I wanted to work during the evening or night hours; a place that has a variety of weapons to choose from with easy access—and most importantly, where physical evidence is routinely destroyed; a place where any '"whistleblowers'" would receive more harassment than I would as the accused, and ideally a place where the victim would be written off as crazy if he has the audacity to accuse me of trying to kill him. It sounds as if a hospital is the perfect place for me!"

Although Special Agent Sackman focuses his attention on the environment of hospitals as an opportunity for the commission of crimes against patients, the reality is that many other venues also provide ample opportunity for pharmaceutical homicides. The luridness of serial murders within hospitals and the betrayal of trust placed in healthcare institutions by vulnerable patients are particularly disheartening and alarming. For this reason, a focus on hospitals as the ideal place for murder is understandable. Yet it may be equally common that people are murdered with pharmaceuticals in their own homes by people who acquired the medications from legitimate sources for therapeutic purposes. The treachery of a person for whom affection is felt, or was at one times felt, may be as profound as the betrayal of responsibility by a licensed healthcare professional. The trusting relationships between friends and family members, along with the sanctuary that a home environment seemingly provides, can create opportunities for pharmaceutical homicide outside healthcare institutions.

Unsafe Practices and Threats to Patient Safety

The medication use system has not historically been designed to promote patient safety. Efficiency of distribution, rather than patient protection, has traditionally been the goal of the medication use system. In the community setting, prescribers customarily have issued prescriptions using Latin words and abbreviations that patients cannot understand. The creative names of the most frequently prescribed drugs have been chosen as a marketing tool to increase product sales, rather than selecting more descriptive names that accurately represent the unique chemical properties of the drugs. The similarity of these exotic and nondescriptive drug names can lead to confusion.

Prescriptions have historically been scribbled semi-legibly on small pieces of paper, or they have been telephoned quickly to a busy pharmacist who transcribes what has been heard onto a note that is later rewritten. Questions that arise about the accuracy or appropriateness of a prescription cannot be easily resolved because a pharmacist usually lacks access to the full patient care record. Contacting the prescriber for clarification is often a futile effort because busy prescribers are usually unavailable. Most prescribers are trying their best to see as many patients as possible so that they can generate adequate revenues. Patients are generally offered an opportunity to consult with a pharmacist when they pick up their medication, but most patients decline this offer. The printed information sheets that pharmacists distribute to patients with medications are often mistaken for sales receipts, and they are often discarded without being read. It is an unsafe medication use system. Concerns for patient safety in the traditional medication use system are justified by the frequency of adverse drug effects and the lack of systematic safeguards.

Technology has somewhat curtailed or dampened the threats to patient safety in the community setting, but it has not reduced them to significant extent. Many patients no longer have a primary care physician, so they rely on urgent care centers or a hospital emergency room for routine treatments, with little continuity of care and no certainty that a useful and comprehensive healthcare record is being created. Electronic prescriptions that are transmitted from the prescriber to the pharmacist prevent patients from ever seeing their prescriptions and recognizing possible errors. The lack of tangible access to the prescription removes one way in which patients can protect themselves from harm. With electronic medication ordering, prescribers select patient names, drug names, directions for use, and other prescription information, from drop-down menus on desktop computers or on handheld electronic devices. There is the constant threat of a prescriber making an incorrect menu choice that is one line above or one line below what is intended by the prescriber. Pharmacy computer systems are programmed to alert the pharmacist to potential problems with a patient's prescriptions, but the alerts are so frequent that pharmacists experience "alert fatigue" diminishing the usefulness of the computer information and threatening to interfere with a meaningful response to alerts that relate to serious problems.

Given the deficiencies of the community-based medication use system, it is not difficult to imagine how strict protocols for medication management can be overlooked, resulting in the unsafe use of pharmaceutical products, either unintentionally or intentionally.

The medication use system in the hospital setting also poses threats to patient safety. Patients who are admitted to a hospital are often cared for by hospitalists who are unfamiliar with a patient's medical history and who must learn not only what drug therapy has and has not worked in the past but also how the patient prefers to use medications. The electronic healthcare record has created barriers between healthcare professionals who no longer directly communicate with each other because they must focus on information obtained from a computer screen. Hospital pharmacists are accustomed to unusual medication orders because hospitalized patients are critically ill, and they often require individualized patient-specific therapy that differs from the standard approach; thus, there may be a reluctance to challenge a medication order that is somewhat outside the norm for patient care.

Medications are usually obtained from the hospital's central pharmacy, which is often located at a distance from the patient care areas. To provide immediate access, many medications can be obtained by nursing staff from decentralized automated dispensing units that are designed to limit medication availability to those situations in which patients truly need medication quickly. These dispensing units are also designed so that they do not create unnecessary barriers to access for critically important patient care. Nurses can develop workarounds that allow access to medications in an automated dispensing unit without oversight or control by the pharmacy department.

If a prescribed medication is not needed for several hours, it may be processed through the pharmacy department's economically efficient robotic system that has limited human oversight. In the hospital setting, nurses administer medications to patients, and nurses stand as the final check to assure patient safety. However, staffing shortages can result in the frequent use of "travel nurses" or "floating nurses" who are skilled and motivated but may not be familiar with the medications used on a particular medical service. There may be a tendency to think that something unusual must be acceptable because somewhere earlier in the chain of order entry, order processing, and medication delivery, any potential problem would have already been resolved.

The medication use system is unsafe due to these threats to quality. Both community practice settings and institutional practice settings are fraught with threats to patient safety. There is a need for additional safety checks to protect patients from harm.

The complexities and challenges of caring for ill patients, all of whom require unique and personalized treatments, create inevitable situations in which a commitment to patient safety standards may fall through the cracks. For some healthcare professionals, it is embarrassing, or at least uncomfortable, to acknowledge that their practices may at times threaten patient safety. Hospitals and other healthcare institutions may be slow to recognize that the care they provide is less than perfectly safe. The "can-do" attitude of healthcare professionals and healthcare organizations can lead to overconfidence that masks the risk of error in patient care.

Against a headwind of denial and self-protectionism, a strong movement advocating greater attention to patient safety has become prominent within the healthcare community. The modern patient safety movement was catalyzed in late 1999 when the Institute of Medicine (IOM) published a report titled "To Err Is Human."[6]

Institute of Medicine Report

The IOM Report is credited with having started a patient safety movement that emerged in 2000 and continues today. Several observations of the IOM Report are particularly instructive, and they are quoted here:

> The common initial reaction when an error occurs is to find and blame someone. However, even apparently single events or errors are due most often to the convergence of multiple contributing factors. Blaming an individual does not change these factors and the same error is likely to recur. Preventing errors and improving safety for patients require a systems approach in order to modify the conditions that contribute to errors. People working in health care are among the most educated and dedicated workers in any industry. The problem is not bad people; the problem is that the system needs to be made safer. (IOM Report, p. 49)

The IOM Report also emphasizes the importance of finding productive forward-looking solutions, rather than using counterproductive backward-looking punishment.

> Current responses to errors tend to focus on the active errors by punishing individuals (e.g., firing or suing them), retraining or other responses aimed at preventing recurrence of the active error. Although a punitive response may be appropriate under some cases (e.g., deliberate misfeasance), it is not an effective way to prevent recurrence. Because large system failures represent latent failures coming together in unexpected ways, they appear to be unique in retrospect. Since the same mix of factors is unlikely to occur again, efforts to prevent specific active errors are not likely to make the system any safer. (IOM Report, p. 56)

This advice instructs not only that blaming and punishing erring individuals is pointless but also that an in-depth investigation of a single error is of limited value. Such an approach might yield a large amount of information about an inadvertent error, and it may prevent that error from occurring again, but other potential errors could be ignored. Taking a systems view requires consideration of all types of errors that might occur, not just those errors that have occurred.

The IOM Report focuses almost entirely on the system of healthcare, and the possibility that healthcare practitioners within the system can be the victims of poor system design.

Although almost all accidents result from human error, it is now recognized that these errors are usually induced by faulty systems that "set people up" to fail. Correction of these system failures is the key to safe performance of individuals. System design—how an organization works, its processes and procedures—is an institutional responsibility. Only the institution can redesign its systems for safety; the great majority of effort in improving safety should focus on safe systems, and the health care organization itself should be held responsible for safety. (IOM Report, p. 169)

As the foundational primer for the patient safety movement, the IOM Report focuses almost exclusively on "forgive and remember" system improvements that de-emphasize individual responsibility for patient safety. This perspective is understandably appropriate for inadvertent human errors of a kind that anyone could make in a system that lacks adequate support and resources to promote error prevention.

On the other hand, this is an approach that can create challenges with the identification of criminally motivated pharmaceutical murderers. It is an approach that positions pharmaceutical homicide beyond the reach of system-oriented patient safety programs. Systems don't commit crimes—people commit crimes. Focusing on system inadequacies, rather than on individual actions, may lead to criminality going unnoticed.

Patient Safety in Practice

Despite unspoken opposition from some healthcare organizations and from defensive healthcare professionals, the patient safety movement has endured. The systems approach to patient safety has softened the threats that were initially perceived by insecure and/or intimidated individual professionals and healthcare institutions. Techniques such as "root cause analysis" and "failure mode and effects analysis" have emphasized how systems can set up individuals to fail. The consequence of an identified system failure will usually be conditional forgiveness of an erring person and the implementation of system-wide improvements. The patient safety movement has stressed the necessity of creating a "just culture," where individuals are not scapegoated for system failures that the individuals were powerless to prevent.

One of the key aspects of the patient safety movement has been an emphasis on evidence-based data analysis. A warm, self-congratulatory feeling that patients must be safe because maximal efforts are being made to keep patients safe has given way to a focus on empirical data that actually measure patient safety. Through the recording and examination of data, it is possible to discover "signals" that identify threats to patient safety. The aggregation of data can expose trends that threaten patient safety, allowing a richer level of analysis than would be possible based on individual observation and memory. Aggregated data provide a starting point for an investigation. Data are not conclusive of any inappropriate activity.

Of the many types of medical care available in the treatment of patients, medications are particularly well disposed to evidence-based analysis. Researchers and practitioners have collaborated effectively to evaluate the correlation between structure, process, and outcomes within clinical practice by examining patterns of institutional medication use. "Structure" refers to the availability of resources that have the potential to improve patient outcomes. Human resources, information technology, and administrative support are examples of structure. "Process" refers to the application of resources to address challenges in patient care. Effective processes can be established through the development and implementation of policies and procedures that reflect best practices for the overall institution or for a group of practitioners within the institution. "Outcomes" refers to the results produced using the available resources, through the application of existing processes. Death, disease, disability, discomfort, and dissatisfaction are sometimes referred to as the "Five Ds" that can be monitored to determine whether outcomes are improving within an institution. It is outcomes that really matter, but structure and process are closely related to outcomes. Improvements made in structures and process of drug therapy can elevate the quality of outcomes for institutionalized patients.

Among the "Five Ds" designating outcomes that can be monitored and evaluated, death is obviously the most significant adverse outcome. It is final and irreversible. Life and death are mutually exclusive. Life and death are sometimes referred to as dichotomous variables or nominal variables. Determining the cause of a person's death is both a medical exercise and a legal exercise. When a person has died, it is necessary to look backward and determine whether the death was caused by the actions of a person who was in a position of responsibility for the deceased individual. This is an application of patient safety principles that moves beyond the system failure approach. While a minimal level of preventable outcomes related to dissatisfaction, disease, disability, or discomfort might be considered as inevitable and remediable, or even tolerable, preventable death is never an acceptable outcome.

There must be regulatory consequences following an action by an individual that causes the death of another individual, particularly when the individual's harmful action is intentional. Pharmaceutical homicide is both a tragic individual crime and a catastrophe for the medication use system that has failed to prevent it. While inadvertent error may be forgiven, criminality must be punished. All humans make occasional mistakes, and inadvertent human errors can be addressed through system improvements. Not all humans commit murder, and pharmaceutical homicide must be dealt with through proportional punishment. The victims of crimes, and their survivors, deserve to have perpetrators held legally accountable for their criminal misdeeds.

Conclusion

Pharmaceutical homicide is a patient safety orphan that is crying out for adoption by the now well-established patient safety movement. Incorporating pharmaceutical homicide into the mainstream of patient safety activities can help determine whether murder with medications is an infrequent event or whether, instead, the reported incidence of pharmaceutical homicide is merely the tip of a horrifying iceberg. There may be a naïve belief within the field of patient safety that pharmaceutical homicide is such a rare and unusual event that it is not possible to detect or prevent it. It has often been said that "seeing is believing." This familiar phrase could explain why many of those who have not seen pharmaceutical homicide do not believe that it happens often enough to actively look for it. But absence of evidence is not evidence of absence. It is also true that "believing is seeing." People tend not to acknowledge they have seen something if they aren't looking for it because they don't believe that it exists. Pharmaceutical homicide is real. Once the established patient safety systems acknowledge pharmaceutical homicide as a significant threat that must be aggressively sought out and immediately dealt with, medication use will be made considerably safer.

Key Takeaways

- People are a significant component of any healthcare system. A focus on "the system" to identify threats to patient safety makes perfect sense in theory, because it is well known that system failures can lead to adverse outcomes for patients. Inadequate equipment, communication barriers, weak leadership, and outdated policies and procedures are examples of system factors that set up healthcare team members to fail. On the other hand, no system can function effectively if healthcare professionals actively seek ways to game the system or if they develop workarounds that undermine the system. Systems can be thwarted by people who are part of the system. The people in the system must support the system just as the system must support the people in the system. Blaming the system after an adverse event has occurred, and forgiving the people who have erred, is appropriate only when the people were trying hard rather than hardly trying. It is an inconvenient truth that not all members of the healthcare team are motivated to help others rather than to harm them. Any assessment of the healthcare system must consider the possibility that a person who was motivated by ill will has interfered with system safeguards to the detriment of patients and others. System disruptors must be removed from the system to preserve system integrity and to promote patient safety.

- The concept of a "just culture" in healthcare must incorporate justice for victims of crimes. In a just culture, people must take those actions that are morally right and fair. It is unfair and morally wrong to criminalize behaviors that could not be avoided due to the imperfection of the human condition. A just culture focuses on behavioral choices and not only on the fact of error or the harm caused by a behavior. Justice is both a legal and a medical concept. The evaluation of healthcare systems must include assessment of aberrant individual conduct even if no adverse outcome has been identified. Waiting for an adverse outcome to occur does not protect patients. It is consistent with the healthcare concept of a just culture, and it is also consistent with the legal principle of justice, for suspicions of potentially harmful activity by healthcare team members to be reported and examined even if no harm has occurred.
- The risk of pharmaceutical homicide is present in any healthcare setting where medications are used. The classification of risk usually incorporates the probability of harm and the magnitude of harm. If harm is unlikely to occur and the consequences are minimal when harm does occur, then the risk is considered low. For harms that are very likely to occur and that are very consequential when they do occur, the risk is considered high. In between low and high risks there are two other possibilities that are often referred to as moderate risks. These risks are either highly probable but of low magnitude, or they are of low probability but high magnitude. Pharmaceutical homicide likely falls into this latter category of moderate risk. Fortunately, pharmaceutical homicide is somewhat unusual (at least this is the current belief—nobody really knows because nobody is systematically recording, reporting, aggregating, and evaluating data). Unfortunately, pharmaceutical homicide is hugely consequential. This is why

pharmaceutical homicide should be classified as a moderate risk. Incorporating this moderate risk into patient safety programs is a necessity in any healthcare setting.

References

1. Johnstone RE, Katz RL, Stanley TH. Homicides using muscle relaxants, opioids, and anesthetic drugs: anesthesiologist assistance in their investigation and prosecution. *Anesthesiology.* 2011 Mar;114(3):713-716.

2. Menshawey R, Menshawey E. Brave Clarice-healthcare serial killers, patterns, motives, and solutions. *Forensic Sci Med Pathol.* 2023 Sep;19(3):452–463.

3. Kizer KW, Yorker BC. Health care serial murder: a patient safety orphan. *Jt Comm J Qual Patient Saf.* 2010 Apr;36(4):186–191.

4. Sackman B, Vecchione M, Schmetterer J. *Behind the Murder Curtain.* New York, NY: Post Hill Press; 2020.

5. Sullivan MK. Serial murder in healthcare. *Nurs Manage.* 2009 Jun;40(6):32–36.

6. *To Err is Human: Building a Safer Health System.* Washington, DC: Institute of Medicine; 1999.

Chapter 2

Foundations of Pharmaceutical Forensics

Medications have been used as implements for the commission of crimes for decades, even for centuries. While all murders are horrifying, it is particularly appalling for a valuable product that is intended for the most beneficial of purposes to be used instead as an instrument of harm. Pharmaceutical crimes may be surprising, shocking, outrageous, and unthinkable, but they should not be considered uncommon. They have been extensively documented and widely reported throughout history. Criminals will use whatever weapon they have available to commit their crimes, and medications are often widely available. The most heinous crime that can be committed with pharmaceuticals is homicide. People can kill other people with pharmaceuticals. The legal process for achieving justice following the commission of pharmaceutical crimes is the same as the legal process for addressing any other crime. There are no special rules in criminal law for pharmaceutical crimes, although the nature of pharmaceutical products when they are used as murder weapons may lead to nuanced applications of conventional criminal laws.

A Brief Review of the Pharmaceutical Homicide Literature

There is a significant body of literature regarding the crime of pharmaceutical homicide. One of the most interesting narratives is found in a book titled, *The Case of the Murderous Dr. Cream: The Hunt for a Victorian Era Serial Killer*, by Dean Jobb (2021).[1] This book describes how in 1892, Dr. Thomas Neill Cream was hanged in London following a criminal career that extended from Canada to the United States and eventually to England. As suspicions arose regarding Dr. Cream's criminal conduct, he simply moved on to a different location where he was not well known. Relocation was an effective way to avoid justice in the late 1800s, because communication about one's criminal acts often did not travel along with one's person. The book's author explains that Dr. Cream was a qualified gynecologist/abortionist who often would botch the procedures he conducted, and who then gave his victims capsules containing a mixture of cocaine, morphine, and strychnine as a supposed remedy for their postsurgical complications. The victims did not live to tell the story of the harm that had been caused to them by Dr. Cream' poor surgical technique. His botched procedures were effectively covered up through pharmaceutical homicide.

Chicago pharmacists played a key role in the first conviction of Dr. Cream for murder. After fleeing the City of Toronto, where he was suspected of having committed several murders, Dr. Cream set up a practice in Northern Illinois. At that time, prescriptions were often written without directions for use, so it was difficult for a pharmacist to know the intended purpose of a prescribed medication. Following the death of one of Dr. Cream's patients, the pharmacist who had prepared a medication that had been ingested by that patient reported to police that Dr. Cream was blackmailing him to remain silent about the contents of the prescription. Although no charges were filed against Dr. Cream on this occasion, the pharmacist's complaint brought Dr. Cream to the attention of law enforcement. One year later, the husband of a woman with whom Dr. Cream was having an affair died from strychnine poisoning. Dr. Cream blamed the pharmacist who prepared the medication. The police conducted a thorough investigation, including an examination of the pharmacy's practices and procedures for medication compounding. No illegal practices were discovered at the pharmacy. However, the investigation resulted in the conviction of Dr. Cream for the crime of second-degree murder. For unknown reasons, Dr. Cream was released from the Illinois State Penitentiary after several years, and he quickly moved to England, where he continued committing pharmaceutical homicides for which he was eventually convicted and executed.

Similar pharmaceutical crimes in a more modern context are described in the book, *Prescription for Murder: The True Story of Dr. Harold Frederick Shipman*, written by Brian Whittle and Jean Ritchie.[2] The authors describe the murderous career of an English family practitioner who is thought to have killed over 200 of his patients. Most of the patients were elderly and in failing health. Their deaths were attributed to "old age" by Dr. Shipman in the death certificates that he signed. The cluster of deaths associated with Dr. Shipman's patients, and the large number of cremation forms submitted for his patients, raised concerns in the mind of the local coroner. The matter was referred to the police, who investigated and found no evidence of wrongdoing. This investigation was later criticized as having been hasty and poorly conducted.

The end of Dr. Shipman's pharmaceutical homicides came when he forged a will that designated him as the beneficiary of a patient whom he had killed. The patient's family contested the will. The patient's body was exhumed, and the results of an autopsy showed morphine levels that implicated Dr. Shipman as a murderer. Dr. Shipman was convicted of murdering 15 of his patients. He committed suicide in prison. The pharmacist who supplied medications to Dr. Shipman was absolved of criminal responsibility, although she was "severely censured" by the licensing agency. The licensing agency concluded that the pharmacist had allowed herself to be charmed by Dr. Shipman and that she had "made serious lapses" in allowing Dr. Shipman to acquire large quantities of morphine. Nevertheless, the pharmacist was permitted to continue practicing pharmacy.

Dr. Sheri Fink's book *Five Days at Memorial*[3] tells a fascinating story of alleged pharmaceutical homicide. The book describes the chaos that existed at Memorial Hospital in New Orleans in the aftermath of Hurricane Katrina. The hurricane virtually destroyed many areas of New Orleans in August 2005. The book focuses on the skilled nursing and rehabilitation floor of the hospital, where patients were allegedly murdered because the healthcare professionals at the hospital believed that the challenges of caring for the patients were too great. The author describes the lack of communication within the hospital; the failure of utilities such as water, sewer, and HVAC; and the lack of leadership support experienced by the healthcare professionals on this service over a period of five chaotic days. A physician was investigated for having administered large doses of morphine and midazolam to patients, allegedly without a therapeutic need for the drugs, allegedly resulting in the deaths of the patients.

Local prosecutors in New Orleans convened a special grand jury to hear the evidence against the physician. By the time the grand jury was convened, public opinion was supportive of the physician for having done what was deemed to be necessary and was considered to be forgivable during a time of crisis. People who lived in New Orleans were well aware of the circumstances they had faced during and after Katrina, and they were not inclined to apply ordinary expectations to extraordinary situations. Postmortem analysis of the cause of death was unclear for the patients who allegedly were the victims of an intentional killing. Some experts concluded that the deaths should be classified as homicide and not as palliative care. Other experts explained that it is impossible to do a scientific analysis of a cadaver that has been in 100-degree heat for ten days. The grand jury declined to indict the physician.

One major obstacle for the prosecution in this New Orleans case was the absence of explicit records for controlled substance distribution and administration that usually are available in a criminal investigation. The pharmacist at the hospital testified that he had been fearful of looters when he went back and forth between the pharmacy and the patient care areas, in the dark and in the heat. The pharmacist had gathered vials of morphine and midazolam and had given the drugs to nurses to use "on the honor system." This highly unusual, and highly illegal, approach to controlled substance distribution was understood to be a necessary accommodation to extraordinary circumstances. Louisiana law was later amended to add provisions recognizing that standards of healthcare practice should be evaluated based on the enormous challenges faced by hospital staff during a "once in a lifetime" natural disaster.

Although each of these three books describes very different circumstances, the result in each situation is that the legal system addressed the criminal liability of the alleged perpetrator of a pharmaceutical crime. Justice was served through the application of recognized legal principles within a recognized procedural framework under the law. An understanding of the basic principles of criminal law can facilitate an appreciation for how officers of the law respond to allegations of pharmaceutical crimes.

Visual Media and Portrayals of Pharmaceutical Homicide

A developing trend in public demand for streaming video expanded during the COVID-19 global pandemic, and filmmakers did their best to meet the demand. One subject that several filmmakers apparently considered to be highly marketable was lurid stories of a murderous nurse whose crimes went undetected for a long period of time during which hospitalized patients died at an unprecedented rate for seemingly inexplicable reasons. Prior to this cluster of "healthcare killers" video productions, there had been several true crime television shows over the previous decade that were either documentaries describing actual healthcare serial murders or were fictional stories that entertained the audience with the audacious message that treatment provided by a healthcare professional could result in a patient's death from an intentional drug overdose.

The most widely publicized of the recent creative efforts was a 2022 film sarcastically called "The Good Nurse." It stars Eddie Redmayne as the notorious serial killer nurse Charles Cullen, and Jessica Chastain as the nurse who was Cullen's "professional friend" and who heroically discovered Cullen's murderous misdeeds. The film sympathetically describes how Chastain's character collaborated with law enforcement, to bring Cullen to justice almost single-handedly. As could be expected, the commercial production turned out to be a generously idealized film. Although the movie purported to be "based on a true story," it tells a significantly fictionalized tale, with numerous fanciful but nevertheless entertaining scenes portraying edge-of-your-seat suspense and challenging interpersonal conflicts. Several documentaries describing the less inspiring, but more historically accurate, "truth behind the movie" were subsequently released.

Two similar streaming productions were released in 2023. The Lifetime movie "A Nurse to Die For," and the four-episode Netflix series "The Nurse" both tell chilling stories of homicide committed with legitimately obtained and clinically useful medications in a healthcare setting. The fourth season of the extremely popular FX series "Fargo" has a subplot involving Nurse Oraetta Mayflower (played by actor Jessie Buckley), who commits pharmaceutical homicide to further her personal interests. A compelling aspect of this storyline is that Nurse Mayfield becomes very aggressive in her threats toward her accusers when she is periodically unmasked as a serial killer. She consistently warns hospital administrators and other healthcare professionals that she will publicize the criminal acts that she has committed in the healthcare institutions where she has worked, accusing everyone else of having been the perpetrator. This menacing approach results in her dismissal from employment without any embarrassing (to the hospital) criminal charges being filed.

The increase in the number of streaming video programs that use pharmaceutical homicide as entertainment has caused concern among healthcare scholars who study this tragic problem. On the one hand, some commentators are concerned that an increase in public exposure to the subject could normalize pharmaceutical homicide and reduce the level of outrage when it is discovered. On the other hand, some analysts view this increased coverage as a strong and positive patient safety message that will encourage patients and their family members to question suspicious actions taken by healthcare professionals.

What Is a Crime?

Actions that threaten, cause harm to, or otherwise endanger the property, health, safety, or moral welfare of people are considered crimes. A crime is an act against the public interest, and those who are alleged to have committed crimes are prosecuted by a public representative. The public representat ve may be a state attorney or a local prosecutor or a federal prosecutor. The prosecutor works for the public, and not for the victim, although the interests of the victim are usually considered by the prosecutor.

Civil wrongs, such as professional malpractice, are different from crimes. A single wrongful act by a professional person may expose the actor to both criminal and civil legal proceedings. Yet, while a criminal proceeding is maintained by a public official such as a government prosecutor, a civil proceeding is generally brought by one private individual against another private individual, usually through a private attorney. The purpose of criminal prosecution is punishment, while the purpose of civil litigation is dispute resolution and compensation.

The formal public response to alleged crimes is nonsystematic. Police, prosecutors, courts, and prisons function separately from each other. Most crimes are treated as local law enforcement issues. The level of resources available to address crimes can vary greatly from one locality to another. There is considerable flexibility in the response to crimes by law enforcement, leading to selectivity with regard to cases that are prosecuted. Sometimes, the huge volume of criminal cases overwhelms available resources, leading to inequities in the way crimes are prioritized.

The principle of proportionality requires that "the punishment fit the crime." When the criminal justice system fails to meet this goal, citizens may become cynical and lose their respect for the system. The law provides guidance on the scope of the sentence that must be applied to perpetrators of a crime. The goal is that everyone is treated essentially the same. Because lawyers differ in their ability to present an effective defense of their clients, it is possible that two people who have committed the same crime will not be given the same punishment due to differences in lawyering skills. The criminal justice system attempts to promote fairness, but it is far from a perfect system.

Most people comply with legal standards and avoid criminal violations out of respect for their fellow citizens. They expect reciprocity through compliance with legal standards by others who reside in their community. Some people comply with laws reluctantly, based on a rational calculation of their own self-interest and the potential costs to them of noncompliance. Criminal laws establish a basic expectation for personal behavior in a civilized society.

Actus Reus: The Guilty Act

An evil thought cannot be considered a crime without a guilty act. If one thinks, "I wish that person was dead," this thought by itself is not sufficient for there to be a crime. An explicit physical act, or in some situations the failure to act when action is legally required, must be established for there to be a crime. The requirement for an "actus reus" (the physical element of a crime) usually means that there must be clear evidence of a voluntary bodily act, or voluntary failure to act, of which the actor was aware and which could have been prevented by the actor.

The analysis of "actus reus" often requires consideration of voluntariness. For example, a sudden reflexive action may not suffice as an actus reus. Likewise, an action taken during a time of acute physical stress, such as acts that occur immediately following a gunshot, may not be considered a sufficient actus reus to support criminal charges. A knee-jerk reflex may not be sufficient to be considered a voluntary act.

Under some circumstances, a medical condition such as a seizure disorder may negate the requirement that there be an actus reus as an essential element of a crime. Suppose a motorist drives through a red light and causes a fatal accident. If the motorist was seizing at the time of the accident, then the actus reus element may not exist. On the other hand, suppose also that the motorist was aware of the seizure disorder, for which medication had been prescribed, yet the motorist intentionally refused to use the prescribed medication. In this situation, the refusal to use the medication could be considered the actus reus, even though the failure to observe the red light might not qualify as an actus reus. The act of intentionally refusing to use necessary medication could support criminal charges.

For an actus reus to be considered an element of a crime, it must have caused the undesired result. By applying what is known as the "but for" test, the evidence must show that "but for" the action or inaction of the defendant, the harm would not have occurred. If the victim would have suffered harm regardless of the alleged perpetrator's action/inaction, then the "but for" test fails, and the perpetrator is not the cause of harm to the victim. Under the "thin skull" rule, persons with unusual vulnerabilities can still be considered victims of crimes, even if they are harmed in a manner that would not have caused harm to most other people.

Mens Rea: The Guilty Mind

A harmful act cannot be considered a crime without a guilty mind. Unintentional lapses do happen. As a general rule, unpreventable accidents are not considered crimes. The basic requirement of "mens rea" (the mental element of a crime) is that the criminal suspect has acted with an intent to cause harm. Intent is usually defined as including awareness and a substantial certainty of causing harm. Under what is known as the "willful blindness" rule, actual knowledge is not required. A person who acts with conscious awareness that they are creating a substantial risk of harm to another, and who chooses to expose another to that risk of harm, has the required mens rea for the commission of a crime, regardless of any hope that the actor may have had that harm would not occur.

For there to be mens rea, ill will and malice toward a victim are not necessary. However, mere negligence is not sufficient to establish mens rea. Malice may be difficult to prove, and, if malice was an essential element of establishing mens rea, it would significantly reduce the number of crimes committed. On the other hand, punishing negligence could lead to over-deterrence by significantly increasing the number of crimes committed because anyone who made a mistake would be considered a criminal. People would likely decline to participate in necessary but risky activities like driving a school bus because any inadvertent error they make could result in criminal charges. Mens rea requires proof of intent, beyond simple negligence, but it does not require malicious intent.

A finding of recklessness may suffice for the element of mens rea. The knowing creation of a situation that will inevitably lead to harm may serve as the basis of a mens rea finding. The harmful situation may have been created by another person or institution, and the failure to object by a person who is in a position to object and prevent harm may also serve as the basis of a mens rea finding. It is the conscious awareness of an unreasonable and reducible risk that serves as the basis for a finding of recklessness. Knowledge of both the magnitude and the probability of harm to a potential victim will influence a finding of mens rea.

Crimes of Omission

Sometimes, a statute will specify that the failure to act is a crime. This may be, for example, an element of a "Good Samaritan" law that requires a healthcare professional to come to the aid of a person who needs medical assistance.

More often, an omission is considered a crime when there is a failure to act in compliance with a legal duty established by a "special relationship." Parents and children are in such a special relationship with each other, leading to the criminal responsibility of a parent who fails to act in a way that is necessary for the protection of a child. Other relationships can be legally established by contract, such as the responsibility of a lifeguard to attempt the rescue of a drowning swimmer.

Professional relationships in healthcare, such as those between a healthcare professional and a patient, may lead to the commission of a crime based on the omission of care. This may happen, for example, when a nursing home fails to properly care for a resident, and the resident suffers harm as the result of neglect. It may happen when a pharmacist makes an error with a prescription but covers up the error and the failure to notify the patient or the prescriber of the error results in harm to the patient.

Mistake of Law or Fact

A person who commits a crime may be able to escape criminal liability if the person was relying on an official statement of the law that later is determined to be invalid or erroneous. If this were not the case, then government agencies could entrap citizens into committing crimes by intentionally providing the public with erroneous information. Likewise, a mistake of fact may serve as the basis for exoneration of a person who has technically committed a crime.

For example, assume that a pharmacist checks a government website and sees clearly that the website lists a prescriber as having a valid state license to practice and a current DEA registration. Based on this information, the pharmacist decides to honor the prescriber's prescription for a controlled substance. If it later turns out that the information was inaccurate, then the pharmacist has made a mistake of law by considering the prescription to be valid, and the pharmacist has made a mistake of fact by determining the licensure and registration issues to be non-problematic. These understandable mistakes, caused by inaccuracies contained within information provided by the government, may negate any crime committed by the pharmacist.

Infractions, Misdemeanors, and Felonies

Not all crimes are of the same level of magnitude. Although there is considerable variation among jurisdictions, "infractions" tend to be the least serious crimes, while "felonies" tend to be the most serious crimes. "Misdemeanors" fall in between. There are levels of severity within each of these types of crimes.

An infraction usually leads to a ticket being handed to a violator, resulting in a fine and no time in jail and also no appearance in court. As long as the ticket is paid, the infraction has been resolved and no further penalty will be applied to the commission of the minor crime.

A misdemeanor usually can result in up to a year in a local jail rather than in a state prison. Misdemeanors may result in no incarceration at all. Prosecutors have considerable discretion in deciding how to respond to a misdemeanor charge and what kind of plea bargain to negotiate with the offender.

A felony is usually punishable by a prison sentence of more than a year. Felonies are crimes that are viewed as particularly heinous by society. These crimes include murder, burglary, rape, and arson. Judges are often guided by statute in the punishment that they may mete out to a convicted felon.

Murder

The crime of murder occurs when one person kills another person with no justification. Murder has been recognized as a crime throughout history. Punishment of the crime of murder has always been particularly severe. Murder is both intrinsically wrong and creates economic costs for society. Most people convicted of murder are incarcerated for long periods. Perhaps they are incarcerated for the remainder of their lives. Capital punishment for murder exists in some states, although it is controversial.

A prosecution for murder must establish that there was an unlawful killing of a human by another human with malice aforethought. Not all killings are unlawful. For example, killing in time of war is considered lawful. Legal cases have demonstrated how the definition of death may vary, depending on interpretations of science as applied to facts. A person who shoots another person may be charged with attempted murder if the victim does not die. That charge can be upgraded to murder if the victim later dies. Generally, cessation of all brain function marks the death of a person. Some courts apply the "year and a day" rule, limiting murder to deaths that occur within one year following harm caused by one person to another.

The requirement that "murder" result in the death of a human excludes from the crime of murder those actions taken against a person who is already dead. This is a commonly asked law school question. If an assassin shoots a person in bed, thinking that the person is sleeping when the person is already dead, the shooting cannot be a murder. Likewise, when a health professional administers what would be considered a lethal dose of medication in an attempt to resuscitate a patient who has already expired, the administration of this lethal dose cannot be considered murder.

The requirement that "murder" result in the death of another also excludes suicide from the crime of murder because killing oneself does not affect "another."

Malice aforethought does not require a lengthy period of preparation prior to commission of the crime of murder. Rather, a murderer may have developed malice aforethought in the fleeting moment prior to committing the act resulting in the death of another person.

Most jurisdictions distinguish between first-degree murder, which is associated with aggravating factors, and second-degree murder, which lacks the aggravating factors.

Manslaughter

Manslaughter is a less serious crime than murder, although both crimes result in the death of another person. The difference is generally based on a lower level of culpability that is associated with manslaughter as opposed to murder.

In most jurisdictions, there are two levels of manslaughter: voluntary and involuntary.

The main difference between voluntary manslaughter and murder is the presence of mitigating circumstances. After discovering that one's spouse is having an affair, a person might intentionally kill the spouse's lover. This type of killing is sometimes referred to as "heat of passion" killing, and it may lead to a manslaughter charge. Aside from the circumstances caused by discovery of the affair, it is essentially murder.

Involuntary manslaughter occurs when one person kills another person while committing an unlawful act. For example, when one person assaults another person in a bar, and the victim hits his head on a table causing death. This assault will likely be considered involuntary manslaughter if the victim did not initiate the altercation. It is important to distinguish such a situation from accidental death, when a person dies through the fault of no one. A child who runs into the street and is killed by a cautious motorist is not the victim of manslaughter. It is a terrible tragedy, but no crime has been committed.

Negligent Homicide

A negligent homicide is less serious than either murder or manslaughter, but it still results in exposure to criminal liability. Many cases of negligent homicide are caused by recklessness or inattentiveness by a person who means no harm but who is distracted or otherwise unaware of facts that should be apparent. A motorist who forgets that a child is in the car and who leaves the child unattended in the parked car on a hot day may be charged with negligent homicide if the child dies from the heat. Drivers who fail to slow down during a rainstorm, or who drive too fast on icy roads, may be charged with negligent homicide if their negligence, although unintentional, leads to the death of another person.

Healthcare professionals who fail to conform to the standard of care may be charged with negligent homicide for resulting deaths of patients. This is rare, but it is not impossible.

Prosecutors are usually careful not to overcharge those whose negligent conduct has led to the death of another person. There may be little point in bringing a criminal action against a person who already faces personal liability litigation and the prospect of living with the knowledge that a death has resulted from their 'careless actions. There are limits to what criminal prosecution can accomplish in circumstances where the perpetrator is consumed with grief and regret.

Felony Murder

Felony murder is a legal pretense that was developed to increase the exposure of an offender to the crime of murder, even when there is no evidence of intent to kill. A felony murder has occurred when, during the commission of a felony such as theft, a perpetrator incidentally kills another person. The felony murder rule may be applied to any participant in the original felony, exposing all participants to a charge of murder when a victim has been incidentally killed during the commission of the underlying felony.

The theory behind felony murder is that intent to commit one crime can be transferred to another crime. The penalties for felony murder are often equivalent to those for premeditated murder since the requisite intent has been transferred from the original felony.

A conviction of felony murder requires proof that the underlying felony presented a foreseeable danger to life, and there must be a direct link between the underlying felony and the victim's death. The underlying felony must be inherently dangerous. For example, there would be no case of felony murder against a health professional who commits grand theft by misleading patients regarding the value of unapproved herbal drugs sold by the health professional for the treatment of cancer. Misleading information about the efficacy of herbals is not inherently dangerous. If the patient dies from using the unapproved herbal drugs, there would be no direct connection with the grand theft felony.

On the other hand, there have been cases in which a physician or pharmacist has been charged with felony murder following their alleged illegal prescribing or dispensing of controlled substances, resulting in the death of the person who used the drugs. Violation of controlled substance laws is the underlying felony. When patients overdose and die from illegally prescribed and/or dispensed controlled substances, the physician or pharmacist may be charged with felony murder, due to the direct connection between the drugs and the patient's death.

Attempted Murder

Attempted murder is a crime that can be prosecuted before harm occurs, relieving the police of the need to wait until the victim has died before stepping in and arresting the perpetrator for murder. A conviction of attempted murder requires that there be "substantial steps toward the commission of the crime" and that the steps are "strongly corroborative of criminal purpose." The element of mens rea requires that there be evidence of intent to commit an act that would have resulted in the commission of murder. The element of actus reus requires that some act has been committed in furtherance of the crime.

A defense of "abandonment" is usually available for a person who has considered the commission of murder, but who had second thoughts and stopped short of completing the crime. However, the impossibility of success cannot be used as a defense to the crime of attempted murder. People who irrationally develop a logistically impossible plan to kill another person may still be guilty of attempted murder even if the plan is fundamentally flawed.

If there is evidence of uncertainty regarding a person's intentions to commit murder, then there may be a situation of "mere preparation" rather than attempt. For example, upon learning that a child has been assaulted, a parent may grab a handgun and run out of the house looking for the assailant, saying "I'm going to kill him." Minutes later, the parent returns home without having found the assailant. There is no attempted murder.

The Necessity Defense

A person accused of murder may say, "I had no choice." This is a claim of necessity, and it may be a defense to a charge of murder.

Self-defense is the classic claim of necessity. To effectively assert self-defense following the killing of another person, the person claiming the defense must show that deadly force was immediately necessary for self-protection, or for the protection of another person, from unlawful force used by the deceased.

A very controversial assertion of the necessity defense would occur when medical evidence shows that a pregnant woman will almost surely die unless her pregnancy is terminated, and a physician performs an abortion to save the life of the woman. The physician might claim necessity as justification for the procedure. Because of the politics of abortion, the response to this claim of necessity will vary from one geographic area to another. Pharmacists who are involved with the use of abortifacient medications should be aware of the applicability of this controversial defense.

Insanity is another type of necessity defense that may be used by those who claim not to be responsible for murder as moral agents, because they lack mental capacity. The traditional approach to recognizing this necessity defense is the "not guilty by reason of insanity" plea. If this defense is allowed, the result is for a person to be committed to a psychiatric hospital and then released when the psychiatric condition has been effectively treated, or perhaps never being released if an effective treatment is not possible. In some jurisdictions, this type of necessity defense has been replaced with a plea such as "guilty but mentally ill," resulting in the defendant being incarcerated in a prison hospital for a specified period of time that corresponds with the time that a sane perpetrator would be incarcerated in prison if convicted of the crime.

Mass Murder

According to the FBI, a "mass murder" occurs at a single location, over a brief period of time, during which four or more people are killed by the murderer. Many mass murders end with the suicide of the murderer. Mass murderers tend to be social outcasts who have no support network among family or friends. The FBI has stated that the vast majority of mass murderers are male, and they are not clinically psychotic. Mass murderers tend to be paranoid, and they display acute behavioral or social disorders. They may display psychopathic tendencies, such as being cruel, manipulative, and lacking in compassion.

Most mass murderers can be considered "ticking time bombs," who see their lives as completely falling apart. An irreparable loss, such as being fired from a job or having a romantic relationship end, can push these individuals over the edge to the point where they think that they have nothing to lose. Losing control over their lives can lead mass murderers to blame anyone and everyone for their failures and can lead them to take the lives of others as revenge for the harm that has been caused to them.

The prevention of mass murder is usually addressed through "first responder" training of those who work in schools, government buildings, and other public places where mass murder is likely to occur. A response by law enforcement is usually too late to prevent a mass murder.

Some mass murders fit the definition of "genocide," which occurs when there is systematic destruction of all, or a significant part, of a racial, religious, ethnic, or national group. Such mass murders are also known as "crimes against humanity."

Serial Killings

According to the FBI, serial killing differs from mass murders in that there is a period of time between the murders. The occasions on which murders occur are separated by what is often referred to as a "cooling-off period." Under federal law, the FBI is allowed to assist local authorities in the investigation of serial killings, when the following definition is met: "A series of three or more killings, not less than one of which was committed within the United States, having common characteristics, such as to suggest the reasonable possibility that the crimes were committed by the same actor or actors."

Serial killers are not necessarily dysfunctional loners. Many of them live in plain sight within their communities, with the appearance of normal lives. Although most serial killers are males, serial killers span all racial groups. Most serial killers have a very limited geographic area of operation. They conduct their killing within a comfort zone defined by an anchor point, such as a residence or place of employment. Serial killers do not necessarily feel compelled to continue killing. Some stop before they are caught, and they may never be caught. First-time serial killers are inexperienced, and they make mistakes. As time passes, they become more confident and make fewer mistakes.

Profiling the Serial Killer

The idea that a serial killer can be "profiled" so that law enforcement officers know where to look for a suspect seems to be more prevalent in Hollywood scripts than in FBI reality. One characteristic that is common to serial killers is psychopathy. The FBI defines psychopathy as a personality disorder manifested in people who use a mixture of charm, manipulation, intimidation, and occasionally violence to control others, as a means to satisfy their own selfish needs. All psychopaths do not become serial killers. Rather, serial killers may possess some or many of the traits consistent with psychopathy.

Interpersonal traits of serial killers include glibness, superficial charm, a grandiose sense of self-worth, pathological lying, and the manipulation of others. Their emotional traits include a lack of remorse and/or guilt, shallow affect, a lack of empathy, and failure to accept responsibility. Lifestyle behaviors include stimulation-seeking, early-childhood behavior problems, and juvenile delinquency.

For the most part, serial murder involves strangers with no visible relationship between the offender and the victim. This reality creates challenges for law enforcement, since the traditional investigation of murder focuses on those persons whose relationships are closest to the victim.

Regardless of the motive, serial killers commit their crimes because they want to. A serial killer's motive may evolve both within a single murder and throughout a series of murders. Control is a motive common to serial killers, who feel empowered and strengthened when they kill their victims.

Challenges with Serial Killings

One of the most significant challenges with serial killings is the identification of them. This is particularly the case when a serial killer operates within a geographic area served by multiple law enforcement agencies or when the victims are of an age or physical condition where death is not considered unnatural.

Any suspicion that "things just don't seem right" should be pursued because patterns of a serial killing may be difficult to discern unless particular care is taken to evaluate each death within the framework of other deaths.

Trend analysis is difficult when data are not managed systematically. If reports of individual deaths are not completed thoroughly and uploaded into a database, then the relationships between two or more deaths may be difficult to identify. Computerized analytical resources can disclose commonalities between deaths, based on factors such as victim characteristics, timing, and cause of death.

Leadership is critical. A series of similar but unexplained deaths may cause law enforcement personnel to feel helplessly inept in identifying the perpetrator. Strong leaders can establish good working relationships both within law enforcement and between law enforcement agencies and other groups affected by the deaths.

Pharmacy Profession and Accusations of Homicide

Pharmacy case law has contributed to a legal distinction between negligence and criminality. The tradition in Anglo-American common law shows a historic lack of differentiation between professional negligence and criminal liability. Malpractice and criminality were at one time viewed as being the same category of legal offense.

One illustrative prosecution is reported in an early British pharmacy case from 1828, called "Tessymond's Case."[4] The facts of the case showed that a "chymist" was indicted for manslaughter in causing the death of an infant child when laudanum (tincture of opium) was dispensed instead of the much less concentrated drug paregoric (camphorated tincture of opium) that had been ordered. There was evidence that the bottles of the two products were very similar. Confusing one bottle for the other was apparently an inadvertent error committed by the "chymist." Nevertheless, the judge instructed the jury, "If a party is guilty of negligence, and death results, the party guilty of that negligence is also guilty of manslaughter. If you think there was negligence on the part of the prisoner, you will find him guilty—if not, you must acquit him." The jury found the "chymist" guilty, and the court sentenced him to pay a fine of 5 pounds.

Well over a century later, in a California case from 1956 called "People v. Stuart,"[5] the Supreme Court of California ruled to the contrary. The defendant pharmacist had compounded a medication for a child, using a stock bottle labeled "sodium citrate." In fact, the bottle contained sodium nitrite. The case did not explain how this mislabeling had occurred. The child died and the pharmacist was convicted of manslaughter. On appeal, the court noted that "no evidence whatever was introduced that would justify an inference that defendant knew or should have known that the bottle labeled sodium citrate contained sodium nitrite." The court acknowledged that intentionally using the wrong product would meet the conditions necessary for manslaughter. The court then said, "When, as in this case, however, the defendant did not know, and could not reasonably be expected to know, that the sodium citrate bottle contained sodium nitrite, those conditions are not met and there is therefore lacking the culpability necessary to make the act an unlawful act." The conviction of the pharmacist was reversed. The prevailing view in modern case law is that simple negligence in pharmacy practice leading to the death of a patient does not support charges of murder or manslaughter against a pharmacist, although recklessness in the creation and maintenance of a dysfunctional pharmacy practice system may serve as the basis to change that result.

A pharmacist's professional expertise may be relevant to the penalty that a pharmacist is given after the commission of a crime. A very unusual case shows how a pharmacist with knowledge of his own actions can be successfully prosecuted after exposing others to a serious risk of death.[6]

The pharmacist who was the defendant in this case had been licensed for thirty-six years. According to the court, he grew irate over what he considered to be substandard care and excessive billing at a New York hospital, based on his personal experience. The pharmacist decided to retaliate by dispersing elemental mercury throughout the hospital, knowing it to be a neurotoxin that can cause death. The pharmacist's stated goal was to "cause panic at the hospital and an attendant loss of business when people became fearful of gaining treatment there." The pharmacist deposited mercury at the hospital on four separate occasions over a period of one year. Fortunately, nobody was harmed by the mercury. The pharmacist was caught and pled guilty to the use of a chemical weapon. He was sentenced to 168 months in prison. He appealed, because the length of his sentence had been increased based on his alleged application of professional skills as a pharmacist in the commission of a crime. One of many factors that can be used by a judge to increase the sentence of a person who has been convicted of a crime is the use of professional knowledge and skill. The pharmacist argued that although he possessed a relevant special skill, there was no evidence that he had actually used his special skill in the commission of his offenses. The court disagreed, noting that the pharmacist "used his special knowledge of chemicals to facilitate his offense because the special skills increased his chances of succeeding." The increased penalty based on the pharmacist's special skills was affirmed.

Conclusion

Everyone is victimized when a crime is committed. An individual perpetrator may be identified, and an individual victim may be specifically linked to the perpetrator's crimes, yet all members of a community are wronged by a perpetrator's criminality because public expectations for civil behavior have been violated. A public representative, either elected by the public or appointed by an elected public official, will charge the perpetrator and will pursue the prosecution of the perpetrator. There are many different types of crimes. Some crimes are more serious than others, and the penalties for the more serious crimes are correspondingly more severe. Some crimes are spur-of-the-moment acts, while other crimes are premeditated. It is generally true that the greater the perpetrator's intent to harm can be established, the more likely it is that the public will insist on retribution through the criminal justice system.

Key Takeaways

- Remember that crimes are an affront to society. When a crime is committed, everyone is the victim, because an ordered society depends on rules being followed by each individual to protect all other individuals. Don't be a spectator when a crime is being committed. It does not matter that you may not be at risk or in danger. Report what you see to law enforcement personnel and allow them to do their job. Justice cannot be served when people who have information about a crime decide not to get involved. Private lawsuits are somewhat different because a system has been established by the government to allow citizens to settle their grievances without the need to resort to retaliation that may escalate and cause unintended harm. Criminal prosecutions are not like private lawsuits because everyone has an interest in preserving a safe society.

- Consider the intent of a potential perpetrator in evaluating whether a crime has been committed. Most crimes result from an intentional act that accompanies a guilty frame of mind. There are exceptions to this general rule, but the basic principle is that inadvertent accidents are not crimes while intentional acts that cause injury are crimes. Be alert to the possibility that a dysfunctional system is so flawed that injury to a person is inevitable. Under these circumstances, the failure to rectify a system failure may qualify as an intentional act leading to a crime, if harm results.
- Remember that murder is the most serious of all crimes. It is a crime that cannot be undone. Pharmaceutical products can be deadly when they are used with the intent to kill. Be sure to familiarize yourself with the FBI definitions of mass murder and serial murder. If you see any suspicious activities that could meet the FBI criteria, then discuss what you see with a supervisor or a trusted colleague. Raising concerns about murder can be a difficult step to take, and it should not be taken without the support of others. Failing to act in the face of incriminating information is irresponsible.

References

1. Jobb D. *The Case of the Murderous Dr. Cream: The Hunt for a Victorian Era Serial Killer.* Chapel Hill, NC: Algonquin Books; 2021.

2. Whittie B, Ritchie J. *Prescription for Murder: The True Story of Dr. Harold Frederick Shipman*. New York, NY: Little Brown; 2005.

3. Fink S. *Five Days at Memorial: Life and Death in a Storm-Ravaged Hospital.* New York, NY Crown Publishers; 2016.

4. Tessymond's Case, 1 Lewin's Crown Cases, 169 (1828).

5. People v. Stuart, 302 P.2d 5 (Cal. 1956).

6. United States v. Kimber, 777 F.3d 553 (2nd Cir. 2015).

Chapter 3

Pharmaceutical Homicide Investigations

Suspects who are accused of committing a crime are presumed to be innocent until they are proven guilty. A person who is prosecuted for the commission of a crime must be proven guilty beyond a reasonable doubt for there to be a conviction. These two basic principles of criminal law are foundational to the concept of justice in a democratic society. The burden of proof is borne by the government in criminal proceedings. The government generally has significant resources to utilize in the prosecution of a suspect who has been accused of a crime. The accused generally has more limited resources. The government has discretion to pursue those prosecutions for which there is substantial evidence of a suspect's guilt, and to abandon cases that would be difficult to prove due to the absence of sufficient evidence of guilt. The vast majority of criminal cases are disposed of through a process of plea bargaining, where the defendant agrees to plead guilty (or "no contest" in some jurisdictions) and accept a lesser penalty than would be applicable if the case were to proceed to trial and result in a guilty verdict.

Justice Does Not Always Prevail

The criminal justice system is far from perfect. The Innocence Project estimates that as much as 10% of those suspects who are convicted of a serious crime are actually innocent. Hundreds of convicted felons have been exonerated of their crimes through the efforts of the Innocence Project and other governmental and nongovernmental agencies that pursue justice for incarcerated persons. At the same time, there are many serious crimes that go unsolved, with countless criminals literally "getting away with murder." According to the FBI, approximately 40% of murders are not "cleared." In the jargon of the agency, a crime is "cleared" when law enforcement has gathered enough evidence to support an arrest, to determine an appropriate charge, and then to submit the offender for prosecution.

The criminal justice system is a search for truth, and truth can only be found through investigation that produces evidence. Investigators piece together the evidence, bit by bit, to support a story that prosecutors can describe to juries as a representation of the truth. Judges determine whether the evidence is credible. Juries are not allowed to consider speculation, rumor, or innuendo, as opposed to facts. It is up to the jury to decide whether the facts, as admitted into evidence, show guilt beyond a reasonable doubt.

The evidence to support a conviction need not be direct. It may be circumstantial. Some investigations produce what is often referred to as "smoking gun" direct evidence. This is a phrase that was coined for situations in which a law enforcement officer witnessed a shooting, and the officer immediately confiscated and preserved the weapon as evidence of guilt. The gun might not have truly been "smoking," but the identification of the gun as the murder weapon was beyond question. The "smoking gun" today may be DNA evidence, or fingerprints, or hair, or other tangible proof that irrefutably links a defendant to the time and place of a crime.

On the other hand, circumstantial evidence requires no "smoking gun" confirmation. Instead, a judge and jury are required to make inferences or indirect judgments about what must have happened based on a variety of interrelated circumstances that are discovered through investigation. Facts related to motive, means, and opportunity may be sufficient to serve as circumstantial evidence in a criminal trial. Circumstantial evidence cannot be based on conjecture, guesswork, and coincidence. Circumstantial evidence must be based on fact.

A decades-old criminal case serves as an appropriate factual background for a discussion of the evidentiary basis required to support the crime of pharmaceutical homicide. This case report includes relevant legal reasoning to provide an illustration of how circumstantial evidence may create suspicions of criminality yet fail to support conviction of a crime.

A Pharmacist's Murder Conviction Is Reversed (Twice)

This case is of particular interest because it describes how a pharmacist was twice convicted of first-degree murder in the poisoning of his wife and how the convictions were twice reversed on appeal. The most important aspects of the case are the quality of the circumstantial evidence used by the government to obtain the two convictions, and the alternative explanations of the evidence that were utilized by the appellate courts in reversing the convictions. Things are often not as clear as they may seem. The lack of clarity in the evidence (the existence of a reasonable doubt) led to the pharmacist's convictions twice being reversed on appeal.

This case is from the 1940s. It provides an interesting perspective on hospital pharmacy during that era, when most drugs were obtained by a nurse from a "drug room," with little or no supervision by a pharmacist. There may not even have been a pharmacist employed by the hospital. If the "drug room" did not have a medication deemed necessary by a patient's attending physician, then the attending physician wrote a prescription. A friend or family member would take the prescription to a community pharmacy, have the prescription filled at that pharmacy, and then bring the medication to the hospital for use by the nursing staff in caring for the patient under the prescriber's supervision.

This case is based on accusations of strychnine poisoning. In the late 1800s and early 1900s, strychnine was used as a medication. It was not unusual to find this product in stock at a pharmacy. It is derived from the "nux vomica" plant. There are many medication containers with this label in pharmacy museums. While strychnine was used historically for a variety of human ailments, its primary use was as a cardiac or bowel stimulant, and as a means to enhance physical performance through increased muscle contraction. It is fortunate that today there are much better remedies for these conditions than strychnine.

Although the hospital practices described in this legal case are outdated, the principles of law from many decades ago remain unchanged today. The defendant pharmacist stood accused of a capital offense, meaning that he could be executed if he was found guilty. Courts are very cautious about the sufficiency of evidence to support conviction of a capital offense. There is no way to undo a legal error once a convict has been executed.

In reading the (somewhat antiquated) language of the court in this case, consider these questions:

- How persuasive must the evidence be to convince a jury that a defendant has committed a crime beyond a reasonable doubt?
- When does circumstantial evidence cross the line from suspicion to confirmation based on the reasonableness of the prosecutor's presentation of facts?
- How can the factual evidence of an alleged murder with medication be preserved for later review and analysis?
- When there is an unresolved disagreement between experts, how can a jury determine the truth of what has happened in a criminal case?

Pharmacist's First Conviction and Reversal on Appeal

The defendant pharmacist was convicted by a jury of murdering his wife. From this conviction the pharmacist appealed.[1] The primary issue throughout the appeal was one of timing and not of causation. The evidence clearly indicated that the wife had died from strychnine poisoning. There was conflicting evidence concerning whether the strychnine had been ingested by the wife on December 7 at her home prior to her being hospitalized, or on December 8 or 9 during her hospitalization. The prosecutor argued that the wife died from ingestion of strychnine during her hospitalization, resulting from the pharmacist (the husband) having provided to the hospital nursing staff a medication that was laced with strychnine. There was no evidence that the pharmacist defendant could possibly have had any connection with the wife ingesting strychnine at home on December 7, if any such ingestion ever occurred at home, because the pharmacist was not present at home with the wife at that time. The inability of the prosecutor to prove that the wife was poisoned during her hospitalization would mean exoneration of the pharmacist, because it was only during the hospitalization that there was any evidence of an opportunity for the pharmacist to have poisoned his wife.

The language provided in italics is quoted directly from the appellate court's opinion reversing the pharmacist's conviction. Note that the prosecution is referred to as "The People."

The defendant stands convicted of murder in the first degree upon an indictment which charges that on or about the 7th, 8th, and 9th days of December 1943, in the County of Kings, the defendant willfully, feloniously and of malice aforethought poisoned his wife, by giving and administering to her a quantity of poison, to wit, strychnine, and as a result of said poisoning the wife died on December 9, 1943.

A close examination of the record has led us to conclude that errors occurred upon the trial, the cumulative effect of which may well have led to the judgment of conviction and thus prejudiced the defendant's rights. In connection with the following summary of evidence the fact should be noted that the judgment of conviction rests upon circumstantial evidence—a process of decision by which a court or jury may reason from circumstances which are known or proved, to establish by inference the reality of the principal fact.

The defendant is a pharmacist who for a period of years had been employed at a drugstore in Brooklyn. He married the decedent in 1940 when she was twenty years old, and he was thirteen years her senior. Although the record does not tell us whether during the three years of their life together a child was born of the marriage, it does appear that the decedent was pregnant at the time of her death and that her pregnancy was not accompanied by unusual illness.

At about nine o'clock on the night of December 7, 1943, when the defendant was on duty at his place of business and the decedent was alone in their apartment she was called upon by her sister. At that time there were no indications that the decedent was ill. Within an hour after the sister left the decedent, a neighbor who lived on the same floor heard a strange noise which led her to open a door leading into the outside hallway. As she did so she saw the decedent standing in the doorway of the apartment apparently in distress. Upon going to her assistance, she noted that the decedent's body had stiffened, her face was drawn, "her eyes were like big saucers, very big, and she kept cringing like that, shivering, her body shaking." Her hands were clenched and drawn in toward her chest and her arms were bent from the elbows. After the neighbor had summoned the defendant by telephone, the decedent's sister, and the decedent's attending physician, she was aided by two other neighbors in placing the decedent on a bed. Although the decedent was conscious her legs had stiffened with toes turned in and her hands were in a claw-like position with fingers, wrists and elbows bent. When the doctor arrived, he found the decedent in a convulsion. Thereafter the defendant arrived at a time when his wife was suffering a second convulsion. According to the doctor's testimony the defendant was "'very anxious'," he "'wanted to help her'," and urged the doctor to "'call a consultant'." When he suggested someone unknown to the doctor the latter suggested "'I would like to get my own man, if it is possible.'" Thereupon the attending physician called in consultation a second physician who arrived when the decedent was suffering a third convulsion. As a result of their consultation the doctors ordered the decedent removed to Beth-El Hospital where she arrived before midnight on December 7th.

At this point in the narrative it should be said that, although the doctors who had been in attendance upon the decedent at her apartment the night of December 7th reached the conclusion (on a later date) that her illness on December 7th had been due to strychnine poisoning, and although the indictment charged that defendant administered strychnine to the decedent "on or about the 7th, 8th and 9th days of December, 1943," the prosecution made no effort by direct or circumstantial evidence to prove that the defendant caused poison in any form to be administered to the decedent on or before December 7th.

Although the hospital chart of December 8th shows that on decedent's first day in the hospital she suffered two convulsions, the attending physicians expressed the opinion that on that day her condition showed improvement. However, in the late afternoon a consultation of three doctors prescribed for her two new types of medication—one was hytakerol, a medicine in tablet form containing a highly concentrated preparation of calcium; the other medicine was a liquid containing calcium chloride and elixir of lactate pepsin. The liquid medicine was to be put up in five or six bottles and administered by giving the patient the contents of one bottle every four hours. Concededly neither of the two medications then prescribed contained a poisonous ingredient which would cause death.

After the prescription for the two new medications had been written upon a single piece of paper one of the doctors handed it to the defendant and said to him: "I think you can get this hytakerol at a local drugstore, and while you are about it you might as well make up the calcium chloride and the elixir of lactate pepsin there, too." With the prescription in hand the defendant left his wife's hospital room accompanied by his brother-in-law who drove him first to the drugstore where he purchased the hytakerol tablets. The defendant was then driven to the drugstore where he was employed, at which place he told his brother-in-law to wait outside. Upon entering the drugstore, the defendant spoke of his wife's illness and told his employer and the prescription clerk that he had come in to prepare a prescription for her. He then went to the prescription counter in the rear of the store where, after asking the prescription clerk to help him, he prepared the liquid medicine which was put into six 6-ounce bottles.

As to what transpired while the defendant was compounding the prescription the testimony of both the owner and the prescription clerk shows that on that night the drugstore was very busy. While the defendant was at work at the prescription counter the proprietor frequently passed back and forth near him. Meantime the prescription clerk aided him to the extent of preparing labels for the six bottles. In doing so he stood at the defendant's side although he was not present when all six bottles were filled. From the owner's testimony it also appears that when he first acquired the drugstore there was on hand—kept with other poisons in a small cabinet near the prescription counter—a quantity of powdered strychnine which was "never used"; also, soluble strychnine sulphate in tablet form known as "triturate tablets." The owner did not recall that in preparing the prescription the defendant used any utensil to grind strychnine tablets or to dissolve them. There is no evidence that any bottle from the poison cabinet containing strychnine was opened on the night of December 8th; nor is there any evidence that the content of any bottle containing strychnine was reduced on that date.

When the defendant had completed preparation of the prescription he returned with his brother-in-law to the hospital and entered his wife's room at about 10:30 P.M. (December 8th). He then delivered the six bottles of "pinkish medicine" to the nurse then on duty who placed them on a window ledge with other medicine and promptly administered to the decedent the contents of one of the bottles. Four hours later—at 2:30 A.M. (December 9th)—the nurse next on duty administered to the decedent the contents of the second bottle of medicine—which medication is claimed by the People to have contained the strychnine which caused decedent's death. At 3:00 A.M. (December 9th) the decedent suffered a convulsion. She died at 4:00 A.M. on that date.

After directing the removal of the body to the hospital morgue the attending nurse disposed of the six bottles which had been brought by the defendant to his wife's room—two of the bottles being empty, the remaining four bottles being full. The disposal thus made of the six bottles was in accord with usual hospital practice where special medication is prescribed for a patient. It is not claimed by the prosecution that the disposal thus made of the bottles was in any way dictated by the defendant. As no chemical analysis was ever made of the contents of any of the six bottles there was no direct proof that any one of them contained strychnine.

The body of the decedent, which had been buried on December 9, 1943, without embalming, was exhumed on May 12, 1944, when a post-mortem examination revealed that her organs contained 3.7 grains of strychnine—an amount three times the minimum lethal dosage.

The trial judge explained to the jury—"In order for the prosecution to prevail in this case you must find beyond a reasonable doubt that the strychnine poison from which she allegedly died was taken at the hospital and at no other place; for if the prosecution has failed to satisfy you beyond a reasonable doubt that the poison was administered to her after the pinkish medicine was brought to the hospital, the defendant must be acquitted."

The issue of fact thus defined by the trial court was not decided by the jury on direct evidence. The record contains no direct proof, as we have seen, that there was strychnine in any one of the six bottles of "pinkish medicine" which the defendant had prepared and brought to the decedent's room. The jury's decision rests upon the conflicting views expressed by experts—each of whom concededly was qualified—called by the People and by the defendant on the question as to how long ingested strychnine retains its lethal effect. All the experts agreed—and the prosecution offered no evidence to the contrary—that the decedent's illness on the night of December 7th, before she was removed to the hospital, was due to strychnine poisoning. The experts disagreed, however, upon the decisive point as to whether her death in the early hours of December 9th could have resulted from strychnine which the experts agree was in her system on the night of December 7th. Upon that issue the People's experts stated their opinion to be that the strychnine which caused decedent's death was not ingested before she entered the hospital on the night of December 7th—twenty-eight hours before her death—but was in the bottle from which the last medication was administered to her at 2:30 A.M. on December 9th. Opposed to that view the opinion of experts sworn by the defendant was that the decedent's death on December 9th could have resulted from strychnine ingested by her on the night of December 7th. Indeed, there was testimony by one of the defendant's experts that he had known of a case where a patient took a lethal dose of strychnine and lived for thirty-six hours.

[EDITORIAL NOTE: The insufficiency of the evidence of guilt was the primary reason for reversal of the pharmacist's conviction. There were not enough undisputed facts to support a conviction based on circumstantial evidence. A second issue considered by the court also supported reversal of the pharmacist's conviction. That issue related to the instruction given by the judge to the jury regarding the meaning of the phrase "reasonable doubt." In evaluating how the trial judge explained the meaning of that important phrase to the jury, consider whether the judge's explanation would make sense to a typical juror.]

These considerations, standing alone, have exerted strong influence upon our judgment that justice to the defendant's rights requires a new trial. They are reinforced, however, by another incident at the trial which becomes decisive in its cumulative weight. One of the fundamental statutory rights accorded to the defendant is that he "is presumed to be innocent, until the contrary be proved; and in case of reasonable doubt whether his guilt is satisfactorily shown, he is entitled to an acquittal." When the trial judge reached that point where he defined for the jury what was intended by the Legislature's use of the phrase "reasonable doubt" he said – "It is not a doubt based upon sympathy or a whim or prejudice or bias or a caprice, or a sentimentality, or upon a reluctance of a weak-kneed, timid, jellyfish of a juror who is seeking to avoid the performance of a disagreeable duty, namely, to convict another human being of the commission of a serious crime."

While no judge is to be confined to the use of any precise verbiage, it is our thought that to define reasonable doubt by use of such characterization was not conducive to a fair and impartial consideration of the evidence.

The judgment of conviction should be reversed, and a new trial ordered.

The conviction was reversed on appeal, due to the insufficiency of the evidence and due to the judge's confusing definition of "reasonable doubt."

The prosecution chose to retry the pharmacist. This is not a situation that falls into the category of double jeopardy. Had the pharmacist been acquitted by the jury in the first trial, then the prosecution would not have been able to conduct a second trial for the same crime. Prosecutors only have one chance to try a defendant who is acquitted. However, if a defendant is convicted, and if the conviction is reversed on appeal, then the prosecutors may usually conduct a second trial of the defendant for the same crime.

Pharmacist's Second Conviction and Reversal on Appeal

The case was retried before a different jury, and the pharmacist was convicted again for the capital offense of first-degree murder.[2] In this second appeal, from the second murder conviction, the issues were similar, but there are important differences. The destruction of the bottles of "pink liquid" brought to the hospital by the pharmacist made it impossible to verify the contents of them. There was no evidence, either direct or circumstantial, that the bottles contained strychnine. Similarly, the decedent's tissues analyzed by the prosecution's toxicologist had been destroyed and were not available for examination by defense experts. Even the toxicologist's notes had somehow been destroyed and were not available for reevaluation by defense experts. The evidence of guilt was simply too speculative.

Below, in italics, is excerpted language from the second appellate opinion that resulted in reversal of the pharmacist's second murder conviction. The appellate court said:

Proof of guilt of administering poison to another, resulting in death, is always difficult and the instant case constitutes no exception. Unless there be a confession or direct testimony by observers of the act, dependence must be upon circumstances attending the event and then the question, in a capital case, which is presented to us for our consideration is whether the guilt of the accused has been established to a moral certainty by circumstances which not only point to the guilt of the accused but are inconsistent with his innocence.

One of the difficulties here is that there is no direct proof that the defendant had anything to do with the strychnine which it is alleged was administered to his wife, the deceased. There was no proof that he ever purchased or possessed any. As a substitute for such proof, it is pointed out that the defendant was a licensed employed pharmacist and thus had access to the poison. The bottle alleged to have contained it was discarded as refuse in the hospital by the nurse in attendance on the deceased after her death. Thus no one can say with certainty that the bottle contained strychnine. The toxicologist, who was not a physician, testified to the presence of strychnine in the organs of the deceased, other than intestines, when he performed an autopsy and analyses some five months after burial. He also testified that in discovering it, all of the organs supplied him consisting of the brain, lungs, liver, spleen, heart, kidneys, blood, empty stomach, two pieces of rib and a male fetus, were used up and that no material is left. There is thus in existence no tangible evidence which others may check and test which would show the presence or amount of strychnine at any time in the body of the deceased. The "very few notes" made on pieces of paper from time to time during the tests which took about a week, were destroyed after being typed by the toxicologist personally, after he had completed his examination and tests. To put it succinctly, the opinion testimony revolved about the estimate of "the total amount of strychnine in the entire body, exclusive of the gastro-intestinal tract and exclusive of the urine" and was calculated upon a body weight of 132 pounds or approximately "60 kilos." Moreover, the stomach showed too small a trace of strychnine to estimate it. The case against the defendant hung upon the correctness of the estimate and calculation plus the opinion testimony. It is rare when a charge in a capital case may depend upon such an "estimate" and conviction should follow only upon the clearest and unconfused proof.

In addition to the toxicologist, four experts or opinion witnesses were called upon to give testimony. Not one of the five had seen the decedent in life. The doctors who had seen and attended her at home on December 7th and in the hospital on December 8th, before her death in the early morning hours of December 9th, diagnosed her case as one of tetany accompanying pregnancy. That indicated a calcium deficiency. The five opinion witnesses called upon at the trial all agreed that on December 7th, the deceased had ingested strychnine. There is no contention by the People that the accused had anything to do with that. The two opinion witnesses for the defendant gave it as their opinion that the deceased died from the December 7th ingestion. The three opinion witnesses called by the People gave it as their opinion that she did not, but she died from the ingestion of strychnine in the early hours of December 9th at the hospital. There was no strychnine found at either hospital or home. If the deceased died from the ingestion of strychnine in her home on December 7th, the accused was entitled to acquittal of the charge made. If she died from the ingestion of strychnine in the hospital on December 9th, the guilt of the accused depended on whether he had put strychnine in one of the bottles which he brought to the hospital and delivered to the nurse in attendance upon his wife and no part of the contents of which was analyzed because of the conduct of the nurse in disposing of it, to which reference has already been made.

In a case as close as this one, it is clear that it was essential for the trial court to make certain that no error in the admission or exclusion of evidence occurred and that there was no confusion as to facts. Concededly that was not an easy task. It is against the background outlined that we consider some of the facts and some of the rulings made.

The toxicologist who performed the autopsy testified that he estimated from his three analyses of specified grams of brain, liver and of a composite sample of heart, brain, liver and blood that there were 3.7 grains of strychnine in the body of deceased. As we have mentioned earlier, the experts for the defendant gave it as their opinion that death could have been caused by "a quantity of strychnine ingested by her twenty-eight hours before"; that the medication administered in the hospital would have tended to postpone death by delaying convulsions and stopping or slowing down intestinal movements. The experts for the People said that that was impossible; that the deceased must have ingested less than a lethal dose on December 7th and must have practically eliminated it from her system; that death was caused by the ingestion of strychnine at two-thirty on the morning of December 9th. Thus, the finding of guilt depended on which opinion witnesses the jury believed. The defendant's experts gave it as their opinion that the deceased ingested strychnine once—on the 7th day of December. The People's experts gave it as their opinion that she ingested strychnine twice—once on the 7th and again on the 9th. All that was opinion based in the final analysis on the testimony of the toxicologist that on autopsy he found strychnine in the organs of the deceased.

[NOTE: The appellate court was also critical of the trial court's refusal to permit defense counsel to use a standard text in refutation of the toxicologist's opinions. The trial court had indicated that a textbook could be used in support of the expert's opinions, but not to refute the expert's opinions. The appellate court ruled that this approach was not consistent with prior law in New York.]

We think the judgment of conviction must be reversed because of the ruling of the court upon the right of the defendant to cross-examine the expert or opinion witnesses. When the toxicologist was being cross-examined, the following questions were asked of him:

"Q. Now, you said that you got part of your information or knowledge about toxicology from literature; is that right?

A. That's right.

Q. Did you ever read "'Textbook of Physiology'" by Howell?

A. "I've glanced at it."

The court, without more, then ruled that if counsel wished to refer to any textbook or literature, he must show it to the witness and that if the witness agreed with it and adopted it, the witness might then be questioned about it. The court said, "I shall not permit you to read from that book or any other book. If you wish to question this witness regarding any material, any writing, any dissertation or questions or statements contained in that book, you will first refer to the witness; let him read it and if the witness replies that he agrees with it or that he adopts that argument as his own, then I will allow you to refer to it. Otherwise, not."

During the same discussion the court repeated the ruling as follows: "you will first refer the book to this witness and if the witness tells the Court that he agrees with that statement or that writing and adopts that argument as his own, you may then question him regarding such statement or such argument. Otherwise, I shall exclude it."

In this state when an expert witness has given opinion testimony and on cross-examination has testified that a book called to his attention is recognized by him as an authority upon the subject as to which he has given an opinion, he may be confronted with a passage from the book which conflicts with the opinion he has expressed. This is permitted for the purpose of discrediting or weakening his testimony. It has been the custom, in this state at least, to call the attention of an expert witness, upon cross-examination, to books upon the subject, and ask whether or not authors whom he admitted being good authority had not expressed opinions different from that which was given by him upon the stand. The reference to books in such cases is not made for the purpose of making the statements in the books evidence before a jury, but solely for the purpose of ascertaining the weight to be given to the testimony of the witness.

[EDITORIAL NOTE: One final point was made by the appellate court in reversing the pharmacist's conviction. That point related to the pharmacist having borrowed a toxicology book from a university professor and the inference that this act of borrowing a book was evidence that the pharmacist intended to murder his wife. The trial court had allowed this fact into evidence and had instructed the jury that it was possible to infer from the pharmacist's borrowing of the book that the pharmacist had murderous intent. The appellate court ruled that the borrowing of the book was too remote from the wife's death to be considered as evidence of the crime of murder.]

There is another matter to which we shall refer since there must be another trial. The People called as a witness a professor in the Brooklyn College of Pharmacy. He had not been a witness on the first trial. He testified that three or four months after he had loaned the defendant a book on toxicology written by Underhill and Koppanyi, he read an article in a newspaper in which the defendant's name was mentioned. There was also mention in the article of the date of the wife's death. That recalled to him the fact that the defendant had visited him and asked the witness to loan him his notes so that the defendant might take the State Board examination to become a pharmacist in Florida. The witness loaned the defendant the book instead. A book was shown to the teacher which he said was an exact copy of the book he had loaned. That copy was then received as evidence over an objection. The assistant district attorney read at length from the exhibit under the headings as to symptoms of strychnine poisoning, and from headings entitled: "Fatal Dose," "Fatal Period," "Post-Mortem Appearances" and "Treatment of Nux Vomica Poisoning."

Apparently, the professor had communicated with the District Attorney subsequent to the first trial which occurred in February 1946.

During his explanation to the jury, the Trial Judge said: "You may only consider on this point, if you find the defendant borrowed the book, whether he did so for the purpose of planning and acquiring knowledge with respect to strychnine poisoning, and you may consider that the borrowing of this book at the time it is alleged to have been given to the defendant, if not too remote to the subsequent death of the defendant's wife by strychnine poisoning, was such conduct or action on the part of the defendant which you may consider on the question of intent, preparation, premeditation or motive to commit the offense charged."

Borrowing of the book by the defendant was not evidence of a motive for the commission of the crime by him. He was not a layman seeking a book on poisons. He was a duly licensed pharmacist who would not have been licensed unless he had studied toxicology. Moreover, there is no proof that he did not borrow the book with the intention of taking an examination in Florida. Motive means the reason why a thing is done and a borrowing of the book by the defendant could not be found to be a reason why he may have killed his wife. Hence the quoted words of the explanation to the jury were incorrect and must be taken to have unduly prejudiced the defendant with the jury, since the court had earlier told them that the presence or absence of motive was a potent or impelling circumstance which could "render important aid when, without it, the intent with which the alleged criminal act was committed would remain in doubt."

The judgment of conviction should be reversed, and a new trial ordered.

At this point, after a second reversal of a second conviction, the prosecution apparently caved in. There is no public record of any further legal proceedings against the pharmacist, leading to the conclusion that a third trial of the pharmacist for murder was deemed not to be an efficient use of public resources.

Was the pharmacist guilty or innocent? It must be one or the other. But that fact is impossible to know from the public record. The two appellate court reversals of the pharmacist's two convictions do not establish guilt or innocence. These convictions and reversals show only that the government (The People) failed to prove the pharmacist guilty, not that the pharmacist was innocent. The evidence presented by the prosecution was insufficient. The investigation of the alleged crime had not produced adequate facts to support a first-degree murder case based on circumstantial evidence. From a legal perspective, the pharmacist was innocent, because he had not been proven guilty.

Challenges of Criminal Investigation

As the case excerpted above demonstrates, pharmaceutical homicide is a difficult crime to investigate and a difficult crime to prosecute. It is all about the strength of the evidence, and the evidence must be discovered through investigation. A noted forensic pharmacist, John H. Trestrail, III, RPh, ABAT, provides insightful guidance on the methods to use in the investigation of a suspected pharmaceutical homicide.[3]

Pharmacist Trestrail explains that unlike bullets and knives and blunt instruments, drugs don't leave visible signs of trauma. There may not even be a crime scene. Or it may be nearly impossible to identify the scene of a pharmaceutical crime. The victim may have no available means to defend themselves from a pharmaceutical crime because it is impossible to live without eating, drinking, and breathing.

Pharmaceuticals may be weapons of choice because even after an unsuccessful first attempt at murder, there is usually an opportunity to try again. Intended victims may not even be aware of an attempt on their life. A pharmaceutical weapon may be overlooked at a crime scene, or it may lead to a murder looking like suicide.

Pharmaceutical homicides are usually done in secret. There are no accomplices who are willing to serve as witnesses and implicate the perpetrator as a means of self-protection. Most pharmaceutical homicides are well-thought-out. They are rarely crimes of passion brought about by a moment of reactive anger. Rational preplanning facilitates an effective cover-up. The investigator must step into the shoes of the murderer and figure out how a rational planner would have organized a pharmaceutical homicide. To catch a criminal, an investigator must think like a criminal.

Investigating the Incident

On those occasions when pharmaceutical homicide is suspected or when there is no other explanation and pharmaceutical homicide must be ruled out, a thorough investigation is required. The initial focus must be on the victim. Who is this person? Where did this person live? Why was this person here? Who else knows about this person's lifestyle and background? What evidence of pharmaceutical overdose is visible at the crime scene (drugs, injection devices, empty containers, vomit, or other bodily fluids)?

The focus must then shift to the availability of pharmaceuticals that could serve as murder weapons. How might a drug have been administered to the victim? Where are potentially weaponized pharmaceuticals stored or prepared? How are these pharmaceuticals distributed? What records are kept of these pharmaceuticals and where are the records maintained?

The first responders, and all other subsequent witnesses at the scene, must be thoroughly interviewed, and their statements must be preserved for follow-up questioning. Specific questions must be asked and answered. What did the victim eat or drink prior to the appearance of symptoms? Did others consume the same substances as those that the victim ate or drank? Were any of the substances that were consumed by the victim unusual for that person?

Any possibly relevant evidence must be confiscated, classified, and preserved in the condition it was found. This would include the remains of any food or drink, all prescription or non-prescription drugs discovered at the place of residence or the place in which healthcare was provided, as well as empty containers that may have held suspicious substances, such as glasses, bottles, utensils, or syringes. All soiled linens or clothing must be preserved as they were found.

Investigating the Environment

Sometimes, the suspected pharmaceutical homicide incident will itself seem inexplicable, yet the circumstances surrounding the incident can provide information that brings into view certain aspects of the incident that would otherwise be of little concern. There may be people who are familiar with the circumstances and environment who have felt for a period of time that "this is quite unusual." While some of these feelings may ultimately turn out to be irrelevant, they nevertheless must be pursued. The approach taken to the investigation of circumstances and environment will differ depending on whether the suspected pharmaceutical homicide occurred in an organized healthcare setting or in the community setting outside a healthcare institution.

The legal case of the pharmacist accused of murdering his wife is a perfect example of how an incomplete investigation can hinder a criminal prosecution. The conclusion that the patient died from strychnine poisoning was subject to challenge based on the toxicologist's failure to preserve tissue samples for retesting by defense experts, and by the lack of access to the toxicologist's lab notes for reanalysis by defense experts. It is the prosecution's burden to prove the case. When key prosecutorial evidence is not subject to examination by defense counsel, a criminal case is difficult to prove. The defense can raise a reasonable doubt based on the absence of evidence. What the prosecutor needs is strong circumstantial evidence to buttress weak direct evidence.

The lack of any circumstantial evidence obtained from the pharmacist's home forced the prosecutor to focus on the hospital as the crime scene. The court in the second appeal recognized that the case was a "close" one and that for this reason there must be "no confusion of facts." The experts disagreed about the timing of the strychnine poisoning. Some experts expressed the opinion that the wife could have been poisoned at home on December 7. The problem that this evidence presented for the prosecution was that the pharmacist was not at home when the wife was visited by her sister on December 7, and the wife appeared to be in good health at that time. The pharmacist was still not at home an hour later when a neighbor discovered the wife in an emergency situation.

The wife's physician appeared on the scene before the pharmacist arrived, and the pharmacist seemed to be saddened. The pharmacist insisted that a specialist physician be summoned. This is not behavior that points toward the pharmacist as the culprit. In fact, it is evidence to the contrary. Had the home been thoroughly investigated, then perhaps additional evidence would have been discovered. Perhaps an investigation of the relationship between the pharmacist and his wife would have produced evidence of discord or of suicidal intention. That investigation apparently did not occur, because no evidence of suspicious discoveries in the home, or suspicious matters related to the couple's lives, was presented by the prosecution. The events that transpired on December 7 remain a mystery. The victim's home may have been a crime scene, but proving that to a jury beyond a reasonable doubt was impossible without evidence.

Focusing on the hospital as the crime scene presented additional challenges for the prosecution. There had, at one time, been direct evidence of the pharmacist's guilt or innocence. The contents of the bottles of "pinkish medicine" brought to the hospital by the pharmacist could have either implicated or exculpated the pharmacist as a first-degree murderer. However, consistent with hospital policy, these bottles were thrown out. The failure to preserve this evidence either destroyed the prosecution's case, or it destroyed the pharmacist's defense. This approach is contrary to policies at many hospitals today. Evidence should be retained for further investigation when an unexplained and unexpected patient death occurs. It is a component of quality assurance activities. Nevertheless, it is a policy that is often not complied with. The mandate to efficiently clean up after one patient admission has ended, to make room for another patient admission, is understandable from a healthcare perspective and from a financial perspective. Unfortunately, it is a problematic mandate from an investigative and prosecutorial perspective. Suspicious and/or unexplained patient deaths must be investigated.

A Medical Examiner Is Charged with Murdering His Wife

The many challenges that prosecutors face following an indefinite murder investigation are further exemplified by a Florida case in which a medical examiner (ME) was charged with murdering his wife. At dawn on the day of the wife's death, the ME left home for the pathology clinic where he worked. During a 7 a.m. meeting, the ME expressed concern over his wife's fitful night's sleep, her complaint of chest pain and left arm pain, her chronic reluctance to seek medical attention, and his inability to obtain a blood sample for testing despite two attempts at inserting a needle into her arm.

The ME asked a staff paramedic to visit the home to check on the wife. At about 10 a.m. when the paramedic arrived, the wife was unresponsive and could not be revived. The paramedic estimated that the wife had died 30 minutes to an hour before he arrived. Later estimations by others ranged from 30 minutes to 3 hours.

It is the practice in Florida, following an unattended death, for the body to be transported to the nearest ME for autopsy. In this case, the husband was the nearest ME. The ME directed that his wife's body be taken to a funeral home because the wife had on many occasions expressed her desire not to be autopsied. Later that day, the ME's colleagues counseled that an autopsy would be appropriate under the circumstances, and the ME readily agreed, dismissing his earlier decision as having been influenced by grief. By that time, however, the body had already been embalmed in preparation for transport to Iowa for burial in the wife's family cemetery.

Arrangements were made for an independent forensic pathologist to perform an autopsy. Meanwhile, state law enforcement received an anonymous phone call reporting that the ME had murdered his wife.

The independent forensic pathologist undertook the autopsy with special care and thoroughness. Substantial pieces of toxicological evidence—blood, fluids, hair, fingernails, and other tissue samples—were taken from the embalmed body and were surrendered to state law enforcement. The autopsy "failed to reveal a convincing anatomic cause of death and indicated that no toxicological substances of note were recovered." The cause of death was ruled as "sudden unexpected death due to undetermined natural causes." Under pressure from state authorities who were still investigating a charge of murder, the pathologist later omitted the word "natural" from his conclusion.

After two state attorneys reviewed the case and determined that the evidence warranted no criminal prosecution, the Governor of Florida appointed a third prosecutor, and gave the case a "high priority." Medical and legal experts probing the death theorized that the wife may have been killed by a "perfect poison" such as potassium chloride. While potassium chloride can cause immediate death from a lethal dose, it is difficult to detect a lethal dose of potassium after death.

Litigation in Iowa

The State of Florida filed a legal action in Iowa seeking disinterment of the wife's body to search for evidence supporting its theory that the ME murdered his wife by injecting her with a lethal dose of potassium.[4] The family opposed the disinterment, arguing that a second autopsy would not furnish sufficient probative evidence that the ME had killed his wife.

Florida law enforcement authorities had referred the case to a private Pennsylvania toxicologist whose laboratory was known for pioneering new methods of detecting and measuring toxic substances. The Supreme Court of Iowa ultimately considered the State of Florida's request for disinterment and noted that the Pennsylvania toxicologist had labored under the mistaken impression that a physician in Florida had earlier found evidence of possible potassium poisoning. The potassium poisoning theory had, in fact, merely come out of investigatory discussions, and it had no scientific basis when it was proposed.

Florida authorities provided the toxicologist with fluid extracted from a lower chamber of the wife's heart. The fluid to be analyzed contained a mixture of blood and embalming fluid. To determine the percent of blood in the sample, the toxicologist began by testing for iron—theorizing that blood contains iron and that embalming fluid does not. The normal iron level would have been 450–520 mg/L, with 485 being the midpoint. The iron level in the tested fluid was 171 mg/L, indicating that the specimen was about one-third blood and two-thirds embalming fluid. With this 1:3 ratio in mind, potassium in the specimen was calculated as 38 mmol/L. The toxicologist tripled this figure to account for the dilution factor, resulting in an extended calculation showing that the potassium level in the wife's blood was 114 mmol/L. The expected range of potassium in a normal individual's blood is 42–52 mmol/L. From these calculations, the toxicologist concluded that a lethal dose of potassium had been administered to the wife, causing her death.

The wife's family provided the court with evidence from four pathologists. These pathologists from several university medical centers in the Upper Midwest sharply disagreed with the toxicologist's conclusions and with the

State of Florida's reliance on them. The experts all agreed that postmortem diffusion of potassium in the body precludes drawing accurate conclusions from potassium levels in the blood or other tissues of deceased persons. They explained that at death, blood cells naturally rupture, releasing potassium into the bloodstream. Potassium also diffuses from muscle and other tissue into the vasculature. These factors call into question the testing of fluids drawn shortly after death, and they also suggest that a second autopsy could produce erroneous results because diffusion occurring over the course of several years would have equalized the potassium levels in various parts of the body. Moreover, the pathologists challenged the toxicologist's assumption that the specimen tested was one-third blood and the assumption that the wife had normal iron levels when she might have suffered from anemia.

The pathologists' concerns were corroborated by a Florida pathologist who believed that no meaningful conclusions could be drawn without comparing the potassium levels in the wife's tissues with potassium levels in other embalmed bodies. The Iowa court noted that this pathologist's view had not been embraced by those involved in the Florida investigation, and he had not played any role in the investigation for several years.

The Iowa Supreme Court referred to the Pennsylvania toxicologist's theory as "novel and untested." The court wrote approvingly of the testimony of the family's experts who concluded that the toxicologist's theory had no validation in the scientific community. The court explained that Iowa statutes require the proponent of disinterment to show by the greater weight of the evidence that disinterment will yield proof of criminal culpability. The court concluded that the rights of the family members to oppose disinterment substantially outweighed the State of Florida's dubious proof that disinterment and a second autopsy would furnish probative evidence that the ME was criminally responsible for his wife's death. The State of Florida's request for disinterment and a second autopsy was denied.

Litigation in Florida

Undaunted by the denial of a second autopsy, the State of Florida decided nonetheless to prosecute the ME for murdering his wife.[5] However, the prosecutor switched to succinylcholine as the alleged murder weapon, rather than potassium chloride. The defense again challenged the scientific basis of the evidence.

After the Iowa debacle, Florida officials turned once again to the private laboratory in Pennsylvania, but this time they relied on a different toxicologist from that laboratory. The new toxicologist was recommended by the original toxicologist whose methods had been discredited by evidence presented to the

Supreme Court of Iowa. The Florida court had ruled that the original toxicologist's testimony would be inadmissible because it was based on methods and processes that were not generally recognized in the scientific community.

The new toxicologist had developed a novel laboratory procedure that he used to detect quaternary ammonium compounds in biological specimens. He used this procedure to test all of the embalmed tissues that had been obtained by the original forensic pathologist on the day of the wife's death. The new toxicologist used three different tests looking for evidence of succinylmonocholine, which is a metabolite formed by the decay of succinylcholine. The first test detected succinylmonocholine in the wife's kidney, brain, and lung specimens. The second test detected succinylmonocholine in the wife's spleen, kidney, lung, and fat specimens. The third test detected succinylmonocholine in the wife's kidney and brain specimens.

Based on the evidence provided by this second toxicologist, the original independent forensic pathologist changed the cause of death on the wife's death certificate that he had issued nine years earlier. The cause of death was changed from "sudden unexpected death due to undetermined causes" to "homicide due to succinylcholine poisoning."

Relying on this new death certificate, the State of Florida proceeded with the murder prosecution. The jury was presented with evidence from the new toxicologist's tests, as well as evidence from an FBI lab that had tested all of the tissue samples three months after the new toxicologist's tests and had detected levels of succinylmonocholine only in the kidney specimen. The jury convicted the ME of first-degree murder and sentenced the ME to life in prison. From this conviction the ME appealed.

The key issue on appeal was the sufficiency and validity of the scientific evidence. The Florida Court of Appeals noted testimony from defense experts who claimed that the new toxicologist's novel method of analysis had not been validated and that method validation is a prerequisite to acceptance in the scientific community.

The defense experts explained that the FBI lab had not reproduced the findings of the second toxicologist because that lab detected succinylmonocholine in only one specimen. They maintained that this was significant because the state-of-the art instrumentation used by the second toxicologist and the FBI lab were extremely sensitive and capable of detecting compounds in very minute trace concentrations. The experts explained that if succinylmonocholine were present, then it would be detected in all tissue samples, yet it was not detected in many of the tissue samples that were examined.

The defense experts testified that, in their opinion, succinylmonocholine could not be detected within the tissues after two years when the tissues had been embalmed ninety minutes after death and immediately preserved in a freezer. Moreover, they agreed that there was no reasonable explanation why succinylmonocholine was found in the brain, spleen, lung, and fatty tissue at the second toxicologist's lab but could not be found by the FBI lab in the same tissue sixty-one days later. If the compound degraded quickly between the two lab tests, then this was inconsistent with the tests being positive in the first place.

The defense experts also testified that there was no scientific literature or published study demonstrating that succinylmonocholine is not routinely found in embalmed tissue, or that succinic acid and choline, both of which are endogenous to the human body, cannot combine to form succinylmonocholine.

One of the defense experts testified that the second toxicologist's lab had not implemented a quality assurance program to ensure sample integrity and to prevent contamination. She noted that there had been a positive reading for succinylmonocholine when the lab ran a blank sample. She also noted that because of poor recordkeeping, there was no way to identify the samples that were tested during particular analytical runs. The lack of quality controls was significant because there was another criminal case in which the lab had tested tissue samples that were known to contain succinylcholine. The possibility of cross-contamination could not be eliminated.

The Court of Appeals of Florida reversed the murder conviction. The court concluded that the state had failed to establish by independent and impartial proof that the testing procedures used by the two labs were generally accepted in the relevant scientific community. The case was remanded for a new trial. Rather than conduct a second trial, the state and the ME agreed that he would plead guilty to manslaughter and accept a sentence of time already served. The ME died a decade later from lung cancer.

This case illustrates the importance of an immediate investigation of any unexpected death. Once a body has been embalmed or cremated, critical evidence that can convict or exonerate a suspect is no longer available. Unproven scientific methods that purport to establish guilt or innocence will not withstand judicial scrutiny. Immediate investigations of suspected pharmaceutical homicides can support a theory of criminality with facts that match the theory. Retaining evidence such as blood, urine, mucous, hair, fingernails, and skin scrapings, before internal organs are altered or destroyed, can facilitate a just resolution of a suspicious death.

Conclusion

In a democratic system of government, a defendant is presumed innocent until proven guilty. Guilt must be determined beyond a reasonable doubt. The determination of guilt is based on evidence and the interpretation of that evidence by a judge and/or jury. Exculpatory evidence is presented by the accused person's attorney. Incriminating evidence is presented by the prosecuting attorney. The evidence must be factual. The facts must be obtained through investigations that preserve both direct and circumstantial evidence for later consideration at trial. Justice is served when a thorough investigation has been conducted by an expert who understands the science and the circumstances of the alleged criminality.

Key Takeaways

- Be an investigator. Maintain an awareness of things that are happening within your sphere of practice. When a patient suffers harm that is unexpected or surprising, then take a step back and ask yourself why this might have occurred. Talk with others to find out whether they share your concerns. Make a mental note of who was involved with a patient's care when the surprising outcome occurred. In an institutional practice setting, if you can't find a reasonable explanation, then report your concerns to the hospital's Morbidity and Mortality (M&M) Committee where adverse outcomes are regularly discussed. In a community practice setting, report your concerns to the pharmacy's Continuous Quality Improvement (CQI) program. In the absence of any formal committee to receive a report, talk with a trusted colleague and a manager. If your concerns can't be resolved, then consult with your corporate risk management department or consult with your malpractice insurance company.
- Recognize that the truth exists only for a fleeting moment. What remains after an incident of patient harm are only memories that facilitate a re-creation of the truth. But human memories are notoriously unreliable. Preserve the facts. Don't trust your memory or any other person's memory. Any physical objects that may be relevant to a continued investigation should be retained and stored in a place where they will not be contaminated. Written and graphic records should be retained as well, including "sticky notes," photographs of whiteboard announcements, and any other informal records that will not be maintained by the medical records department. Comments

made by personnel should be preserved also, noting the date and time when the comments were made.

- Don't rely on assumptions. Patient care is a team responsibility. There are many members of the healthcare team who respect each other and who work together to produce positive outcomes for patients. One of the responsibilities of team members is to consult with others on the team when some aspect of a patient's care may be contrary to the patient's best interests. During a consultation, changes may be made to a plan of care based on new ideas presented by a team member. There may be a temptation to view this teamwork as a cohesive, well-oiled, process of patient care, where errors are efficiently detected and rectified before any harm is done to a patient. This viewpoint is a mirage. Unfortunately, healthcare is not free from error, despite the best efforts of all healthcare team members. Assuming that all must be well with a patient's care because so many team members are involved is a dangerous approach. Reject the impulse to assume that all is well. Investigate anything that is out of the ordinary, even if it may seem futile to do so. Sometimes, secrets exist not far under the surface of a seemingly innocuous situation, and these secrets are discovered only when someone looks for them.

References

1. People v. Feldman, 71 N.E.2d 433 (N.Y. 1947).

2. People v. Feldman, 83 N.E.2d 913 (N.Y. 1949).

3. Trestrail JH, III. *Criminal Poisoning: Investigational Guide for Law Enforcement, Toxicologists, Forensic Scientists, and Attorneys.* 2nd ed. Humana Press; 2007.

4. In re the Matter of Kay Marie Sybers, William A Sybers, 583 N.W.2d 890 (Iowa 1998).

5. Sybers v. State of Florida, 841 So.2d 532 (Fla. App. 2003).

Chapter 4

The Forensic Pharmacy Expert

The term "forensic pharmacy" can have different meanings. It is a relatively new term that applies primarily to any area of pharmacy law for which perpetrators can be punished with incarceration or fines or financial penalties. It is a relatively small slice of the pharmacy law pie. But it is an important slice. Any use of a pharmaceutical product in the commission of a crime is a subject that can be addressed through the application of the principles of forensic pharmacy. These crimes are particularly significant for pharmacists because the physical object with which the crime was committed, or attempted, has usually been provided through pharmacy channels. For a criminal to take a beneficial product, that is intended to relieve suffering, and to use that product for a destructive purpose, is shocking and horrific. It is one of the worst crimes imaginable.

A History of Forensic Pharmacy

Despite the relatively recent emergence of forensic pharmacy as a recognized field of study and of pharmacy practice, there is a history of forensic pharmacy that dates back to ancient times, because crimes at that time were often committed using poisons that were intended for use as medicinal remedies. It's all a matter of appropriate dosing, and what is sometimes referred to as the "Goldilocks Principle" that determines whether the amount of drug used is too little (subtherapeutic), or too much (toxic), or is just right (therapeutic). As the metaphor of Goldilocks fable suggests, what is needed in pharmacotherapy is not an underdose, and not an overdose, but just the right dose of medication for each patient.

In many parts of the ancient world, there were specially qualified people who could prepare medications and recommend the amount of a preparation that would be necessary to achieve a therapeutic effect. These were the first pharmacists (also referred to as "druggists" or "apothecaries" or "chemists"). These same remedies also served as toxins that could be used for murderous purposes at higher doses. Some of the pharmacists who prepared the medications were regularly called upon to determine whether an unexpected death was due to an overdose of a medication with which they were familiar. These were the first forensic pharmacists. At that time, poisons were as readily accessible as knives and clubs and other murder weapons, but poisons were far less likely to be detected after a murder had been committed. Forensic pharmacists found themselves busy in the application of their crime detection skills, in support of those public officials who enforced societal expectations for permissible behaviors through adherence to local laws. The crime of murder was as significant then as it is today, but the various means to detect a murder and to support the prosecution of a murderer were not as available then as they are now.

Pharmacy law is a broader field than forensic pharmacy, and it is formally taught as a comprehensive area of academic interest in schools of pharmacy. The subject of pharmacy law covers the requirements of administrative agencies, such as the FDA, the DEA, and state licensing boards. It also covers the potential for pharmacist exposure to malpractice liability and the basic principles of pharmacy risk management that can provide protection from claims of negligent practices that have resulted in harm to a patient. Most areas of pharmacy law deal with the development and implementation of systems to facilitate regulatory compliance. Forensic pharmacy fits into this framework when a failure to comply with pharmacy laws carries with it the potential for criminal liability and other punitive action. Administrative discipline and malpractice liability both have punitive components, and forensic pharmacy deals with those as well, although in a more forceful and consequential way. The concept of pharmacy "jurisprudence" is also used in a broader sense that includes all areas of pharmacy law, with a particular emphasis on the theoretical constructs that explain the purpose and rationale for pharmacy laws.

There are no uniformly recognized credentials that are required for a person to be an expert in forensic pharmacy. Most people who work in the field of forensic pharmacy have a professional degree in pharmacy and a pharmacy license, although they may instead have studied pharmacology or another scientific discipline related to the pharmacy profession. Some people in forensic pharmacy have supplemented their basic education with a degree in law or in toxicology, although this additional training is not necessarily the best way to acquire expertise in forensic pharmacy. Most pharmacists who have achieved at a high level in clinical practice, and who have an interest in learning more about the field of forensic pharmacy, can acquire the level of expertise they need to pursue forensic pharmacy without additional formal education.

Generalist Approach and Specialist Approach

There are aspects of virtually every area in pharmacy practice that require the application of forensic principles to the clinical evaluation of patient care or to the assessment of a prescription order. In this sense, one might say that "every pharmacist is a forensic pharmacist." This is a broad view that is accepted, but not without some limitations, by many of the experts who have formally studied the field of forensic pharmacy. Peter Anderson, a respected forensic pharmacist, noted in his article "The Broad Field of Forensic Pharmacy" that "almost every pharmacist does some type of forensic work whether he or she recognizes it or not."[1] For example, pharmacists routinely screen controlled substance prescriptions to detect the crimes of forgery and drug dealing. Pharmacists monitor patients' medication use for signs of criminal drug diversion, conduct prospective drug use review to detect possible healthcare fraud, and help identify drugs that high school teachers confiscate from their students to determine whether criminals are targeting children as customers for the purchase of illicit substances.

On the other hand, Anderson recognizes that some pharmacists practice in a specialty area that is more focused directly on forensics than on the many legal aspects of clinical practice that are present in virtually every community pharmacy and institutional pharmacy. These specialists in forensic pharmacy often work closely with government agencies or with private attorneys. They may consult with prosecutors or with defense attorneys in criminal cases. The forensic expertise of pharmacists is of particular value in legal cases related to charges of intentional poisoning, date rape, driving under the influence of controlled substances, or suspected suicide. Forensic pharmacists may support investigations by coroners in small towns where there is no qualified medical examiner with formal training. In this situation, the pharmacist may be the only person with a background in healthcare who can provide information about the role that drugs may have played in causing a person's death. Alternatively, pharmacists may function as key members of a large forensic team in a major city within a well-staffed medical examiner's office. As members of such a forensic team, pharmacists can dive deeply into questions related to adverse drug effects, based on postmortem analysis and available medical records. Specialists in forensic pharmacy may be few in number, but they are greatly appreciated for what they do. Anderson lists over a dozen pharmacists who have served as officers of professional organizations in the field of forensic science.

Anderson's description of a forensic pharmacist's role is supported by Pharmacist Jeannette Wick in her article "Forensic Pharmacy: Can You Prove It?"[2] As was the case with Anderson's broad description of forensics in clinical pharmacy practice, Wick explains that "Regulation by state and federal law forces pharmacists to engage, knowingly or unknowingly, in forensic work almost daily." Also consistent with Anderson, Wick describes how specialty forensic pharmacy practitioners serve as "consultants to attorneys, claims adjusters, detectives/investigators, and other forensic specialists." Wick notes that pharmacists can be particularly useful in evaluating legal cases based on allegations of drug-induced violence or elder abuse.

Most pharmacists involved in the field of forensics function in a consultant role. They provide their professional expertise when periodically called upon to do so, based on a perceived need to prove or disprove an allegation of unlawful activity. Within the consultant role as a forensic pharmacy specialist, pharmacists can provide the greatest assistance when they are willing to testify in court as an expert witness regarding the evidence they have reviewed and the conclusions they have drawn from the evidence. Consultants known as "non-testifying experts" may also be of value to litigants, but it is a forensic pharmacist's willingness to testify and the ability to testify persuasively that are of greatest value as a consultant in litigation based on allegations that a pharmaceutically related crime has been committed.

Qualifications of the Testifying Expert

Judges are often referred to as the "gatekeepers" of evidence provided to a jury. It is the judge's responsibility to ensure that juries consider the guilt or innocence of an alleged criminal defendant based on valid and scientifically supportable evidence. An expert witness must be professionally qualified to provide the testimony that is presented to a jury. The testimony itself must be based on a reliable foundation. Although experts provide what are referred to as "opinions," these opinions cannot be speculative theories based on personal experience rather than being based on established professional principles. Expert testimony must be based on well-founded opinions that reflect accepted science and established facts.

Pharmacists are generally allowed to testify as to the known characteristics of drugs as well as the specific effects of a particular drug for a particular patient. Pharmacists are generally not allowed to testify about the standard of care for a physician or other healthcare professional who is not a pharmacist. Pharmacists are also generally not allowed to testify that a drug caused a patient's death, although they may be permitted to testify that a patient could die from a drug that was used in a particular way.

General rules about pharmacist testimony are evolving. Courts will examine the training of a pharmacist who is offered as an expert on a particular issue, and the courts will judge a pharmacist's qualifications on a case-by-case basis.

Pharmacist Expertise in Alcohol Metabolism

The trial judge in one interesting legal case decided to exclude a pharmacist from testifying as an expert regarding the science of alcohol absorption, metabolism, and elimination.[3] The defendant had been accused of driving under the influence of alcohol. The judge was not well informed about the pharmacy profession. He allowed his preconceived notions about pharmacy to influence his ruling on the admissibility of expert testimony by a pharmacist. He was not willing to learn more about the expertise of pharmacists. Here is the confusing language that the trial judge used to justify his ruling that a pharmacist was unqualified to testify as an expert witness in the case:

> I don't find that the pharmacist satisfies the requirement for the court to accept him as an expert to testify in this area. I just have a really difficult time believing that any pharmacist in any drug store could walk into a courtroom and testify in an operating-while-intoxicated case as an expert on the issue, and that is the position that he has taken. He has been, he has testified 20 times, he said. He hasn't been trained with respect to anything except the various machines. He's studied pharmacy. He's studied pharmo, pharmokinetics. So have a lot of other people. I don't find him to be an expert. [Note: This language contains no typos. It is a direct quote from the ill-informed judge.]

The defendant was convicted, and he appealed his conviction based on the trial court's refusal to allow expert witness testimony by the expert pharmacist whom he had retained. The appellate court noted the basic rule about scientific testimony: "For a witness to qualify as an expert, the subject matter of the witness's testimony must be distinctly related to some scientific field, business, or profession beyond the knowledge of the average person, and the witness must have sufficient skill, knowledge, or experience in that area so that the opinion will aid the trier of fact."

At the defendant's trial, the defense attorney has asked the pharmacist: "Have you had the occasion to study the effects and ingestion of alcohol and the issues of absorption and burnoff?" The pharmacist responded: "That's what we call pharmacokinetics. That's what every pharmacist studies if they want to get a pharmacy degree. So, the idea is looking at absorption, elimination, how the drugs are eliminated, not just looking at the routes but in clinical pharmacology we quantify routes as we call it. Some still call it clinical pharmacology or pharmacokinetics, toxicokinetics, depending on whether you are monitoring a toxic effect."

The appellate court accepted this explanation and concluded that the pharmacist's proposed testimony was "related to a scientific field—pharmacokinetics." The court also concluded that the pharmacist "had sufficient knowledge and experience in this area that would have helped the trier of fact." The appellate court ruled that the trial court had erred in disallowing trial testimony by the expert pharmacist. The defendant's conviction was reversed, and the case was remanded to the trial court for a retrial with the jury being permitted to hear the pharmacist's testimony. There is no public record of the result, likely meaning that the case was dismissed or that the defendant entered into a plea agreement involving a lesser crime.

The result in this case does not support recognition of all pharmacists as experts in every type of criminal case. It does support recognizing pharmacists who have appropriate training and experience, as qualified experts in criminal cases that involve subject matter within a specialty field of expertise that the pharmacist has pursued professionally.

Pharmacist Expertise in Toxicology

A similar result occurred in a legal case involving a pharmacist who had completed residency training as well as a fellowship in toxicology.[4] The pharmacist was presented to the court as an expert regarding the toxic effects of a drug that had been prescribed for a patient. The pharmacist had worked at a poison center for many years. The pharmacist's qualifications as an expert were challenged because he was not a medical doctor and therefore it was argued that the pharmacist could not be considered a medical expert. The court said: "One cannot seriously argue that a licensed pharmacist and clinical toxicologist is not a medical expert." The court ruled that the pharmacist was qualified to testify regarding the toxicity of drugs. This ruling likely would not have applied to every pharmacist, but it did apply to the pharmacist whose credentials supported a high level of expertise in toxicology.

Pharmacist Expert Sued for Alleged Improper Testimony

A pharmacist's qualifications as an expert witness can be challenged by a criminal defendant following exoneration of the defendant. In a South Carolina case, a woman was convicted of "homicide by child abuse" in the death of her child.[5] The convicted mother had administered to her child an overdose of hydroxyzine that had been prescribed for the child to treat eczema. A pharmacist was retained by the government as a "forensic expert." The pharmacist advised the criminal investigator and the prosecutor that the facts showed a case of "chemical restraint" rather than "intentional poisoning." Nevertheless, the manner of death was determined to be "homicide." The mother contended that she had misunderstood the dosing instructions and that, due to this misunderstanding, she had dosed the child with one-half tablespoonful of medication when one-half teaspoonful had been prescribed. The mother alleged that the death of her child was the result of a tragic mistake and was not the result of child abuse through use of a chemical restraint.

The mother was convicted, but the conviction was overturned by the appellate court based on the absence of any intent to commit harm. The appellate court agreed with the mother's explanation of the overdose as being a tragic mistake. Following her release from prison, the mother sued the investigator, the prosecutor, and the pharmacist for malicious prosecution. She alleged that the pharmacist was particularly well positioned to measure the volume of liquid remaining in the medication bottle, and to conclude that the precise missing amount of medication supported the explanation of a tablespoonful/teaspoonful error. Moreover, the pharmacist allegedly was in a position to advise prosecutors that the toxicology report of the hydroxyzine in the child's tissues was consistent with the inadvertent error theory rather than with the intentional overdose theory.

Here is what the court had to say about the mother's case against the pharmacist (the mother is referred to as the "plaintiff" and the pharmacist is the "defendant"):

> Plaintiff alleges that the defendant operates a business through which she offers consultation services in the analysis and interpretation of toxicology reports. Plaintiff alleges that the defendant, a pharmacist, is also employed as the director of the forensic laboratory for the County Sheriff's Office. Plaintiff alleges that the pharmacist is not a physician, and that she violated South Carolina law when she opined and then testified as to the cause and manner of death of the child since this conclusion was a medical opinion and beyond her education or expertise. Plaintiff alleges that the defendant also violated established South Carolina law when she communicated to the investigator and prosecutor that the child had died of a drug overdose and that plaintiff used the medication to chemically restrain the child, since such conclusions are also medical judgments and well beyond the expertise of a pharmacist.
>
> Plaintiff alleges that the concentration of hydroxyzine in the child's system and the amount of drug that remained in the medicine bottle was consistent with the child mistakenly taking one-half tablespoon dosages of the prescribed medication, not one-half teaspoon dosages, and that the defendant knew that the amount of hydroxyzine in the child's system was consistent with the child having received one-half tablespoon dosages of the medication, but nevertheless actively participated with the investigator and prosecutor in plaintiff's prosecution for homicide by child abuse, which required the state to prove that plaintiff recklessly disregarded the well-being of her child. Plaintiff alleges that the defendant offered highly misleading information to the Court during trial in support of the chemical restraint theory, including that it was unusual for a child to be prescribed hydroxyzine although it has been approved by the FDA for pediatric use.

The case against the pharmacist was dismissed, based on the court's reasoning that the pharmacist had merely provided advice to the prosecutor and to the investigator. The decision to charge the mother with homicide by child abuse was not made by the pharmacist. Nevertheless, this case is worthy of consideration by any pharmacist who provides consulting services to prosecuting attorneys and criminal investigators. The pharmacist consultant's job is to investigate the evidence and not to reach conclusions about what crime to charge based on that evidence. Conclusions about criminal charges can be made by government law enforcement officials after consideration of the factual information provided by a pharmacist. The government will decide what crime to charge, if any. In this case, the mother's claims against the prosecutor and the criminal investigator were also dismissed, based on government immunity.

Quality of Expert Witness's Testimony

Judges are gatekeepers not only of expert witness qualifications. They are also gatekeepers of the quality of expert witness testimony. Judge Richard Posner, a highly regarded judge on the U.S. Court of Appeals for the Seventh Circuit, once said—"the courtroom is not the place for scientific guesswork, even of the inspired sort. Law lags science: it does not lead it." Judge Posner explained, in this oft-quoted sentence, that an expert witness's testimony must be based on fact and not on conjecture. Even well-qualified experts must discipline themselves to provide only useful information for consideration by a jury.

The leading legal case that explains the parameters of allowable expert witness testimony is the "Daubert" case from the Supreme Court of the United States.[7]

The Daubert case was a pharmaceutical case. The plaintiffs were the parents of a child who had been born with birth defects. The parents claimed that their child's birth defects were caused by an anti-nauseant drug that was taken by the mother during her pregnancy. The drug had been manufactured and marketed by the defendant, that is, the pharmaceutical manufacturer. The pharmaceutical manufacturer contended that the child's birth defects were not caused by the drug. The plaintiffs had the burden of proving their allegations against the drug manufacturer.

The scientific evidence was inconclusive. Clinical trials with pregnant women are not ethical, so the evidence was epidemiological. Most scientific experts concluded there was no evidence that the children born to mothers who took the anti-nauseant drug were any more likely to have birth defects than the children born to mothers who did not take the anti-nauseant drug. Several studies showed slightly elevated levels of birth defects in drug-exposed children based on the raw data, but these elevated levels were not statistically significant.

The plaintiffs attempted to rely on the testimony of experts who lacked the qualifications necessary to survive the judge's gatekeeping review. The plaintiffs were able to identify only one expert who was qualified by scientific training and experience, and who was willing to testify that the drug caused the birth defects. The trial judge had determined that the expert's proposed testimony was not credible. Without that testimony, the plaintiff's case would fail. The case was appealed to the Supreme Court of the United States where the trial court's original ruling was upheld. In making this ruling, the Supreme Court established what has become known as the "Daubert Rule" of admissibility of scientific testimony.

Here is what the court said in the Daubert case:

> There are differences between the quest for truth in the courtroom and the quest for truth in the laboratory. Scientific conclusions are subject to perpetual revision. Law, on the other hand, must resolve disputes finally and quickly. The scientific project is advanced by broad and wide-ranging consideration of a multitude of hypotheses, for those that are incorrect will eventually be shown to be so, and that in itself is an advance. Conjectures that are probably wrong are of little use, however, in the project of reaching a quick, final, and binding legal judgment often of great consequence about a particular set of events in the past. We recognize that, in practice, a gatekeeping role for the judge, no matter how flexible, inevitably on occasion will prevent the jury from learning of authentic insights and innovations. That, nevertheless, is the balance that is struck by Rules of Evidence designed not for the exhaustive search for cosmic understanding but for the particularized resolution of legal disputes.

The court's reference to the Rules of Evidence was to Rule 702 of the Federal Rules of Evidence, which states:

> If scientific, technical, or other specialized knowledge will assist the trier of fact to understand the evidence or to determine a fact in issue, a witness qualified as an expert by knowledge, skill, experience, training, or education, may testify thereto in the form of an opinion or otherwise, if (1) the testimony is based upon sufficient facts or data, (2) the testimony is the product of reliable principles and methods, and (3) the witness has applied the principles and methods reliably to the facts of the case.

In the Daubert case, the Court elaborated on this rule, noting that scientific testimony or evidence must be both relevant and reliable. Proposed testimony must be supported by appropriate validation, that is, "good grounds," based on what is known, and not on speculation. In short, the requirement that an expert's testimony pertain to "scientific knowledge" establishes a standard of evidentiary reliability. In determining whether to admit expert scientific testimony, the trial court must determine whether the expert's testimony is based on scientific knowledge that will assist the trier of fact in understanding or determining a fact in issue.

The Court offered these general guidelines for the evaluation of expert testimony:

- Ordinarily, a key question to be answered in determining whether a theory or technique is scientific knowledge that will assist the trier of fact is whether it can be (and has been) tested.
- Another pertinent consideration is whether the theory or technique has been subjected to peer review and publication.
- Additionally, in the case of a particular scientific technique, the court ordinarily should consider the known or potential rate of error, and the existence and maintenance of standards controlling the technique's operation.
- Finally, "general acceptance" can yet have a bearing on the inquiry.

In offering these guidelines, the court emphasized that it was not formulating a rigid test or checklist. The court relied instead on the ability of federal judges to properly determine admissibility. The Supreme Court explained that the Federal Rules of Evidence, especially Rule 702, assign to the trial judge the task of ensuring that an expert's testimony both rests on a reliable foundation and is relevant to the task at hand. Reliability relates to the reproducibility of the results. A study that can be reproduced by others using the same techniques is reliable. A study that cannot be reproduced is not reliable. Relevance means that the information offered by the expert contributes something necessary to the understanding of a solution to a problem. Information that is confusing, rather than clarifying, is not relevant.

If a judge concludes that the scientific evidence proposed by a qualified scientific expert for presentation to a jury is either not reliable or is not relevant, then the proposed testimony will not be allowed, even if the qualifications of the expert are sufficient. A judge may rule that some of the proposed testimony is allowable, while other aspects of the proposed testimony are not allowable. These determinations are usually made prior to trial, and the pretrial rulings made by the judge are enforced by the judge during the trial.

A Court Considers the Admissibility of a Pharmacist's Proposed Expert Testimony

To illustrate how a court evaluates the reliability and relevance of an expert witness's proposed testimony, it is useful to examine the language from a legal case in which the court limited the content of a pharmacist's expert witness testimony.

A lawsuit had been filed by a group of government agencies (the plaintiffs) against a group of corporate pharmacies (the defendants), alleging that the pharmacies did not meet their legal responsibilities to screen opioid prescriptions.[8] The lawsuit relied on the testimony of a pharmacist serving as an expert witness for the plaintiffs.

The court reviewed a report submitted by the pharmacist that contained opinions concerning the defendants' conduct with respect to: "maintaining effective policies and practices to guard against the diversion of prescription opioids, their failure to maintain and adhere to well-established pharmacy standards of care, and their dispensing of opioids into Lake and Trumbull Counties despite obvious and significant red flags."

Relying on numerous authoritative sources, the pharmacist had identified a set of "red flag" warning signals that pharmacies could use to identify potentially illegitimate prescriptions.

The presence of a red flag, the pharmacist explained, raises a responsibility on the part of both pharmacies and pharmacists to "determine if a prescription is valid and issued for a legitimate medical purpose by a practitioner authorized by law while acting in the usual course of his professional practice." The pharmacist expressed the opinion that the defendants had failed to fulfill this responsibility. According to the pharmacist, effective steps to address a red flag warning must include: (1) investigating the prescription and (2) documenting either a resolution of the red flag or a refusal to fill the prescription.

The pharmacist's report summarized his key opinions as follows:

- Defendants' local stores filled thousands of prescriptions presenting red flags without evidence of resolving those red flags.
- Defendants and their pharmacists have a corresponding responsibility to only fill prescriptions for controlled substances that are issued for a

legitimate medical purpose by an individual practitioner acting in the usual course of their professional practice.

- Defendants failed to provide their pharmacists with data, information, and the tools necessary to assist their pharmacists in fulfilling their corresponding responsibility duties, including but not limited to, utilizing dispensing data to identify patterns, trends, and practitioners possibly involved in diversion as well as to recognize and resolve red flags. The subsequent result of the failure to provide such data, information, and tools was the diversion of significant quantities of controlled substances, particularly opioids, outside of the closed distribution and dispensing system for controlled substances.

The defendant pharmacies sought to exclude or limit the pharmacist's testimony on three grounds. First, they contended that the pharmacist's "red flag" metrics for identifying potentially suspicious prescriptions were unreliable and untested. Second, the defendants argued that the court should bar the pharmacist from testifying that flagged prescriptions were not written for a legitimate medical purpose. Third, the defendants claimed that the pharmacist was not qualified as an expert and lacked a reliable basis to express opinions regarding any statistical link or correlation between flagged prescriptions and diversion. The court addressed each argument below.

Reliability of Methodology to Identify "Red Flag" Prescriptions

The court first considered challenges to the pharmacist's methodology in the identification of "red flags." Here is the language of the court:

> The pharmacist identifies certain "red flags" that pharmacies could use to identify potentially suspicious prescriptions. For example, if a "patient was dispensed opioid prescriptions written by at least 3 different prescribers such that all the opioid prescriptions were written in a 45-day period," those prescriptions are suspicious because they present indicia of doctor-shopping to obtain illicit opioids. Similarly, if a "patient was dispensed an opioid, a benzodiazepine and a muscle relaxer on the same day and all the prescriptions were written by the same prescriber," those prescriptions are suspicious because the combination of those three drugs suggests likely abuse. The pharmacist opines that the presence of a "red flag" is a warning signal that pharmacies and pharmacists must investigate to determine if the prescription is, in fact, valid and issued for a legitimate medical purpose.

Defendants argue the pharmacist's flagging methodology is unreliable because it is applied "mechanistically" and draws "bright line tests," regardless of context or other information about the prescription or prescriber. Defendants further object that the pharmacist has not tested whether his methodology, in fact, accurately flags illegitimate prescriptions.

As an example of "the arbitrary and irrational nature" of the pharmacist's methodology, the defendants point to his designation of a patient traveling more than 25 miles to see her prescriber as a "red flag" metric (suggesting possible pharmacy shopping to obtain illicit opioids). Defendants observe that the pharmacist admitted in his deposition that 25 miles is not a uniform standard of care requirement, and other pharmacists might reasonably determine that 20 miles or 30 miles is an appropriate "red flag" metric. That other pharmacists might apply differing "red flag" metrics, however, in no way suggests the pharmacist's choice of 25 miles is "arbitrary" or "irrational." As discussed, the pharmacist identifies "red flags" that pharmacists could use to identify potentially suspicious prescriptions. He does not contend that pharmacists must use his exact "red flag" metrics, or that pharmacists could not reasonably come up with differing metrics to effectively flag potentially illegitimate prescriptions. As the defendants point out, the pharmacist testified "pharmacists could properly use their professional and independent judgment to apply different standard of care tests." Indeed, simple common sense suggests it is reasonable for a pharmacist to be at least a little suspicious about a patient who seeks to fill an opioid prescription at a pharmacy distant from her home, and the further the patient travels to fill an opioid prescription the brighter the "red flag" becomes.

Here, the pharmacist's extensive experience in the practice and regulation of pharmacy provides a reliable basis for him to testify regarding different "red flag" metrics that are available to pharmacists to flag potentially illegitimate prescriptions. The pharmacist's report cites to various sources supporting his "red flag" criteria, including the defendants' own policies and DEA and court opinions. The Court has carefully reviewed the relevant portions of the pharmacist's report and finds that his sources, coupled with his extensive relevant experience in pharmacy practice and regulation, create a reliable foundation for each of his red flags.

The Court finds that, in determining whether the defendants employed effective measures to investigate and resolve "red flag"

> warning signs, it would be helpful to the finder of fact to hear evidence about the number of potentially suspicious prescriptions that the pharmacist's metrics would have flagged, and the different "red flag" metrics that a pharmacy could choose to employ. Accordingly, the Court concludes the pharmacist' "red flagging" methodology is reliable and would aid the jury's determination of material issues in the case. The Court therefore denies the defendants' motion to exclude the pharmacist's opinions on this ground.

Opinion That Flagged Prescriptions Were Illegitimate

Having denied the defendants' motion to exclude the pharmacist's opinions on "red flag" identification methods, the court turned its attention to the defendants' challenge to the pharmacist's opinions on prescription legitimacy. Here is the language of the court:

> Defendants assert the pharmacist lacks a reliable basis to opine that prescriptions flagged by his methodology were, in fact, not written for a legitimate medical purpose. As the defendants point out, the pharmacist agreed in deposition that, if a prescription meets one of his "red flag" designations, this does not necessarily mean the prescription was written for an illegitimate purpose. Defendants ask the Court to clarify that, at trial, the pharmacist may not testify—and plaintiffs may not argue—that prescriptions flagged by his methodology were not written for a legitimate medical purpose.
>
> Plaintiffs do not respond directly to the defendants' arguments. Rather, Plaintiffs assert the pharmacist does not intend to testify about specific, individual prescriptions that were not written for a legitimate medical purpose. But the defendants do not ask the Court to limit the pharmacist's testimony regarding specific prescriptions. Instead, Defendants assert the pharmacist has not established a sufficient foundation to opine that his flagging methodology, in fact, identifies illegitimate prescriptions. In other words, the defendants seek to preclude testimony that, because a prescription is "red-flagged," it has to be the case that it was not written for a legitimate medical purpose.
>
> Plaintiffs explain that the pharmacist intends to opine that Defendants' systematic dispensing of "red-flagged" prescriptions, in the aggregate, led to increased dispensing of illegitimate prescriptions. Plaintiffs further state: "It is sufficient for the pharmacist to make conclusions about the consequences of the sheer magnitude of 'red flag' prescriptions overall." Again, this argument does not directly

address the defendants' assertion that the pharmacist should be precluded from opining that "red-flagged" prescriptions were definitely not written for a legitimate medical purpose, or even that some of them must not have been.

The Court concludes the plaintiffs have not shown the pharmacist is sufficiently qualified to express opinions regarding actual consequences—as opposed to likely consequences—of the defendants' alleged conduct, even in the aggregate. On this record, the Court will preclude the pharmacist from opining that "red-flagged" prescriptions were not written for a legitimate medical purpose. While the pharmacist's methodology reliably supports his opinions that "red-flagged" prescriptions were potentially illegitimate, the pharmacist may not opine that the mere presence of a red flag, without more, in fact means a prescription is illegitimate.

Opinions regarding Actual Diversion Caused by Defendants' Dispensing of "Red-Flagged" Opioid Prescriptions

Finally, the court considered arguments by the defendants that the pharmacist cannot reliably testify regarding the cause of diversion as a result of filling "red flag" prescriptions. Here is the language of the court:

> Defendants argue the pharmacist is not qualified and lacks a reliable basis to opine that the defendants' dispensing of "red-flagged" opioid prescriptions, in fact, caused actual diversion. More specifically, the defendants ask the Court to exclude the pharmacist's opinions that: (1) a "statistical link" exists between flagged prescriptions and the rate of opioid diversion; and (2) "opioids dispensed pursuant to flagged prescriptions were diverted at a higher rate than other prescription opioids that were not flagged.
>
> In support of their motion, the defendants do not cite or discuss any particular opinions set out in the pharmacist's report. Rather, the defendants point to the pharmacist's deposition testimony that a "significant number of the prescriptions identified by his red flags were not for legitimate purposes and were diverted." Defendants contend the pharmacist is not qualified to state this opinion and seek to preclude him from testifying about any "statistical link" or correlation between the number of "red-flagged" prescriptions and the rate of opioid diversion.
>
> The record amply demonstrates the pharmacist has specialized experience and expertise to reliably state how, in his opinion, the

> defendants' pharmacy practices, procedures, and standards of care resulted in systematic failures to guard against diversion. Further, as the plaintiffs assert (and the defendants do not refute), this expertise also qualifies him to express opinions regarding the likely consequences of the defendants' alleged conduct—that is, that dispensing "red flag" prescriptions without conducting adequate investigation or due diligence is likely to lead to diversion. However, the pharmacist is neither a statistician nor an epidemiologist. The fact that he may be qualified to testify as to likely consequences (e.g., that the defendants' dispensing practices created a greater likelihood that prescriptions were diverted) does not show he has the requisite expertise to opine that the defendants' conduct, in fact, definitely resulted in diversion (or a "significant" or specific amount of diversion) of opioids.
>
> Plaintiffs have not shown the pharmacist is qualified to offer expert opinions regarding a statistical link or causal correlation between the number of "red-flagged" prescriptions and actual diversion of opioids, or that "red-flagged" prescriptions, in fact, were diverted at a higher rate than other prescription opioids.

For the reasons explained by the court in this case, the defendants' Motion to Exclude the Opinions and Testimony of the pharmacist was granted in part and denied in part. The pharmacist was not allowed to offer expert opinions regarding a statistical link or causal correlation between the number of red-flagged prescriptions and the actual diversion of opioids, or that a significant amount (or any number) of prescriptions identified by his "red flag" algorithms were, in fact, definitely illegitimate or actually diverted. The pharmacist was allowed to testify regarding his method for identifying "red flags." The court's ruling means that the pharmacist was allowed to testify, but that the substance of the pharmacist's testimony would be limited.

Just the Facts, Please

Sometimes, a pharmacist will be asked to testify to facts, but not to opinions. A so-called "fact witness" can describe what has happened but should not make any interpretations about the legal significance of what happened or about the implications of anything that has happened. A woman in the State of Washington died from an overdose of medications, and her husband was found guilty of first-degree premeditated murder.[9] The prosecution contended that the husband ground up a lethal dose of hydrocodone and mixed it into an ice cream drink that he made for his wife. The husband was having an affair with his high school sweetheart at the time of the wife's death. The high school sweetheart lived in New York, and their romance had rekindled during trips by the husband to New York.

The toxicology report detected hydrocodone, cyclobenzaprine, and trazodone in the wife's tissues. The medical examiner concluded that the hydrocodone level was ten times that of a toxic level, and, in his opinion, "the death was caused by hydrocodone toxicity in combination with the presence of the other drugs and exposure to the other drugs."

A pharmacist from the family's pharmacy testified that the wife had been prescribed small quantities of hydrocodone over the seventeen years prior to her death, but she had not received the drug recently. The wife had never been prescribed either cyclobenzaprine or trazodone. On the other hand, shortly before the wife's death, the husband had been prescribed 24 tablets of hydrocodone, along with cyclobenzaprine and trazodone. Pharmacy records also indicated that the husband had been prescribed sildenafil at times corresponding with his visits to New York.

Based on this pharmacist's testimony, and on other fact evidence, a data analyst for a local law enforcement agency testified using language that conveyed his opinion that the husband had murdered his wife. The data analyst used a slide show to present his testimony to the jury, and one slide was titled, "Pathway to Premeditation." This testimony was the basis of the husband's appeal of his first-degree murder conviction. The husband contended that it is the jury's role to determine guilt or innocence and that the witness's stated opinion of the husband's premeditation had unconstitutionally invaded the province of the jury. Whether an action undertaken by a defendant was premeditated must be left up to the jury and not to an expert witness.

Conclusion

The field of forensic pharmacy provides many opportunities for pharmacists to consult with various parties who have a level of involvement with the investigation, prosecution, or defense of alleged crimes or other unlawful conduct. Courts have recognized the expertise of pharmacists as expert witnesses in litigation. The testimony offered by pharmacists, or any other scientific expert, must be relevant and reliable. Judges serve as the gatekeepers of trial testimony to assure that expert witnesses provide information that will assist the court and jury in achieving a just result.

Key Takeaways

- *Stay within your pharmacy lane.* Do not try to "outlawyer the lawyers." It won't work. Respect their expertise in the law as you require them to respect your expertise in pharmacy. Do not try to anticipate the direction the lawyers are taking in a line of questioning, even if you can tell that they are heading toward a dead end. Let them go wherever they want to go, and you can follow their lead. You may need to help them if they ask a question like: "How do pharmacists prescribe medications?" Be forgiving of a question like this. You will have to explain that pharmacists do not generally prescribe medications, although some pharmacists do function as prescribers. This is an opportunity to further explain the role of pharmacists generally and, more specifically, the role of pharmacists as it relates to the consultation you have done with regard to a particular legal matter.

- *Be respectful and cooperative.* Even if a person who is questioning you becomes visibly upset with your answers, do not become upset yourself. Stay cool. Judges and juries will identify with your professional demeanor and will be negatively affected by the examiner's antagonism. On the other hand, you are not expected to be meek or timid. Be firm about your opinions and about the scientific basis of your opinions. If the opinion you offer is solid and cannot be refuted, then the person who is examining you may resort to an attack on you rather than on your testimony. This is a mistake by the examiner. It will not be well received by the judge or the jury. Don't make a similar mistake by responding with your own attack on the examiner.
- *Answer the question you have been asked.* Pay close attention to the question and ask for clarification if the question is not clear. Think before you answer. Always tell the truth. Do not continue to provide additional information that goes beyond answering the question you have been asked. For example, an examiner may say something like, "there was a problem with the prescription, wasn't there?" If the answer is yes, then be sure to explain the problem. You can say something like "Yes. There was a drug–drug interaction between two incompatible drugs." An examiner may ask that you provide a "yes or no" answer, which you should be prepared to do. Judges will then allow you to explain the answer. Take your time and do not let yourself be rushed into a simple answer to a complex question, even if the examiner obviously wants to move on to other subjects. If you do not know the answer to a question, then just admit that you do not know. Never make up an answer or provide unfounded speculation when you have no basis for providing an accurate answer.

References

1. Anderson PD. The broad field of forensic pharmacy. J Pharm Pract. 2012; 25(1):7-12.

2. Wick JY. Forensic pharmacy: can you prove it? Consult Pharm. 2013; 28(7):418-424.

3. Hastings v. State, 58 N.E.3d 919 (Ind.App. 2016).

4. Fusco v. Shannon, 63 A.3d 145 (Md.App. 2013).

5. Avery v. McCall Tanner, 2014 WL 5365731 (D. S.C. Oct. 21, 2014).

6. Rosen v. Ciba-Geigy Corporation, 78 F.3d 316 (7th Cir. 1996).

7. Daubert v. Merrell Dow Pharmaceuticals, Inc., 509 U.S. 579 (1993).

8. In re National Opiate Litigation, 2021 WL 4146672 (N.D. Ohio Sept. 13, 2021).

9. State of Washington v. Pettis, 2024 WL 3874378 (Wa.App. 2024).

Chapter 5

Notorious Pharmaceutical Serial Murderers

Healthcare professionals are no less likely than anyone else to commit crimes. It is naïve to think otherwise. Simply because a person has formally made a commitment to serving the needs of others does not mean that the person will avoid intentionally harming others or will avoid intentionally placing others at risk of death. When concerns arise after the unexpected death of a patient in a healthcare institution, nobody should be considered above suspicion. The status of a healthcare professional as a licensed expert in the healing arts does not preclude the possibility that the healthcare professional will commit a crime. In fact, there are some crimes that are considered "crimes of opportunity" in the healthcare professions, because the means for the commission of the crimes are readily available only to healthcare professionals.

Criminality in Healthcare

Crimes of opportunity in healthcare include healthcare fraud, controlled substance diversion, and sexual abuse. The responsibility for the coding of procedures for billing purposes, authority over the distribution of medications, and unsupervised access to patients, all provide healthcare professionals with the means to commit crimes. Even more egregious is the use of beneficial medications, acquired through the pharmacy department, for harmful purposes. In the most extreme example of such crimes, healthcare professionals have been found guilty of murdering patients through the administration of lethal doses of medications.

The Hippocratic Oath reflects an awareness that nefarious actions may be undertaken by healthcare professionals, and this understanding reflects the reality that such condemnable activity was well known in ancient times. Many centuries ago, the Greek physician Hippocrates instructed that all medical healers must commit to the basic principle, "I will follow that system of regimen which, according to my ability and judgment, I consider for the benefit of my patients, and abstain from whatever is deleterious and mischievous." More specifically, the Hippocratic Oath states, "I will give no deadly medicine to anyone if asked, nor suggest any such counsel." These two sections of the Hippocratic Oath have often been summarized with the more contemporary statement, "First, do no harm," although that language does not appear in the Hippocratic Oath. The inference that can be taken from these statements is that known cases of pharmaceutical homicide during the time of Hippocrates required that the statements be made. Why would Hippocrates have made these statements if he had not been aware of the need to make them? The statements renouncing pharmaceutical homicide must have been included in the Hippocratic Oath for a specific reason. They were a response by Hippocrates to murders that had been committed by people who were entrusted to heal others. One can infer from the language used in the Hippocratic Oath that medical healers had, in the past, administered "deadly medicine" to their patients and Hippocrates felt it necessary to clearly forbid any such actions in the future.

History also compels reflection on the crimes committed by Nazi physicians during World War II. On December 9, 1946, in Nuremberg, twenty-three German physicians and medical administrators were put on trial for their willing participation in war crimes, including euthanasia and pseudoscientific "experiments." Sixteen of the defendants were found guilty. Seven were sentenced to death and were executed on June 2, 1948. The most notorious Nazi physician, Dr. Josef Mengele, escaped to South America, where he died in 1979. Dr. Mengele has sometimes been referred to as the "Angel of Death," a moniker that has more recently been applied to other licensed healthcare professionals who have used their professional training to kill people rather than to heal them. Concentration camp inmates called Dr. Mengele "Der Weisse Engel" (The White Angel) because he would wear a white coat while meeting trains arriving at Auschwitz, standing on a pedestal, with one arm pointing to the left and one arm pointing to the right, designating who would be sent to immediate death and who would live (even if only temporarily).

Given this historical background, it is perhaps no surprise that a small number of healthcare professionals continue to commit murder against vulnerable people whom they have sworn to protect from harm. What happened in the past continues to happen today. This reality of murder by healthcare professionals is not often discussed, but it is factual. It is important to learn from the past through analysis of how murders can be, and have been, committed by healthcare professionals. The discussion of these murders is particularly applicable in pharmacy because the murder weapon used by most healthcare killers has been acquired through pharmacy distribution channels.

The remainder of this chapter provides a series of narratives that describe the actions undertaken by some of the most notorious pharmaceutical mass murderers. The murderers described in the biographical sketches that are presented in this chapter can be persuasive evidence for anyone who is skeptical about the significance of pharmaceutical homicide committed by healthcare professionals. It is tempting to disbelieve all of these histories. They are outrageous. They seem implausible. Yet they are true. Ignoring them will not stop them. These stories must be believed, and the reality of them must be confronted so that they can be stopped.

An important aspect of these stories is the criminals' modus operandi. Be prepared to identify the same or similar actions if you encounter them in your practice. Ask yourself—why were the perpetrators not caught sooner? Do you think that other healthcare personnel who were working with the perpetrators were completely unaware of the murders that were occurring? Is murder by medication in a healthcare setting so outlandish that it can't be believed because it is not easily seen? How might healthcare systems adapt to the unfortunate reality of pharmaceutical homicide in the healthcare setting, to better protect patients from the evil motives of criminal healthcare professionals?

Charles Cullen—Staff Nurse

Charles Cullen graduated from a New Jersey nursing school in 1987. He began working on a burn unit at a local hospital. His first murder victim was a 72-year-old patient whom Cullen killed using a lethal injection of lidocaine in 1988. During his time at this first hospital, Cullen murdered at least five other patients. Hospital authorities began to investigate their suspicions that something was terribly amiss and that Cullen was poisoning patients. Cullen was fired in 1992. The hospital's investigation disclosed that the contents of IV bags had been contaminated with drugs that could be lethal to patients. The investigation concluded that Cullen was likely responsible for this contamination and for the patient deaths. By the time the investigators' conclusion was reached, Cullen had left the hospital, and no further action was taken as a result of the investigation.

Shortly after he left the first hospital, Cullen obtained employment at a second hospital, where he continued his murderous ways, working on the coronary care unit. It was later determined that Cullen used digoxin as his murder weapon at this hospital. Suspicions were raised about Cullen's potentially criminal behaviors when a patient reported that a "sneaky male nurse" (Cullen) had injected her with a medication. Cullen was investigated and he passed a polygraph test. The elderly patient's remarks were dismissed by family members and hospital personnel as being the result of the patient's confusion and misunderstanding of the situation. At the end of 1993, Cullen resigned from this hospital.

In 1994, Cullen began working in the ICU of a third hospital. Cullen received an award for diligence and hard work at this hospital. Nevertheless, he later admitted that he killed five patients with digoxin while on that staff. He quit this job after three years and found employment at a fourth hospital. He was dismissed from this fourth hospital after only a few months based on poor job performance. There is no evidence that Cullen murdered any patients at the fourth hospital.

In late 1998, Cullen began working on the burn unit of a fifth hospital. He murdered three patients with digoxin overdoses at this hospital. In mid-2000, he quit the fifth hospital and took a job at a sixth hospital where he murdered six patients with digoxin overdoses. Cullen left that hospital after one year, because rumors were circulating about his lethal activities, and hospital officials were becoming suspicious of him. Shortly thereafter, the hospital reported Cullen to the State Board of Nursing for "probably unprofessional conduct." The Board of Nursing investigated. After finding what the Board believed to be incriminating evidence against Cullen, the Board turned this incriminating evidence over to the police, but no further action was taken. Cullen continued to maintain his active nursing license.

Cullen then obtained employment at what would be his final hospital. He soon began murdering patients with digoxin, norepinephrine, and dobutamine. In total, Cullen murdered over a dozen patients in less than a year at this hospital. The hospital investigated Cullen and discovered that he was accessing computerized patient information without authorization. In addition, Cullen was removing drugs from automated dispensing units without an order for a patient. The pharmacy department noted that the drug orders transmitted to the pharmacy by Cullen were unusual, contradictory, and irrational. The hospital notified the state police.

A criminal investigation was conducted, and a nurse who was a former colleague of Cullen provided the investigators with incriminating evidence against Cullen. The nurse agreed to wear a wire when she met with Cullen, and at this meeting Cullen provided sufficient information to support his being arrested. During his interrogation by police, Cullen admitted that he had administered between thirty and forty lethal doses of medication to patients over his sixteen-year career. Cullen pled guilty to twenty-two murders, and he was sentenced to eleven consecutive life terms in prison.

State and federal government agencies also launched an investigation into the hospitals where Cullen had worked. The investigation revealed that due to a shortage of nurses, the hospitals were willing to hire virtually any person with a nursing license without conducting background checks. When he was discharged from employment at the hospitals based on suspicions of illegal activity, Cullen was officially allowed to resign, with the hospitals unofficially agreeing that Cullen would be given a reference that omitted any negative commentary about his suspicious behaviors.

Robert Rubane Diaz—ICU Nurse

On March 29, 1981, Robert Rubane Diaz, a registered nurse, began work on the night shift in the cardiac care/intensive care unit (ICU) at a community hospital in Perris, California. In the next three-and-a-half weeks, at least thirteen patients on the night shift suffered violent seizures, which were generally followed by cardiac and respiratory arrest. Nine of these patients died. The nurses who had observed the seizures described them as being similar to grand mal seizures. None of the nurses had previously seen such symptoms in cardiac patients. Following the closure of the ICU at the community hospital, Diaz accepted employment at a second hospital. Within three days, while Diaz was on duty, a patient died at that second hospital after displaying the same symptoms as those observed in the patients who had died at the first hospital. One day later, Diaz was arrested and charged with murdering a total of twelve patients (including two in whom seizures were not observed).

At his trial, the prosecution contended that Diaz had killed the twelve patients by injecting them with massive overdoses of lidocaine. All but one of the deceased patients had been given therapeutic doses of lidocaine while in the hospital's ICU. The prosecution's evidence showed that Diaz assisted in the care of the patients before their seizures and, thus, was in a position to administer fatal doses of lidocaine; that on several occasions Diaz exhibited unusual behavior on nights when patients died; that the patients' symptoms were consistent with having been given large overdoses of lidocaine; that the patients' tissues or blood had unusually high concentrations of lidocaine; that syringes containing high concentrations of lidocaine were found in the hospital; and that lidocaine was found in Diaz's home.

The defense contended that some of the deaths resulted from natural causes, while others were caused by adverse reactions to medications administered for therapeutic purposes.

Although the deceased patients had suffered from serious medical problems, many of them were not regarded as terminally ill. The evidence presented at trial did not suggest that the deaths were "mercy killings." The prosecution did not argue such a theory at trial; nor did it suggest any other motive for the slayings.

Diaz was convicted of the crime of murder, and he was sentenced to death. He appealed his conviction. His arguments on appeal challenged the validity of the scientific testimony presented to the jury and the circumstantial nature of the evidence. Nobody had actually seen Diaz administer lethal doses of medications to patients.

In his appeal, Diaz contended that the testimony of the prosecution's experts was invalid. Specifically, he argued that the trial court should have excluded the experts' testimony that (1) inferred amounts of lidocaine present in the patients' bodies at death from amounts found in tissues tested long after death; (2) inferred amounts of lidocaine in entire organs from quantities found in small samples of organs; (3) inferred, from average organ weights, the quantity of lidocaine in the organs of decedents; (4) inferred amounts of lidocaine in the patients' entire body from amounts found in the patients' "central compartment" (the internal organs from which tissue samples were taken); and (5) inferred, from amounts of lidocaine found in the blood and tissues, that before death the patients received massive overdoses of lidocaine.

Because each of the twelve patients had been seriously ill at the time of death, there was initially no suspicion of foul play. Understandably, therefore, autopsies of most of the patients were not considered necessary, and ten of the twelve patients were embalmed and buried. As the number of deaths at the hospital mounted, and as authorities became suspicious that the patients had not died from natural causes, the bodies of the patients that had already been buried were exhumed, autopsied, and tested for lidocaine and other drugs. The bodies of the last two patients to have died had not yet been embalmed when the autopsies began, and they were also examined and tested.

Because of the embalming, blood samples were unavailable for any of the patients except the last two. Accordingly, prosecution experts took tissue samples from the patients' internal organs (heart, brain, liver, lungs, kidneys, and, in some cases, the vitreous humor) and measured the quantity of lidocaine found in these samples. Based on these calculations, the experts concluded that each of the patients had been given a massive overdose of lidocaine. Although all of the patients had been given therapeutic doses of lidocaine during their hospitalization, according to prosecution experts, the amount of lidocaine found in the tissue samples far exceeded the level that could be attributed to the therapeutic doses.

Lending additional support to the prosecution experts' conclusions was the presence, in some patients, of relatively small quantities of a metabolite into which lidocaine may decay, indicating that the lidocaine poisoning resulted from administration of a large overdose shortly before death and not from the buildup of lidocaine therapeutically administered over a period of time.

The Supreme Court of California said, "If we make the not-unreasonable assumption that all fatal overdoses were administered by the same person, defendant must be the killer. The patients were poisoned at night, in the hospital's ICU, where the presence of a stranger certainly would have attracted the staff's attention. At least two nurses were on duty on each of the nights when overdoses were administered, but defendant was the only nurse who was on duty on all of those nights. None of the other nurses was present on any more than five of the relevant nights. Although no one saw defendant inject the fatal overdoses, in each of the twelve instances he had the opportunity to do so, and many of the victims started having seizures soon after defendant announced that he was about to give them medication."

The Supreme Court of California affirmed the conviction of Robert Rubane Diaz for capital murder. Subsequently, before the execution could be carried out, California abolished capital punishment. Diaz' sentence was reduced to life in prison without parole. He died in prison on August 9, 2010.

Kristen Gilbert—ICU Nurse

Kristen Gilbert was employed as a nurse at a VA Medical Center in Massachusetts from March 1989 through February 1996. She was assigned to Ward C and worked the late afternoon to midnight shift four days per week. Ward C housed chronically ill patients and the hospital's intensive care unit. Gilbert was a popular hospital employee who received high evaluations from her supervisors. Her evaluations indicated that she reacted well to emergencies and that she seemed to know how to manage patients effectively during an emergency. Nobody initially suspected that her adept management of emergencies was due to her having caused the emergencies and that her knowledge of the cause helped her know how to treat the patients who were the subjects of the emergencies.

Beginning in the summer of 1995, Gilbert befriended a hospital police officer whose work schedule roughly corresponded to hers and whose duties required him to respond to medical emergencies in Ward C. By fall, Gilbert was having an affair with the police officer.

In the months following the beginning of her relationship with the hospital police officer, and continuing until she terminated her employment at the VAMC in February 1996, Gilbert's colleagues observed a marked rise in the number of fatalities and emergencies in Ward C. Later data analysis disclosed that the rate of deaths on Ward C tripled during the time Gilbert worked on that service. The death rate declined back to its previous level once Gilbert was removed from that service.

Members of the VAMC pharmacy staff noticed a simultaneous increase in the hospital's procurement of the drug epinephrine during this time. Moreover, epinephrine was constantly reported as missing during the time Gilbert worked on Ward C. These facts and staff perceptions prompted an investigation by the

Office of Healthcare Inspections of the Department of Veterans Affairs. This investigation concluded that there was no evidence that any VAMC employee had intentionally harmed any patients. Eventually, however, a criminal investigation conducted by law enforcement authorities led to Gilbert's arrest.

During the criminal investigation, at times when Gilbert knew the hospital police officer would be answering the telephone, Gilbert made a series of anonymous, threatening calls to the VAMC. During one of these calls, Gilbert made a false bomb threat for which she was convicted. Gilbert also directly harassed and threatened the hospital police officer, who had ended their romantic relationship and had agreed to cooperate with the authorities. She expressed anger toward certain coworkers who cooperated with the criminal investigation and who refused to speak with Gilbert's own private investigator. In addition, Gilbert once attempted to obstruct the criminal investigation by temporarily blocking the hospital police officer's car in his driveway and pleading with the police officer not to keep an appointment with criminal investigators who were looking into the possibility of criminality at the VAMC. After the police officer refused her request, Gilbert followed him and then vandalized his car while he was being interviewed.

The government alleged that in the six-month period following the commencement of her relationship with the police officer, Gilbert killed four Ward C patients and attempted to kill three others, by poisoning them with intravenous injections of epinephrine (and insulin, in the case of one diabetic patient). The government noted that epinephrine, a clear, odorless liquid, is medically indicated for resuscitating patients in a state of cardiac arrest or anaphylactic shock but causes a potentially fatal rapid or irregular heartbeat when administered in excessive doses. The four deaths and three near-deaths all involved some sort of cardiac arrest on the part of the victim.

According to the government, Gilbert committed these crimes using the same modus operandi. She would obtain epinephrine from Ward C's medicine cabinet, enter the patient's hospital room after all other medical personnel had left, and inject the patient with a fatal dose of epinephrine under the pretense of flushing the patient's intravenous line with a saline solution. The government's theory was that, by thus injecting non-prescribed medication into these patients, all of whom suffered from differing degrees of cardiac problems, Gilbert was able to generate an emergency, or "code," in which she plausibly could claim to be responding to naturally occurring cardiac emergencies. Gilbert orchestrated these codes, in the government's view, because they brought her into contact with the hospital police officer, and because they provided her with the attention and excitement that she craved. The government's principal evidence in support of its theory consisted of two admissions Gilbert made to the police officer, and toxicological evidence obtained from patients who Gilbert allegedly murdered.

Kristen Gilbert was found guilty, and she was sentenced to life in prison.

Michael Swango—Physician

Michael Swango, who sometimes used the pseudonyms "Jackson Kirk" and "David Jackson Adams," graduated from medical school at Southern Illinois University. From 1990 to 1997, he practiced medicine in the United States and internationally under false pretenses. After he had been hired by a hospital, Swango would murder, attempt to murder, or assault patients who had been entrusted to his care by using intravenous and intramuscular injections of medications. Swango made false statements and created false patient records to facilitate his murders. For example, he attempted to obtain "do not resuscitate" (DNR) orders for patients whom he intended to murder in order to prevent other institutional staff from making efforts to revive those patients.

After graduation from medical school, Swango worked as an intern at a hospital where he murdered a patient by injecting a lethal dose of potassium chloride. He also administered an intravenous injection of succinylcholine that caused a patient to experience respiratory paralysis, but the patient survived. The hospital's residency review committee voted not to allow Swango to continue in the residency program. Law enforcement authorities initiated a murder investigation of Swango. The investigation did not result in the filing of murder charges against Swango.

Following his dismissal from the residency program, Swango accepted a position as a paramedic with an ambulance service. After a year in this position, Swango was charged with having poisoned coworkers at the ambulance service with arsenic that he placed in the food and drink that he prepared for the coworkers. Swango was convicted of aggravated battery based on these poisonings. He was sentenced to five years in prison.

Following his release from prison, Swango applied for a position at a hospital residency program in Ohio. He falsely explained that his conviction for aggravated battery was based on a barroom brawl. After learning the truth about the conviction, the Ohio hospital rejected Swango's application. A VA Medical Center in South Dakota accepted Swango into its residency program, but later discharged Swango from the program after learning the truth about the aggravated battery conviction.

The following year, Swango was accepted into a residency program at a New York VA Medical Center. Shortly after the residency began, Swango advised physicians and staff at the hospital that a patient's family and attending physician had agreed to a DNR order. Swango recorded this DNR order in the patient's medical record. Two days later, the patient died as the result of Swango's administration of an intravenous epinephrine injection that caused cardiac arrest. Two months after this patient's death, Swango murdered another patient by administering lethal doses of succinylcholine. After two more patients died from succinylcholine administered by Swango, he was terminated from the residency program.

Swango's next position was with a hospital in Zimbabwe. This posting was arranged through a faith-based hospital group. After it was determined that he had poisoned three patients with succinylcholine at this hospital, Swango was suspended from practice in Zimbabwe.

During Swango's time in Zimbabwe, VA Medical Center authorities began to investigate his activities in the residency programs from which he had been dismissed. The investigators discovered evidence that Swango had fraudulently misrepresented the nature of his aggravated battery conviction. The FBI issued a warrant for Swango's arrest for lying on his federal job applications for employment at VA Medical Centers. Swango was arrested on this charge, and he pleaded guilty to it. He was sentenced to three-and-a-half years in prison.

Federal authorities took advantage of this period of imprisonment to accumulate evidence that Swango had murdered patients in the VA Medical Centers. The bodies of patients were exhumed, and toxicology consultants were retained to examine records. Hospital personnel who had worked with Swango were interviewed.

Once the VA Medical Center murder evidence had been obtained and the investigation confirmed that Swango had committed murder, federal authorities told Swango that he faced extradition to Zimbabwe to face charges of murders committed there, which would almost certainly result in Swango's execution. Confronted with this reality, Swango pleaded guilty to murdering three patients, in exchange for a sentence of life in prison without possibility of parole. Swango currently resides in the federal supermax prison in Florence, Colorado.

Terri Rachals—ICU Nurse

Terri Rachals was a nurse employed in the surgical intensive care unit of a hospital in Albany, Georgia. Following an unusual increase in the number of cardiac arrests of patients in the hospital during the latter part of 1985, investigations were conducted by the Georgia Department of Human Resources and the Georgia Bureau of Investigation. As a result of these investigations, Rachals was arrested on charges of murder and aggravated assault. An unexplained cluster of cardiac arrests had occurred with patients being cared for by Rachals. Postmortem examinations indicated that six deaths had resulted from injections of potassium chloride. Six other patients were nearly killed by potassium chloride injections, but they survived. Rachals confessed to investigators that she had intentionally injected the patients with potassium chloride.

Rachals was indicted and was tried on six counts of murder and twenty counts of aggravated assault, alleging the administration of potassium chloride to patients in the intensive care unit. Prosecutors contended that Rachals "felt like a second-class citizen all her life" and that she "sought power and control" through her criminal acts. The defense claimed that Rachals had long suffered from mental illness and that she needed psychiatric care rather than punishment. The evidence of mental illness was apparently persuasive. The jury returned verdicts of "not guilty" on all murder charges and on nineteen counts alleging aggravated assault. Rachals was found "guilty but mentally ill" of aggravated assault, with intent to murder one patient by injecting potassium chloride into a bag of fresh frozen plasma, which was then introduced into a patient's body while the patient was admitted to the ICU. For this one count of aggravated assault, she was sentenced to seventeen years in prison. The "guilty but mentally ill" verdict for Rachals assured that she would be incarcerated and that she would be treated for her mental illness during her incarceration. It also assured that she would be released once she had served her sentence.

On appeal, Rachals argued that the prosecution had presented unreliable evidence to the jury regarding the probability that the deaths resulted from actions undertaken by Rachals as opposed to someone else. The prosecution had presented evidence from which an inference could be made that "Terri Rachals was, by odds of five out of nine, probably guilty." Rachals contended that this was insufficient evidence of her guilt. An epidemiologist had been retained by the prosecution to assist in evaluating the increase in the number of cardiac arrests occurring in the hospital. The epidemiologist went to the hospital and examined the hospital's records for the entire year prior to the cluster of suspicious events. In three of those months, the hospital experienced no cardiac arrests. In two of the months, four cardiac arrests occurred in each month. Accordingly, the epidemiologist testified that the hospital should have between zero and four cardiac arrests in a normal month. However, in the month of November 1985, eleven cardiac arrests occurred during the 3:00 o'clock to 11:00 o'clock shift. The epidemiologist stated that the probability of this occurring "by chance alone is less than one in a trillion." In the month of November, five cardiac arrests occurred in one day.

The epidemiologist listed all cardiac arrest patients for the period that was investigated and the primary nurse on duty with those patients. Rachals was the primary nurse for eleven cardiac arrest patients in the month of November. No other nurse was the primary care nurse for more than one cardiac arrest patient. The epidemiologist charted all twenty-four nurses for that month and the number of cardiac arrests that occurred on their shift and those that occurred when they were not on shift to calculate a "rate ratio." The "rate ratio" for most nurses was around 1, while the "rate ratio" for Rachals was 26.6. The epidemiologist explained that this calculation meant that "it was 26.6 times more likely that a cardiac arrest would occur while Rachals was on duty than when she was not on duty." Rachals' defense attorney contended that this testimony impermissibly invaded the province of the jury, because it essentially told the jury that they must convict Rachals.

The court disagreed with the defense argument and ruled that it was appropriate for the jury to hear the testimony of the epidemiologist. The court reasoned that the number of variables was limited in the controlled hospital situation, and the statistics were not derived from a random sampling. Rather, hospital records established the average number of cardiac arrests for the entire year prior to November 1985, when the dramatic increase in the number of cardiac arrests was noticed. The appeal was denied.

Rachals was imprisoned in 1986 and was released in 2003.

Genene Jones—Pediatric Nurse

Genene Jones was trained as a licensed vocational nurse in Texas. She was hired by a hospital in San Antonio, where she worked only a few months until she was fired for ignoring physician orders because she believed she knew more than the physicians about appropriate patient care. She worked briefly at several other hospitals where she was fired for essentially the same reason. There is no evidence that she murdered any patients at these hospitals.

Jones was eventually hired at a hospital where she was assigned to the pediatric intensive care unit. Jones worked long hours, and she expressed concern that patients would not thrive without the special care that she alone was able to provide. Jones identified closely with favorite pediatric patients, and she refused to carry out physician orders for these patients if she believed that the orders were not in the child's best interests. During her first year at the hospital, Jones skipped training sessions because she viewed them as unnecessary for her. She made several serious medication administration errors, but the head nurse defended Jones due to what the head nurse viewed as Jones' positive attitude and her commitment to quality patient care.

When a new director was hired for the pediatric intensive care unit, he arranged for Jones to take responsibility for the most gravely ill patients, due to the high level of care and concern that Jones displayed. When a child died, Jones would gently prepare the body, sing to it, and personally take the corpse to the morgue. Nobody initially became concerned when children on the unit began dying from conditions that shouldn't have been fatal. Jones was always there to attempt resuscitation in times of emergency. During this time, Jones was actually administering injections of digoxin, heparin, and succinylcholine to create medical crises and to then receive praise for her effective management of the crises. Jones' colleagues began to call her on-duty hours "The Death Shift." Criticisms of Jones were attributed by management to grumbling by less competent nurses who were simply jealous of Jones' expertise.

As the deaths increased, a statistical analysis confirmed an inordinate number of deaths on the pediatric intensive care unit. Hospital administration concluded that a major problem existed, but there was concern about negative publicity for the hospital that might accompany a formal investigation. The hospital decided to replace all licensed vocational nurses on the unit with registered nurses. Due to this change, Jones was allowed to resign her position and the problem was considered to be solved. It was later determined that Jones had murdered between eleven and forty-six infants and children with lethal injections. The exact number was difficult to quantify, because hospital officials either misplaced or destroyed the relevant records.

Jones was then hired by a pediatrician who was opening a pediatric clinic in a nearby town. The pediatrician had worked with Jones at the hospital. The pediatrician had heard rumors about Jones, but she concluded that Jones was the victim of a male-dominated medical patriarchy.

Soon after the clinic opened, with Jones on its staff, seven different children had unexplained seizures while being treated at the clinic. Each child was transported by ambulance to a nearby hospital. From the sheer numbers of children afflicted in the same clinic, the hospital staff thought something odd must be going on, especially since the children always recovered quickly while in the hospital. Eventually a child died on the way to the hospital, and a medical committee began to investigate. The focus of their investigation was the pediatrician and her practices. Realizing that a problem might exist, and that she was being investigated as the possible perpetrator of a crime, the pediatrician conducted her own internal investigation of the clinic.

During her investigation, the pediatrician examined two vials of succinylcholine that were stocked in the clinic. They were both nearly full, but one had pinprick holes through the rubber stopper. When the pediatrician asked Jones about it, Jones denied any wrongdoing and suggested that the pediatrician throw the vials out to avoid questions. The pediatrician's suspicions were aroused, and she turned both bottles over to investigators, who later discovered that the bottles contained no succinylcholine at all. They contained only normal saline. All the succinylcholine had already been removed from the vials. An additional vial of succinylcholine that had been ordered for the clinic was missing.

The body of the child who died was exhumed, and it was determined that her death was due to an overdose of succinylcholine. Jones explained that her motive was to show how desperately inadequate pediatric services were in the area, to justify funding that would expand medical care for children. On February 15, 1984, Jones was convicted of attempted murder and murder. She was given the maximum sentence of ninety-nine years.

Vickie Dawn Jackson—Staff Nurse

Vickie Dawn Jackson was a licensed vocational nurse at a small Texas hospital. She was a serial killer nurse who never confessed yet was sentenced to life in prison based on the evidence of her guilt and a "no contest" plea. Her story is especially noteworthy because of the role a pharmacist played in bringing her to justice. Otherwise, the murders she committed were not significantly different from other murders committed by other healthcare professionals who violated their oath and turned on their patients.

In 2000 and 2001 during Jackson's night shift, twenty-two patients died. Records showed that on other shifts during the same period there was a single death. The hospital had only forty-five beds, and the patients who died had been hospitalized for "minor ailments—including a foot sore, diarrhea or dementia." Deaths were relatively rare in this hospital because critically ill patients were transferred to other hospitals where they could receive more intensive care. In February 2002, a pharmacist noticed that more than twenty bottles of mivacurium chloride were missing. The hospital pharmacist alerted law enforcement, telling them of the unexpected deaths in the hospital and explaining that mivacurium chloride is "used to temporarily paralyze patients during emergency care, stopping the natural breathing process to relax the chest muscles. It can result in death if improperly used."

A police investigation turned up a syringe with traces of the drug. This syringe was found in Jackson's discarded trash. Jackson was suspected of murder, but additional evidence was required to support a prosecution, so the bodies of ten of her patients were exhumed. All autopsies showed traces of mivacurium chloride. Jackson was forced out of her job, and in July 2002 was arrested and indicted for causing ten deaths. At trial, an FBI special agent who had interviewed Jackson testified that Jackson was "angered by patients and their unreasonable demands of her, while other nurses were compassionate and showed humor." Jones entered a "no contest" plea and was sentenced to life in prison.

Following this conviction, the families of the deceased patients sued the hospital, as well as several staff members of the hospital, including the pharmacist who allegedly did not discover the missing mivacurium in time to save the patients from being murdered by Jackson. Many of the nurses and physicians at the hospital were dismissed from the case, based on the court's conclusion that they had no way to know of Jackson's criminal acts. The pharmacist, however, was not dismissed from the case. Here is what the court had to say about the pharmacist (the pharmacist's name has been redacted):

> Defendant [pharmacist] was allegedly hired by the Defendant Hospital to provide pharmaceutical services to the Hospital and as Pharmacist-in-Charge to supervise the Hospital staff with respect to the use and stocking of the drug cart from which Nurse Jackson allegedly obtained her supply of Mivacron. Plaintiffs allege that he had multiple supervisory, management and policy making duties respecting the drugs, drug cart, and drug administering staff. Plaintiffs' pleadings are unclear whether he was hired by the Hospital as an employee or engaged as an independent contractor. But the distinction makes no difference since his alleged duties were performed for the benefit of the hospital in the discharge of its duties to patients such as the decedents.

The court continued:

> The Plaintiffs have not alleged that this Defendant actively participated in Nurse Jackson's actions, knew, or countenanced those actions, or in his official capacity for the hospital actively adopted any policy or procedure mandating or condoning Nurse Jackson's actions. Rather it is his inaction, lack of policy, lack of procedure, lack of supervision, failures to log and report that allowed the drug Mivacron to be available to Nurse Jackson. His liability, if any, rests on the character and degree of knowledge he had (or is charged with) of Nurse Jackson's actions or of the thefts of Mivacron from the drug cart and when he acquired or is charged with such knowledge. I find that the allegations of Plaintiffs against this defendant are sufficiently particular as to his supervisory responsibility and control of the drug cart, the drugs, and their usage as to implicate his inaction as a "moving force" for Nurse Jackson's violations. And coupled with allegations of deliberate indifference, the allegations are sufficient to state a cause of action against him and permit the case to proceed against him.

The pharmacist's motion to dismiss the case was denied. There is no further public record of the case. It is likely that the case was settled out of court. The important message of this case is that pharmacists have responsibilities to monitor the use of potentially lethal medications, particularly when unexpected deaths are occurring. The pharmacist in this case did the right thing in reporting his suspicions to the police. Whether that action was sufficient to avoid malpractice liability as a "moving force" for Jackson's violations is unknown due to settlement of the case.

Lee Roy Hargrave, Jr.—Nurse's Aide

Lee Roy Hargrave Jr. was a nurse's aide at a hospital in Petersburg, Virginia. Hargrave was tried and convicted of murdering one elderly patient by injecting her with a fatal dose of lidocaine. He was initially charged with five other similar killings, but he did not go to trial on those charges. Hargrave appealed his conviction, and the conviction was affirmed by the state Supreme Court. Hargrave then filed a writ of habeas corpus in federal court. Habeas corpus is a "Hail Mary" claim that is filed in federal court and is based on the incarcerated defendant's contention that the state court did not provide the defendant with a fair trial.

Hargrave argued that the trial court should have granted his motion for a change of venue due to the allegedly unfair and biased publicity his arrest had received in the press prior to his trial. He contended that the "pre-trial publicity in his case was so intense and pervasive that it must of necessity be considered prejudicial." However, the federal court noted that the tenor of the newspaper articles presented by the defendant were primarily informative and factual. Although the court admitted that "the slayings themselves were macabre," the court said, "it is difficult to conceive of a situation where a nurse's assistant allegedly injecting a number of elderly patients with a deadly drug would not receive extensive publicity." Viewing the months of coverage by local newspapers, the court felt that it was commendable that the treatment of the story appeared so objective. No coverage of the story in the newspaper articles used inflammatory language. Both the prosecutor and the defense attorney were interviewed by the local media. The federal court found nothing that indicated the jury had been prevented from reaching a fair verdict based solely on the law and on the evidence as they were presented in open court.

Hargrave also contended that the evidence did not support his conviction. Again, the federal court disagreed. The court said, "in the present case there is ample evidence to show that the defendant had the opportunity to administer a lethal dose of lidocaine to the victim while he was alone with her for at least two minutes." The court ruled that Hargrave had the means to commit the murder because he was seen in the treatment room where the lidocaine was stored and where it was found to be missing after the patient's death. Hargrave testified that he had never administered any medication to any patient, yet his statement was contradicted by two former patients who testified that he did administer medications to them even though he was not authorized to do so. After reviewing the evidence, and the definition of murder in Virginia ("any willful, deliberate, and premeditated killing"), the court concluded that the essential elements of the crime of murder had been established beyond a reasonable doubt.

Eyvette Hunter—Floor Nurse

Eyvette Hunter was a registered nurse working at a hospital in Lexington, Kentucky. She was charged in 2022 with murder in the death of a 97-year-old patient to whom she had administered intravenous lorazepam without a physician's order. A short time later, another nurse discovered the patient who was experiencing labored breathing. The patient died from aspiration pneumonia. He had been admitted to the hospital in "excellent health" according to family members as a precautionary measure following a slip and fall. He was due to be discharged from the hospital.

In June of 2023, Hunter was allowed to plead guilty to manslaughter. She was sentenced to five years in prison, and she can never again be employed in a healthcare setting. The patient's family agreed to the plea agreement to avoid the emotional experience of going to trial.

This case differs from many of the other pharmaceutical homicide cases because it appears to have been a single incident. The administration of the unauthorized medication, and the resulting patient death, were noted by hospital clinical staff and were reviewed by quality improvement professionals. While it is impossible to know for sure, this may be a case in which future similar crimes by this perpetrator were prevented through decisive action after discovery of the first criminal incident.

Several aspects of this case suggest that it might have been a precursor to other patient deaths if it had not been detected and firmly addressed with the filing of criminal charges. Nurse Hunter knowingly violated the law by administering a controlled substance to a patient without a physician's order. The patient was elderly and vulnerable. After administering the medication, Hunter did not monitor the patient's response. Hunter reportedly told the family, "I did not intend to harm your dad." Based on other reports of pharmaceutical homicide, these actions could fit the pattern of a nascent hospital serial murderer. Most of the previously identified hospital serial murderers began by taking a single lethal action that they thought was in the best interests of the patient, or at least they justified their actions with this explanation. Hunter's remorse and sorrow may be related to her having been discovered and punished, and they may not necessarily reflect regret for the lethal act that she committed.

On the other hand, it is more comforting to take the view that this was a one-time error of judgment leading to a lifetime of shame. Making inferences of criminal intent toward Hunter may be hugely unfair and inappropriate. While the benefit of doubt will ordinarily be extended to stressed and overwhelmed hospital staff, the protection of patients must take priority.

Efren Saldivar—Respiratory Therapist

Efren Saldivar worked as a respiratory therapist at two hospitals in Southern California. Although he did not graduate from high school, he was able to use his general equivalency diploma to qualify for a respiratory therapist training program, which he completed in 1988. He volunteered to work the aptly named "graveyard shift," where his weapon of choice was the paralytic drug pancuronium. As often happens with healthcare killers who are later referred to as "angels of death," suspicions of Saldivar's murderous tendencies were frequently and openly discussed among his colleagues. Saldivar's coworkers referred to the "magic syringe" that he carried with him.

Saldivar was careful about the patients whom he chose as victims. To avoid arousing suspicions, he murdered only those patients who were close to a natural death. Saldivar applied what he called "ethical criteria" in the choice of his victims. He explained that he felt sorry for patients who were being kept alive under painful and undignified conditions that they would certainly want to avoid if they could and so he helped them by hastening their inevitable deaths. He later admitted that he felt overworked by the large number of patients to whom he had been assigned, and that reducing the workload was his goal, which he admitted was "shameful."

One coworker caught Saldivar attempting to murder a patient, but she did not report what she saw because she and Saldivar were having an affair while on the job. Another coworker broke into Saldivar's locker to pull a prank and was shocked to see syringes and vials of both pancuronium and morphine. Although the coworker was initially fearful to report this information to management, because the prank was a clear violation of hospital rules, the coworker eventually made a report that led to a police investigation.

Saldivar initially confessed to murdering fifty patients. He was fired by the hospital, and his license was suspended. Shortly thereafter, he recanted his confession. The police and the hospital collaborated in their evaluation of over 1,000 deaths that had occurred in the hospital during Saldivar's period of employment. They selected twenty bodies to exhume and analyze for the presence of pancuronium. Unlike succinylcholine, which is a similar paralytic drug that degrades quickly postmortem, pancuronium remains identifiable for many months.

The autopsies found that six cadavers had evidence of lethal pancuronium concentrations. No healthcare practitioner had ordered pancuronium for any of these patients. Facing the prospect of execution, Saldivar entered a plea of guilty to all six murder counts against him, as well as the attempted murder that had been witnessed by his amorous coworker. He was sentenced to seven consecutive life terms in prison without the possibility of parole.

Saldivar admitted that he had killed as many as fifty patients and that his activities had contributed to the deaths of as many as 100 to 200 more patients. The exact number is impossible to know, because Saldivar lost count of his murders, and many of his deceased patients were cremated.

Reta Mays—Nursing Assistant

Reta Mays is a native of West Virginia who served on active duty in Iraq and Kuwait with the West Virginia Army National Guard. She suffered from posttraumatic stress disorder and a history of other emotional conditions. She was employed for a period of time as a corrections officer at a state prison, and she eventually obtained employment as a nursing assistant at a Veterans Administration Medical Center (VAMC). Nursing assistants are not licensed or qualified to administer any medications.

After two years of employment at the VAMC, Mays was assigned to work the night shift. Over a period of just under a year, staff members noticed that many patients were dying due to hypoglycemia, although they were not insulin-dependent diabetics and there was no record of their having received insulin. The VAMC initiated an investigation of eleven such deaths.

After the internal investigation, the VAMC turned the matter over to federal law enforcement authorities. Mays was subjected to lengthy interrogations, but she maintained her innocence. Investigators uncovered evidence that Mays had conducted an internet search of female serial killers, and her Netflix account indicated that she had viewed an episode of the program "Nurses Who Kill" that dealt with insulin overdoses.

Based on the circumstantial evidence that they had discovered, law enforcement focused on Mays as the perpetrator of pharmaceutical homicide. Hard evidence was elusive. There was no surveillance video on which to base murder charges. The VAMC did not track the use of insulin. There was no means through which Mays could be clearly connected with the patient deaths.

The investigators undertook a painstaking review of all 1,200 employees who had worked at the hospital at the time of the patient deaths. Only four employees had been on duty during all of the shifts when the deaths occurred, and Mays was one of them. The other three employees were ruled out through analysis of identification card swipe records and computer access records that placed them at other places in the hospital during the times when the insulin overdoses had been administered.

At trial, it was relatively easy to show that the patients' cause of death was an overdose of insulin. Proving who administered the overdoses was a greater challenge. To meet this evidentiary challenge, the prosecution used an expert in pharmacokinetics. The pharmacokinetics expert was able to identify the type and dose of insulin used as 100 or more units of regular insulin. The pharmacokinetics expert was also able to narrow down the administration window to a few hours, which corresponded with the time when Mays was present with patients.

Faced with the compelling evidence against her, Mays entered a plea of guilty to second-degree murder for intentionally injecting the patients with insulin. She was sentenced to life in prison. The sentencing federal judge referred to her as "the monster that no one sees coming."

Heather Pressdee—Long-Term Care Nurse

Heather Pressdee is a former registered nurse who worked in the rehabilitation unit of five different Pennsylvania long-term care facilities over the span of three years and who was suspected of murdering residents at all five facilities by injecting them with insulin overdoses. Pressdee attended community college to study nursing, but she dropped out and became a veterinary technician. In that role, Pressdee spent fourteen years administering veterinary anesthesia and conducting veterinary euthanasia. Pressdee later returned to community college where she completed her nursing degree, and she was licensed as a registered nurse.

Coworkers at the facility where Pressdee worked became concerned that she was killing residents, and they reported their concerns to facility administration. An internal investigation was begun, and Pressdee was suspended pending the results of the investigation. The internal investigation revealed that there was no identifiable evidence to support the concerns of Pressdee's coworkers.

Pressdee came to the attention of the state department of health in February 2022 when a physician at a local hospital reported concerns about patients who had been transported to the hospital after having been cared for by Pressdee. A criminal referral was made to the state's attorney general in December 2022. Pressdee was arrested in May 2023.

Law enforcement investigators discovered that there had been many suspicious deaths due to hypoglycemia at facilities where Pressdee had worked. Pressdee had been fired from numerous facilities for her abusive behavior toward residents. On her applications for employment at subsequent facilities, she used fictitious names as references for supposed past colleagues, and she listed a relative's telephone number as contact information for the fictitious references.

Text messages sent by Pressdee to her mother included these comments:

- "I'm gonna murder already."
- "I drugged him already and I don't know why he is awake."
- "I may kill this resident. I need to set some sort of boundary with him."

Pressdee entered a plea of guilty to three counts of first-degree murder and 19 counts of criminal intent to commit murder. She was sentenced to three consecutive terms of imprisonment on the first-degree murder charges and up to 760 years in prison for criminal intent to commit murder. Prosecutors stated that they believed she had murdered seventeen residents by administering lethal doses of insulin. The families of the patients have indicated that they will file lawsuits against the facilities for failing to protect the deceased residents from Pressdee's murderous ways.

Conclusion

The purpose of relating these horrifying and heartbreaking stories is to emphasize the reality that seemingly dedicated healthcare professionals can do bad things to their patients. People kill other people. Murderers can use drugs acquired from a pharmacy to commit their ugly deeds. All of the murder weapons used in the crimes described in this chapter were provided innocently by a pharmacy department.

These narratives suggest that perhaps it is time to become less trusting of the safety provided by the healthcare setting, given the facts of the cases described in this chapter. A healthcare setting is not a refuge free from crime. The cases that have been reviewed in this chapter are not isolated cases. There are many more just like them. Nurses are most frequently the culprits of pharmaceutical homicide in a healthcare institution because they have unsupervised access to medications and to patients. Nurses have the means and the opportunity to commit the crime of murder with medication.

Why is this apparent reality of pharmaceutical homicide not discussed openly and frequently in pharmacy and in healthcare? Perhaps because healthcare criminality is disgusting and a difficult subject to confront (this is certainly true—challenging a colleague is risky and uncomfortable). Perhaps because pharmaceutical homicide is viewed as a rare outlier that hardly ever happens (this is certainly not true—as the narratives in this chapter illustrate). Regardless of the discomfort or disbelief that one may experience in reacting to stories of pharmaceutical homicide, the occurrence of pharmaceutical homicide must be the subject of consideration and reflection, even if it is not frequently spoken of.

Patients deserve to have medications dispensed and administered by healthcare professionals who will use them only for beneficial therapeutic purposes. Pharmacists are the gatekeepers of the nation's drug supply, and they must do their best to prevent crimes with the pharmaceutical products that they distribute and monitor.

Key Takeaways

- Avoid naïve feelings about the implausibility of pharmaceutical homicide in the institutional setting. Don't be lulled into a state of complacency thinking that "this can't really be happening" when evidence suggesting the commission of a pharmaceutical crime becomes apparent to you. There is a sad but solid history of murder by medication, with healthcare professionals as the perpetrators. Hippocrates would not have bothered to speak out against healthcare murderers if he had not appreciated the reality of it. Recent experience of pharmaceutical homicide in the institutional setting supports continued vigilance to prevent patient harm of the kind that Hippocrates warned against. Serial killers in the healthcare setting can be emboldened to expand their criminal ways if they are not investigated early on. If a situation seems suspicious, then take a closer look to see what might be happening.
- Don't assume that seemingly competent and caring healthcare professionals are incapable of heinous crimes. The narratives in this chapter describe how suspicions about nefarious activities by healthcare professionals can be disregarded even when formal investigations are undertaken to examine the validity of the suspicions. Anyone who has ready access to pharmaceutical products and to patients, particularly with little direct supervision, may use medications as murder weapons. The perpetrator's motive is the key

to understanding why a person with the means and opportunity would commit such a crime. Look for a motive to help you confirm or contradict your suspicions of criminality.

- If you have suspicions about criminal use of medications, then generate documentation on which to base an evaluation of medication use. This can be done through a formal medication utilization evaluation (MUE) process, or it can be done through a more focused investigation that examines a particular service on which aberrations from the norm have been observed. Let the data speak for itself. You need not accuse anyone of anything illegal. Others will take the data and make their decisions about the significance of what the numbers suggest. You inform; they decide. Don't allow yourself to make empty accusations. Use data to make your point.

References

1. Smith D. 'Did I notice a dark side?': the true story behind serial killer drama The Good Nurse, *The Guardian*. November 3, 2022. **https://www.theguardian.com/film/2022/nov/03/the-good-nurse-true-story-netflix-serial-killer**. McAuliffe C. The serial killer male nurse accused of murdering more than 400 patients. *Ranker.* April 22, 2024. **https://www.ranker.com/list/nurse-charles-cullen/cat-mcauliffe**

2. People v. Diaz, 834 P.2d 1171 (Cal. 1992); DeAtley DK. Angel of death dies in prison, The Press Enterprise. August 12, 2010. **https://www.pressenterprise.com/2010/08/12/angel-of-death-dies-in-prison/**

3. Cutting v. United States, 204 F.Supp.2d 216 (D.Mass. 2002); Cobb G, Gehlbach S. Statistics in the Courtroom. **http://www.stat.ucla.edu/~nchristo/statistics13/article.pdf**

4. Kaufman E. 'Double-O Swango': What happened to Dr. Michael Swango, who left trail of dead patients in Midwest, elsewhere. Mitchell Republic. May 2, 2022. **https://www.mitchellrepublic.com/news/the-vault/double-o-swango-what-happened-to-dr-michael-swango-who-left-trail-of-dead-patients-in-midwest-elsewhere**. Sackman B, Vecchione M, Schmetterer J. *Behind the Murder Curtain.* New York, NY: Post Hill Press; 2020.

5. Rachals v. State, 361 S.E.2d 671 (Ga. App. 1987): Grine J. *Serial Murder in Institutional Settings.* USF Tampa Digital Thesis. July 16, 2023. **https://digitalcommons.usf.edu/cgi/viewcontent.cgi?article=2379&context=etd**

6. Jones v. State, 751 S.W.2d 682 (Texas App. 1988); Elkind P. The death shift. Texas Monthly. August 1983. https://www.texasmonthly.com/true-crime/the-death-shift-2/

7. James v. Nocona General Hospital. United States District Court, N.D. Texas, Wichita Falls Division. Sept 8, 2004. https://casetext.com/case/james-v-nocona-general-hospital-3. Hollandsworth S. Angel of death. Texas Monthly. July 2007. https://www.texasmonthly.com/true-crime/angel-of-death/

8. Hargrave v. Landon, 584 F.Supp. 302 (DC Va. 1984); Staff Writer. "Lidocaine Killer" Hargrave released from prison. *The Progress-Index*. March 3, 2010. https://www.progress-index.com/story/news/2010/03/04/lidocaine-killer-hargrave-released/36483649007/

9. Robbins R. Former Nurse Charged with Murder in Death of 97-Year-Old War Veteran. Medscape. August 24, 2022. https://www.medscape.com/viewarticle/979715?form=fpf; Six T. Former Lexington nurse gets prison time after pleading guilty to elderly patient's death. Lexington Herald Leader. June 8, 2023. https://www.kentucky.com/news/local/crime/article276181451.html

10. Lieberman P. Hospital 'Angel of death' gets life without parole. *Los Angeles Times*. April 18, 2002. https://www.latimes.com/archives/la-xpm-2002-apr-18-mn-38536-story.html; Scoles S. How a Nuclear Weapons Lab Helped Crack a Serial-Killer Case. February 9, 2024. https://undark.org/2024/02/09/wilo-serial-killer-nuclear-lab/

11. United States Department of Justice. Former VA Hospital Nursing Assistant Sentenced to Seven Consecutive Life Sentences for Murdering Seven Veterans and Assault with Intent to Commit Murder of an Eighth. Press Release. May 11, 2021. https://www.justice.gov/usao-ndwv/pr/former-va-hospital-nursing-assistant-sentenced-seven-consecutive-life-sentences; Douglas J. A What unit: The expert evidence involved in the medical serial murder case of Reta Mays. West Virginia Lawyer. 2021; Autumn:38–42.

12. Burke M. Pennsylvania nurse pleads guilty to killing patients with lethal doses of insulin. *NBC News*. May 4, 2024. https://www.nbcnews.com/news/us-news/pennsylvania-nurse-pleads-guilty-killing-patients-lethal-doses-insulin-rcna150366; Pennsylvania Office of Attorney General. Heather Pressdee Criminal Complaint. https://www.attorneygeneral.gov/wp-content/uploads/2023/11/2023-11-02-Heather-PRESSDEE-Criminal-Complaint.pdf

Chapter 6

Unexpected Death? Rule Out Homicide!

When patients are admitted to a hospital, they have a right to expect that they will be treated with care and concern. Hospitalized patients are particularly vulnerable to exploitation and mistreatment because they are in an unfamiliar place where they are dependent on strangers to meet their basic needs. The cultural and societal expectation for patients who are hospitalized is that they must remain patient with a system that is very different from their usual place of residence and not become impatient when frustrating system obstacles arise. In this sense, the term "patient" is used both as a noun (a person who receives medical treatments) and as an adjective (able to good-naturedly accept or tolerate delays, problems, or suffering without becoming annoyed or anxious). Patients are expected to be patient. Patients are unlikely to complain when the care they receive seems to be odd or unusual, because everything seems odd or unusual in a hospital. The vulnerability of hospitalized patients, due to their unfamiliarity with the hospital setting, makes them susceptible to harmful mistreatment, and even lethal mistreatment, by criminally motivated hospital personnel.

Role of Hospital

Historically hospitals were established as safe places where patients could be given shelter, food, and protection from harm. Housing, nutrition, and public safety were not consistently acceptable in many places where people lived during the time when early hospitals were established, and it was an exercise in futility to attempt medical treatment of ill people if their home treatment environment did not lend itself to healing. Until the middle of the twentieth century, hospitals were responsible primarily for creating a safe environment for patient care. Physicians with privileges at the hospitals were responsible for the quantity and quality of healthcare services provided to admitted patients. Nurses and other health professionals employed by the hospital provided patient care based on the orders of physicians. Hospitals were not considered primary healthcare providers. They were essentially comfortable hotels with clean water, sanitary bedding, and nutritious diets (the food was often the object of jokes, because it was healthy rather than palatable). Hospitals were a protected place for patients to stay while they were being cared for by a physician who was responsible for the provision of medical care.

Modern hospitals function very differently. Not only do they provide safe accommodations for patients who have been admitted to the hospital, they also accept primary responsibility for the provision of many types of medical services, and they provide oversight of the activities of health professionals who practice within the institutional environment. The medical staff are overseen by a credentialing committee that evaluates the quality of a physician's practice and authorizes the procedures and treatments that a physician may provide to admitted patients. Peer-review activities are rigorous and are inclusive of all licensed health professionals employed at the hospital. Continuous quality improvement (CQI) programs evaluate patient outcomes and determine how structures and processes can be improved to produce better outcomes from patient care. Morbidity and Mortality (M&M) meetings are convened regularly to address concerns about decision-making and technical aspects of care that may require improvement.

Hospital activities that address potential problems in clinical care may be somewhat constrained by the business side of the institution. After all, to keep the doors open for people who need medical care, hospitals must make money. Even "not for profit" hospitals must minimize their losses and generate surplus revenues to fund the expansion of facilities and personnel. The business of hospitals is overseen from what is often referred to as the "C-Suite," which is a set of plush offices, usually on the hospital's top floor with a stunning view, where administrators with titles starting with the word "Chief" (CEO, COO, CFO, CIO, etc.) conduct their daily business of providing quality care without running the balance sheet into the red. Many of those who occupy the C-Suite are current or former clinicians. All of them want the care provided within the institution to be of the highest quality. Yet they must insist that patient care be efficient as well as cost-effective (optimal minimum resource utilization for best possible care).

One of the key business functions of any hospital is "risk management." Although this department overlaps somewhat with a department called "quality improvement," the goals are fundamentally different. Whereas risk management's role is to reduce the risk of financial loss from legal liability caused by medical errors, quality improvement's corollary role is to provide the resources necessary for healthcare professionals to produce satisfactory medical results for patients.

Any medical error that may result in a patient complaint that could lead to litigation must be documented in an "incident report" that is sent to the risk management department. These reports are carefully guarded. They are not distributed for general review by hospital staff. They are kept secret. Most risk management departments attempt to resolve legal claims quietly to avoid negative publicity. A hospital's reputation in the community is hugely important. A hospital that develops a reputation as being "a place where people go to die" will not remain profitable for long.

A hospital's quality improvement and risk management programs rely on the pharmacy department to produce good outcomes from drug therapy and prevent bad outcomes from it. Pharmacists are responsible for the security of any hospital's drug supply. Pharmaceutical product security may not be the most exciting responsibility for a profession that is rapidly moving into new roles of direct patient care, but it is nevertheless a critically important responsibility.

Patients expect that the medications they receive in a hospital are acquired from reliable sources and accurately distributed pursuant to physician orders that are reviewed for appropriateness by a pharmacist. Patients also expect that medications made available to nursing staff and other hospital personnel are monitored by the pharmacy department to assure their appropriate use. Patients expect that any unlawful use, or intentionally harmful use, of medications distributed by the pharmacy department will be investigated and the distribution of medications for these unlawful purposes will cease.

It is the pharmacy department on which the system relies to assure the safety of drug use within a hospital. When there is an unexpected adverse event that may have been produced from the use of a pharmaceutical product, the responsible pharmacy department will investigate.

Identifying the Cause

Pharmacists routinely conduct both root cause analysis and failure mode and effects analysis in their patient safety reviews that are focused on preventing medication errors. A key factor in any analysis of this type is the consideration of possible causes of recorded medication errors and the correlation of those possible causes with a wide array of potential adverse effects. The investigation of one identified error may lead to recognition of system shortcomings that could lead to other errors in the future or perhaps have already led to other errors in the past. The failure to consider all possibilities can hinder the process. If the cause of an error can be identified, then the system can be repaired to prevent further errors of the same type.

One standard approach to problem-solving in healthcare is the differential diagnosis. Through this process of elimination, various potential causes of a disease or condition can be ruled out, even if the process does not result in the identification of a single disease or condition. The diagnosis of "rule out condition X" means that the clinicians suspect "condition X" as the ailment from which a patient is suffering. To confirm their suspicions, and to validate the diagnosis, they conduct a process designed to rule out, or disprove, their suspicions if they are wrong. The inability to disprove the suspicions can be interpreted as confirmation that the suspicions were correct. If a diagnosis cannot be ruled out, through a deliberate process of considering other possibilities, then the diagnosis is effectively ruled in, and treatment of the identified condition can begin.

When a trend of unexpected fatal adverse drug events occurs in a hospital, it may be appropriate to rule out homicide as a cause. Recent experience with homicidal healthcare professionals justifies this approach. Pharmaceutical homicide in the healthcare setting is no longer impossible to imagine and should be considered as a possibility when there is any suspicious patient death. An unexplained cluster of fatalities, with no clue as to the reason, should prompt those who are investigating the cluster to disprove a suspicion that a murderer may be the cause.

Challenges with Collecting Evidence

Although all large cities (and many small towns) have a long list of "cold case" unsolved murders, the reality is that most murders are solved relatively quickly, if they are solved at all. The television news magazine "48 Hours" bases its title on the reality that if detectives do not find a lead within the first 48 hours of discovering a murder, the chances of solving the crime are reduced dramatically.

The fact that a death was the result of a murder is obvious to the first team of police personnel who arrive at the scene of many crimes. The murder weapon is quickly identified, and the murderer is apprehended within hours or days. By contrast, murders that occur within a healthcare setting are difficult to detect, are rarely investigated, and often cannot be successfully prosecuted due to the lack of incriminating evidence.

Death occurs relatively frequently within a healthcare setting. The death of a patient is less likely to raise immediate suspicions than a death that occurs in the community setting. Most hospital-based clinical care is provided in isolation, with few observers to detect criminal activity. The availability of multiple, potentially lethal, pharmaceutical agents provides the instrumentality for murder, often with no accountability.

After a patient dies, the site of death is usually cleaned within minutes, and the body is removed to a morgue. Efforts to resuscitate a patient may alter a crime scene significantly within a healthcare institution. Investigators often can't re-create what happened before a code was called. Patient privacy issues interfere with investigations, causing further delays in determining whether foul play was involved.

The legal standard of proof for a criminal conviction requires that the jury be convinced "beyond a reasonable doubt" that a crime has occurred. When the accusation is murder, legal proceedings are appropriately cautious with the review of evidence, due to the extreme consequences of a guilty verdict. Many healthcare serial murderers are allowed to plead guilty to lesser offenses due to the difficulty of prosecuting them.

Scope of Problem

How often are patients murdered by a healthcare professional within a healthcare institution? That's a good question, and the best answer is that nobody really knows. It is likely that nobody will ever really know for sure. This frustrating answer then begs the question: If we can't ever know the extent of the problem, then is there any real point in discussing the problem? The best answer to this question is, yes. It is worth discussing, because the only alternative is to allow murderers to continue killing their patients. Murdered patients and their families have the right to a thorough investigation of the circumstances of a patient's death. The public deserves an investigative process that is undertaken aggressively despite its difficulty.

Perhaps another answer to the question of why pharmaceutical homicide should be considered as a possibility, even if the probability of its occurrence cannot be quantified, can be found in the concept of a "never event." As this phrase suggests, a "never event" is an event that should never happen. This concept has been developed by the National Quality Forum and by other patient safety organizations.

Never events are rare and often unquantifiable in the aggregate due to their rarity, but they are very serious, and they are preventable. Never events indicate systematic problems in healthcare safety systems that are significantly influenced by policies and procedures. The investigation of never events is important for public credibility and accountability. A hospital that does not look for never events will likely not see them when they happen and will fail to meet its responsibility to the public.

The appropriate reaction to never events is that there can be no tolerance for them. While there may be a threshold level of forgiveness and understanding for some adverse events, because adverse events are inevitable in the ordinary course of patient care (e.g., misjudging the severity of a drug–drug interaction alert, or failing to prevent a patient's allergic reaction to the first use of a drug when there was no known allergy), there is no tolerance level for never events (e.g., the administration of a drug by IV push when the appropriate administration is IV infusion, or confusing a daily milligram dose with a milligram per kilogram dose).

Even one occasion of a never event warrants extensive remediation, along with the allocation of additional resources as necessary. It does not matter how many patients are murdered by healthcare professionals in a healthcare setting. Murder is a never event. Even one murder of a patient in a healthcare setting is one too many.

Prioritizing Healthcare Homicide

Murders of patients within a healthcare setting are sordid, scandalous, and may even seem fascinating to some from an academic point of view of investigation, given the scope and complexity of the investigation into such matters entails. They have a particularly voyeuristic appeal because they happen within places that are often considered mysterious, impersonal, sterile, and a bit frightening. They warrant attention due to their unusual nature and the obvious betrayal of trust on the part of homicidal healthcare professionals. But the question must be asked: Are murders in a healthcare setting really such a "big deal" that they warrant high prioritization among all of the many other significant problems and challenges facing regulators and administrators who are responsible for protecting patients within healthcare systems? This question begs another question: On the list of patient safety challenges that must be addressed by a hospital, is healthcare murder a priority at all? These are difficult questions to resolve, because the reality is that hospitals must solve the most pressing problems first. The relative infrequency of healthcare murders might place them far down the list of hospital priorities. On the other hand, the massive betrayal of trust that they represent might place them much higher on the list of hospital priorities.

The extraordinary level of trust placed in healthcare professionals by the society at large as well as the individual patients and the public trust in the institutions in which health professionals practice warrant a high priority being placed on the prevention of healthcare homicide. Extraordinary efforts must be made to earn the trust that is placed in health professionals and in healthcare institutions. The public that is being served by a healthcare institution may accept as inevitable the occasional human error that causes harm to a patient. That same public will reject as outrageous even a single event of pharmaceutical homicide within a healthcare institution.

Assuring patients that healthcare professionals employed in hospitals and other institutions do not have a history of behaviors that indicate criminal propensities is a core institutional responsibility. These behaviors could include sexual assault, verbal and physical abuse, the theft of patient property, or the intentional withholding of patient care. The egregious nature of these behaviors justifies placing a high level of importance on assuring the public that healthcare professionals within an institution do not have psychological conditions that might make them dangerous to patients. If individual patients lose trust in healthcare institutions, then they will delay seeking care, and the public health will be adversely affected.

Reducing the Incidence of Healthcare Homicide

In their article addressing the problem of what they refer to as "health care serial murder" (HCSM), Kizer and Yorker suggest concrete steps that would strengthen the weaknesses in healthcare safety systems revealed by the occurrence of HCSM.[1]

First, they suggest that healthcare organizations, accrediting agencies, and regulatory boards should remove the secrecy surrounding HCSM and increase awareness among health professionals and the public that healthcare workers have committed murder in the past and will continue to do so in the future if significant steps are not taken to prevent HCSM. Recognizing that the intentional killing of patients is not a pleasant subject to discuss, Kizer and Yorker stress that the first step in solving any problem is recognizing and admitting that it exists.

Sweeping problems under the rug and ignoring their existence because they are unsavory simply assure that the problems will continue. The adoption of a policy of transparency has helped remove barriers to solving other patient safety problems, and it could do the same with HCSM. That said, it is well known that hospitals are not incentivized to air their dirty laundry. Secrets are kept. Truths are withheld from the public. There are many barriers to the development of institutional programs that address HCSM.

A second point the authors make is that data on HCSM should be reported to a central repository overseen by a governmental or nongovernmental agency. These reported data should be aggregated and maintained by that agency in a searchable database and made available to healthcare institutions and researchers for the purpose of reducing the incidence of HCSM. No such database exists currently. An appropriate agency for the maintenance of a database could be in the area of law enforcement, such as the Federal Bureau of Investigation, or in the area of public health, such as the Centers for Disease Control and Prevention. The Joint Commission or the United States Pharmacopeia can be other options.

A third point is that secrets about a healthcare professional's previous employment often are kept from a later employer when decisions are made about offering employment. Hospitals will cite their fear of being sued for defamation if they convey suspicions about a former employer's performance to a prospective employer. Kizer and Yorker suggest that legal protection be granted to communications of this nature, when there is an honest belief that patient harm has occurred based on evidence and when dismissal from employment has resulted from that evidence. There is a recognized pattern of murderous healthcare professionals being dismissed and moving to a new workplace to commit more murders. This pattern must be disrupted.

The fourth point is that healthcare professionals should be alert to the possibility that a colleague has committed intentional harm toward a patient and should report suspicious circumstances to institutional safety authorities when circumstances arise. Institutions should develop and maintain specific procedures for collecting and maintaining evidence in an objective manner following the submission of such a report.

Last, the authors recommend that institutional systems be reviewed to reduce the likelihood of HCSM. They emphasize that "policies and procedures for use of high-alert medications should be particularly reviewed because administration of non-narcotic medications has been the primary weapon used by health care serial killers in the U.S."

Healthcare institutions have implemented high-security requirements for opioids and for ultra-expensive medications, to prevent their being stolen and diverted from appropriate therapeutic use. Most medications that are used as weapons by healthcare murderers fall into neither category. The authors suggest that medications with the potential for use as weapons by murderers should be placed in the high-security category to enhance the monitoring of their use, even if these products are not controlled substances and are not high-cost drugs and are not in short supply.

Incomplete Records of Healthcare Murders

Nurse Mary Sullivan has extensively studied healthcare murder and reported her observations in the journal *Nursing Management* in 2009.[2] Sullivan reported that as of 2009, 90 criminal prosecutions of healthcare workers had occurred over the previous three decades, with fifty four convictions of murder or attempted murder and five additional plea bargains to lesser crimes. Many culprits had committed multiple murders. The convictions resulted from 317 total confirmed murders (most perpetrators committed multiple murders), although there were 2,113 suspicious deaths that were likely the result of criminal activities that could not be proven as murders.

The most widely used method of murder, according to Sullivan, was drug injection. Most of the deaths occurred in a hospital setting, and the evening or night shift was the preferred work period for murder. Nurses were the most likely personnel to be identified as murderers, although other healthcare professionals were involved as well.

The most difficult cases to prove are those in which the alleged method of killing was administering to the patient a lethal dose of drug that is a part of the medications prescribed for them while they are in the hospital. High levels of a prescribed drug may be the result of impaired metabolism, or they may result from an inadvertent error in the administration of the drug. A toxicology report that includes a drug that has not been prescribed for the patient is the most persuasive evidence of murder.

Lack of Investigative Expertise

Patient safety has become a new field of study within healthcare. It was previously given attention only by a few "radicals" who dared to discuss and investigate what some clinicians considered to be "bad news." Healthcare murder is a field that has similarly been given little attention.

There are few experts on whom reliance can be placed when circumstances of a patient's death seem suspicious and are potentially the result of criminal misconduct by attending healthcare staff. In a healthcare setting, discussions of errors and adverse events are often viewed as being "negative" and "pessimistic." Those who express the need to improve patient safety are encouraged to be more "positive" and more "optimistic." The messenger who conveys the patient safety message is rarely rewarded or welcomed by healthcare institution staff.

Experts in medical record review generally focus on the appropriateness of care and not on discovering inappropriate activities. The medical record will likely not include notations from a murderer, so the traditional investigative approach of records review provides little useful information in support of efforts to identify the crime of murder.

Due to the highly technical nature of patient care information, expert analysis and testimony will be required to support a medical murder conviction. There are only a few forensic experts who are well qualified in this area. Crimes committed with handguns, knives, and blunt instruments can be easily addressed by experts in the field of forensics. Murder with medication requires a different kind of expertise, and forensic pharmacists can provide their expertise to fill the knowledge and practice gap in such events.

First Steps toward a Solution

As difficult as medical murder can be to identify and investigate, there are some steps that can be taken by those who suspect that "something seems wrong here" following the unexpected death of a patient. Here is what Sullivan suggests:

- Preserve and sequester medical devices that may have been used in the treatment of the patient. This would include syringes, drug cups, and, in particular, infusion pumps that can be programmed for drug delivery.
- Assure that the laboratory saves any blood samples or other tissues that may have been tested for any reason. Lab results are important as well, but the samples themselves should be retained for later testing if there are suspicions that can be confirmed or ruled out by additional forensic tests.
- Make a record of every person who was present when the patient died and also of those who were present in the area of patient care within an hour prior to the patient's death. Do not rely on staff scheduling to identify those who may have had access to the patient at critical times. Even family members and other likely innocent people such as chaplains should be included on the list.
- Preserve the patient care record as it exists at the time of the patient's death. If there are informal notes, then they need to be included. Do not rely on the medical records department to save everything.

Working with Risk Management

It is widely recognized that the primary purpose of a hospital's risk management department is to protect the institution from financial loss due to liability for harm to patients. It is a business activity. Healthcare institutions are businesses, and they can't stay in business if they suffer major financial losses due to legal liability.

The risk management department also has an important secondary role, which is to promote patient safety activities that reduce exposure to financial liability. It is important to remember that the risk management's patient safety role is subsidiary to its primary responsibility, which is financial.

Although the risk management department is unlikely to view pharmaceutical homicide prevention as their key responsibility, especially in institutions where turf-guarding is prevalent within the culture, their knowledge and skill with investigation and evidence preservation can make them important allies when suspicions arise following an unusual death of a patient. This may be the case despite initial concerns about discovering something that will raise the risk of liability.

The risk management department may also serve as an appropriate repository for information about a suspicious event, and this will not seem strange or accusatory since records of this kind are often preserved for quality improvement and risk management purposes. In addition, the risk management department may be persuaded to identify a specific person to handle forensic cases, including suspected pharmaceutical homicide.

Circumstances and Culture

An apparent increase in the incidences of medical murder may be both circumstantial and cultural. The circumstances of institutional patient care have created a situation where most patients are critically ill, the census is high, and the opportunity for interaction and reflection is minimal. Personnel who have murderous intentions will have little trouble identifying services that are chaotic (most are at one time or another) and where supervising healthcare professionals are overwhelmed and at times inattentive.

Shift change is a time when opportunities are particularly likely to arise for those health professionals with murderous intent.

A culture of caution may also create opportunities for wrongdoers in an institution. Casual comments about a patient's condition, or about a coworker's performance, are now far less likely to be shared among healthcare colleagues because there are firm rules about when, how, and to whom such remarks may be made. Violating these rules is not worth the risk of disciplinary action, so significant observations about problematic care may be kept to oneself. Patient privacy concerns may lead to reluctance to share information about a specific patient, even with another healthcare professional.

Institutional Caution

Hospitals tend to shut themselves off from the outside world, to preserve patient confidentiality, to protect the integrity of medical care, and for fear of liability. This level of institutional caution and isolation is a real concern, and it is a threat to the discovery of pharmaceutical homicide, as well as a disincentive to openly addressing the consequences of pharmaceutical homicide.

There may be a bias inherent in any hospital that considers itself to be among the best-quality institutions within a community and whose administrators simply cannot believe that anyone on their staff would intentionally kill a patient. The arrogance of self-proclaimed excellence may prevent those in the C-Suite from acknowledging the possibility of criminality by any of their hospital's staff. Administrators may order investigators to back off suspicions of homicide, or they may fail to support the conduct of an investigation when they are certain that there is "nothing to investigate" because they can't believe that anything unlawful would occur in their hospital.

Most healthcare serial killers would have worked at numerous institutions, and their criminality would have long been suspected. A hospital's hypothetical exposure to liability for not informing a subsequent employer of problems at the hospital where a healthcare worker was previously employed is offset by the very real liability from openly admitting patient deaths that could have and should have been prevented. Providing neutral references avoids spreading the word of criminality at the hospital. Providing deceptive and incomplete references also places patients at risk of harm. Hospitals are not likely to engage in an activity that publicizes the hazards to their patients.

Hospitals must prepare in advance for a surprise public disclosure that implicates hospital staff in pharmaceutical homicide. It is important that hospitals not overreact to a perceived public relations crisis with incautious press releases that exacerbate the problem. In an Ohio case where a physician was accused of killing patients with drug overdoses, the hospital issued an initial statement that said: "Following the discovery, the doctor was removed from all patient care, and his employment was terminated. We're working hard to learn all we can about these cases, and we removed 20 other hospital staff from providing further patient care while we gather more facts. This includes a number of nurses who were administering the medication and a number of pharmacists who were also involved in the related patient care." A statement like this that blames hospital staff is unlikely to quell public concerns about dangers to hospitalized patients.

Two months later, the hospital issued a less defensive statement that said: "We have identified a total of 48 nurses and pharmacists whose actions are under review and whose names have been reported to the relevant nursing and pharmacy boards. Out of abundance of caution, we have removed all colleagues who were associated with medication administration for an impacted patient."[3] The cautious approach of the second statement preserves public trust while at the same time it conveys important information. The difficulty of discussing a challenging issue does not justify the failure to cautiously address community concerns about alleged unlawful activities within a hospital.

Motive for Murder

A 2023 article in *Forensic Science, Medicine and Pathology* presents an interesting perspective on why nurses become serial killers within a healthcare setting.[4]

The article first distinguishes between nurses who kill once and nurses who kill and then keep on killing. The one-time killers are often reacting to an unusual situation, in response to a disrespectful statement made about them, or due to another trigger that has pushed them to do the unthinkable without a plan or specific purpose.

Serial killer nurses are different. They think through what they do, and they plan to take advantage of a given opportunity. The article rejects the conclusion that nurses who kill are mentally ill and, therefore, are abnormal. This is too easy an answer, and it excuses the conduct to a certain degree.

The conclusion of the article is that nurses who murder their patients are exercising a level of strength and control that their nursing role does not grant them on a regular basis. According to this assessment, many nurses may feel that their role is subordinate and that they have no choice but to continue powerlessly following the orders of others. Additional factors build on the foundational feeling of powerlessness, and the totality of these factors is what pushes some nurses over the top and into killing as an exercise of gaining ultimate power. The article concludes that the only way to stop this criminality is through incarceration.

Medical Staff Oversight Responsibility

In 2005, the Indiana Court of Appeals addressed allegations that hospital medical staff have oversight responsibility to prevent pharmaceutical homicide by nurses at the hospital.[5] The case under consideration by the court resulted from the conviction of an ICU nurse for the murder of six patients in the defendant hospital. The families of the victims filed a lawsuit against the hospital. They named as defendants in the lawsuit two individual physicians who the families claimed had peer-review responsibilities and who allegedly had committed malpractice by failing to provide proper peer-review that would have identified the ICU nurse as a murderer.

The court noted that, under Indiana law, it is the members of medical staff committees who conduct retrospective medical reviews in a hospital and that these committees are afforded absolute immunity from malpractice litigation. Individual physicians cannot be held liable when the function they allegedly did not perform is by law considered to be a committee function for which immunity has been granted to individual committee members.

The court dismissed the case against the two individual physicians, although the court noted that it did not condone the hospital's lack of attention to a pattern of suspicious deaths. Oversight of medication use is an institutional responsibility and not an individual responsibility. Systematic controls, through the Pharmacy and Therapeutics Committee and the Quality Improvement Committee and through personnel assigned to control both medication utilization administration and antibiotic stewardship, are designed to monitor medication use and to detect potential problems. According to this ruling in Indiana, individual healthcare professionals are not responsible for conducting their own independent investigations of potential problems with institutional medication use, and individual healthcare professionals cannot be held legally liable if an institution fails to meet its oversight responsibilities.

Red Flags of a Healthcare Murderer

It would certainly be useful if there were specific factors that could be monitored because, with such monitoring, one could relatively quickly identify a potential healthcare murderer. Unfortunately, singling out healthcare murderers from among those who are potential culprits is no easier than identifying a specific patient's disease from among the many possible diagnoses. But there are certain factors that have been associated with healthcare murderers. These factors can be referred to as "red flags."

Elizabeth Yardley and David Wilson published their list of red flags to identify healthcare murderers in the November 2014 issue of the *Journal of Investigative Psychology and Offender Profiling*.[6]

Yardley and Wilson caution that a red flag is simply a screen that warrants closer attention. Seldom does a single red flag carry any significance in and of itself. It is a pattern of several red flags that should attract attention and should lead to focused investigation.

The red flags identified by Yardley and Wilson include the following:

- Frequent moves from one hospital to another
- Secretive and difficult personal relationships
- A history of mental instability or depression
- Predicts the day and shift when a patient will die
- Claims to be jinxed because patient died on their shift
- Likes to talk about death/behaves oddly when a patient dies
- Higher incidence of death on their shift
- Seems inordinately enthusiastic about their skills
- Inconsistent statements when asked to explain patient deaths
- Prefers night shifts and other shifts when fewer colleagues are present
- Has been associated with incidents at other hospitals
- Involved with other criminal activities
- Colleagues are anxious and suspicious in their presence

- Craves attention and praise
- Tries to prevent others from checking on their patients
- Stays around during investigations of deaths
- In possession of drugs in pockets or locker
- Has lied about personal information
- Possesses books about poison or serial murder
- Has had disciplinary problems
- Appears to have a personality disorder
- Has a substance abuse problem.

This list of factors may be useful in conducting a process of ruling out homicide. The authors caution that this list should be used with care. Identifying the culprit when there has been a series of suspicious deaths is complicated and cannot be simplified with a list. It may be that focusing on healthcare professionals as possible culprits will not be as effective as focusing on the type of patients who have died or on the manner in which the deaths have occurred. The authors conclude that "the importance of monitoring access to drugs within hospitals cannot be overestimated."

No Rush to Judgment

A British article was published in 1988 in the journal *Intensive and Critical Care Nursing* titled, "Is a Murder Charge an Occupational Hazard of Intensive Care Nursing?"[7] The article makes the point that a media frenzy can follow charges made against a nurse for murder of a patient and that, within this media environment, it is inevitable that a stigma will follow the accused for years, even if the charges are dropped. The author urges caution with investigation of medical murder cases, due to the consequences that can result.

The author suggests that a series of untoward events places an ICU nurse in a uniquely difficult position. There will be pressure to explain the events, and the nurse can easily become the prime suspect. A nurse in this position can be associated with the "crime of being there."

To avoid jumping to erroneous conclusions, the author suggests using data normally applied in the field of epidemiology. Situations that seem convincingly criminal may be unpersuasive when these data are examined. Even persuasive data are simply a beginning. Causality must be determined based on other evidence, together with data.

The author cautions against jumping to conclusions without complete information. When an investigation of a possible medical murder occurs, the suspect should be provided with legal counsel, who can assure that the suspect's rights are respected. Ruling out homicide makes sense, but respecting the rights of those who were involved in caring for the deceased patient is equally as important.

Investigative Methods and Data Analysis

A report published in 2022 by the Royal Statistical Society cautions that statistics and research methods used in the investigation of unexpected deaths must be rigorous in their evaluation of alleged misconduct by healthcare professionals.[8] The article offers three suggestions to assure valid investigative procedures.

The first suggestion is to identify all potential causal factors. Be sure that the facts lead the investigation and do not allow the investigation to lead the facts. An investigation cannot be premised on the assumption that a pharmaceutical homicide has occurred merely because a coincidence appears to be highly unlikely. Other possible explanations must be entertained; for example, changes in the underlying population of patients, changes in the policy on assigning patients to certain medical services, and administrative changes such as staffing levels, training, or case load.

The second suggestion is to take great care in the avoidance of bias. Rumors about the "killer nurse on ward three" should be stifled. While a patient death may be suspicious, and the cause of a patient's death may be a suspicious drug, the temptation to identify a suspicious healthcare professional based on innuendo and gossip must be resisted.

Blinding is essential to proper and defensible conclusions drawn from statistical evidence. Blinding requires that researchers not be told background information about suspected murderers while the data are being evaluated. Once the data analysis has been completed, law enforcement authorities can consider all of the evidence and can decide how to proceed. Blinding can also include withholding from law enforcement the identity of data analyst, to avoid bias that might be introduced due to the reputation of a data analyst for accuracy or fallibility.

Last, the authors suggest that statistics be used with great care. This requires avoiding conclusions based on small data samples that reflect only a brief period of time. The authors caution that "intuition," "rules of thumb," and "standard practices" are not a substitute for rigorous data analysis.

Furthermore, data do not speak for themselves. Data require interpretation by a qualified expert, such as a toxicologist or pathologist, who understands the background from which the data have been gathered.

Notorious Unproven Accusations

Several high-profile cases of alleged pharmaceutical homicide have resulted in acquittals that challenge the saying, "where there's smoke; there's fire." These prosecutions have alleged that proximity to a patient who died was sufficient to support suspicions of criminality. However, in these cases, although there was plenty of smoke, there was no fire. Media coverage of acquittals and dismissals is less comprehensive than media coverage of prosecutions and convictions. The lesson learned from these cases is that criminalizing patient deaths must be done cautiously. "Being there" is not necessarily a crime.

Susan Nellis—Pediatric Nurse[9]

Ontario nurse Susan Nellis was accused in 1981 of poisoning four infants through an intentional digoxin overdose. A cluster of infant deaths at the hospital was attributed to digoxin toxicity based on laboratory analysis. Nellis had responsibility for each of the infants who died. In an attempt to solve the problem, the hospital pharmacy placed digoxin into the same category as controlled substances, with the attendant restrictions that apply to those drugs. Nellis learned that she was to be interviewed by police, and a friend of hers advised that she "lawyer up and say nothing," which Nellis did. Nellis was arrested and charged with murder. After her arrest, the digoxin deaths ended. The court dismissed all four murder charges against Nellis based on the insufficiency of the evidence. The new pharmacy restrictions on access to digoxin were a likely reason for the cessation in digoxin-related deaths. Although Nellis was the only nurse who refused to talk with the police, and this behavior was considered suspicious by the police, the court ruled that seeking legal counsel before being interrogated by police should not be considered as a basis of suspicion. Nellis successfully sued the prosecutor for malicious prosecution. Analysis of the Nellis case a decade later resulted in an observation that the chemical MBT had been used to toughen syringes and medical tubing at the time of the deaths. Scientific evidence demonstrated how MBT could mimic digoxin in autopsies. Additionally, the laboratory test used to measure digoxin levels in the early 1980s had been shown to produce erroneously elevated results. The Nellis case is a classic example of allowing the theory to lead the facts, rather than allowing the facts to lead the theory.

William Husel—ICU Physician[10]

Ohio physician William Husel worked as an intensivist in the ICU where he often treated critically ill patients who were actively dying. The treatment of these patients often required that they be extubated, and Husel used very high doses of fentanyl to assure the patients' physical comfort while their breathing tube was removed. These doses were far larger than the doses used by other physicians during the same procedure. The patients died within minutes of receiving the medication. Two pharmacists at the hospital were alarmed by the large doses of fentanyl ordered by Husel. They reported their concerns to hospital administrators, who turned over the information to local law enforcement. Husel was charged with twenty-five counts of murder. A judge dismissed eleven of these counts due to the lack of evidence. At his trial for the remaining fourteen counts of murder, the question presented to the jury was whether Husel was a murderer or whether he was providing comfort care to dying patients. Over the course of several weeks, the jury heard testimony from numerous physicians and pharmacists. The prosecution focused primarily on the drug and the allegedly excessive doses. The defense focused primarily on the dying patients and the need for caring physicians to protect patients from unnecessary pain at the end of life. The jury found Husel not guilty of any charges. Although it was obvious that the doses of fentanyl ordered by Husel were very high, there was no proof that these doses caused the deaths of the already dying patients.

Jane Bolding—ICU Nurse[11]

Maryland nurse Jane Bolding was tried for murder after colleagues of hers in the ICU noticed an unusual number of CPR incidents with patients under her care. Prosecutors concluded that these patients had died as the result of potassium chloride injections administered by Bolding. After the hospital alerted law enforcement to the suspicions held by Bolding's ICU colleagues, detectives interrogated Bolding for twenty-three hours without letting her sleep before she admitted to the detectives that she had injected two elderly patients with potassium chloride. To support their murder charges, prosecutors utilized a study by the CDC showing that Bolding's patients were 100 times more likely to have cardiac arrests than the patients of other ICU nurses. The CDC study stated, however, that "Statistical analysis cannot answer whether or not intentional acts were committed against patients." The CDC report also said, "No matter how strong, epidemiologic associations of cardiac arrests with nurses attending patients cannot address factors such as exclusive access to patients or intent to do harm."

At trial, the judge ruled that the incriminating statements Bolding had given to the detectives were inadmissible due to the length of the interrogation and due to questions regarding her access to attorneys at that time. The prosecution was left with only statistical evidence to prove the two charges of murder.

After the prosecution rested its case, the judge granted a defense motion for acquittal. The judge noted that two other cases, one in Albany, Georgia, and one in San Antonio, Texas, had resulted in convictions for potassium chloride murders based on statistical evidence, but in both of those cases the prosecution was able to provide additional inculpatory evidence to support the statistics. The statistical evidence, by itself, was insufficient to support a conviction for murder. Statistics can be a starting point, but they are not sufficient evidence in and of themselves.

The clear message of this case is that healthcare institutions should conduct a thorough internal investigation of charges that a healthcare professional has committed pharmaceutical homicide at the healthcare institution. Turning over accusations and speculation to law enforcement and prosecutors may result in the misapplication of law to clinical science.

Filipina Narciso and Leonora Perez—Staff Nurses[12]

During the months of July and August 1975, 35 patients at the Ann Arbor Veterans Administration Medical Center suffered a total of 51 cardiac arrests. An intensive epidemiological and criminal investigation was begun to determine the cause of these unexpected events. The investigation concluded that nine patients had died due to the administration of the paralytic drug pancuronium without that drug having been ordered for them. In June 1976, a grand jury charged nurses Filipina Narciso and Leonora Perez with five counts of murder and ten counts of poisoning, as well as conspiracy to commit these crimes. Following these findings, the United States filed criminal charges against the two nurses. A jury found Narciso and Perez not guilty of murder but guilty of poisoning and conspiracy. Following this conviction, both nurses filed motions for a new trial based on prosecutorial misconduct.

Narciso and Perez were citizens of the Philippines who had come to the United States to practice nursing, in hopes of becoming U.S. citizens. The prosecution and conviction of them were widely publicized both in the United States and in the Philippines. Many supporters of the two nurses believed that Narciso and Perez had been made scapegoats by the American healthcare system and by the American justice system.

In ruling on the nurses' motion for a new trial, the court noted that the testimony presented to the jury had been complex and lengthy, extending over almost three months. The government's case was exceptionally complicated. The government had presented eighty-nine witnesses, including seventeen experts. This massive set of evidence was entirely circumstantial. The government submitted no direct proof of the defendants' guilt on any count.

No witness testified that the defendants ever had pancuronium in their possession. No witness stated that the defendants had ever administered any drug to the victims by injection. Nor was there any evidence that the defendants were any more familiar with pancuronium than any of numerous other staff in the hospital.

The government sought to show through numerous witnesses that certain respiratory failures were criminal in nature and that the defendants had the opportunity to commit the alleged crimes. The government attempted to prove that the defendants were present during the critical time period when, according to expert testimony, the drug must have been injected and that no other staff had been present during that critical time. The government offered no evidence of motive in support of its case against the defendants.

The defendants based their request for a new trial on a series of alleged errors made by the prosecution during pretrial proceedings and during the trial itself. The court focused on the prosecutor's closing argument to the jury. The prosecutor had argued to the jury that the defendants were guilty beyond a reasonable doubt. However, the prosecutor also argued to the jury that the defendants' arguments and facts presented were "worthless." The court concluded that the implication contained in this language was "inescapable though subtle: that the jury should consider what the prosecutor believed to be the defendants' failure to prove themselves innocent." The failure to prove one's own innocence is, of course, not the standard of proof in an American courtroom where defendants are legally innocent until proven guilty. Convictions must be based on the government's proof of guilt and not on a failure by defendants to prove themselves innocent. The prosecutor had argued a false standard to the jury.

The court then stated that the most egregious prosecutorial error in closing argument was in the prosecutor's final remarks. The prosecutor had argued that there were forty-four reasons that justified conviction of the defendants. He first reviewed what he considered to be the forty-three factual circumstances proving guilt beyond a reasonable doubt. He then stated to the jury that the forty-fourth reason was more powerful than the previous forty-three. Admitting to the jury that the forty-fourth reason could not be found in the trial testimony, he explained that the forty-fourth reason was the combination of the previous 43 reasons. According to the judge, the prosecutor said, "What are the odds, ladies and gentlemen, what is the chance, what is the probability that these defendants engaged in these activities and that all of these factors that are incriminating could exist and that the defendants would still nevertheless be innocent?"

The court concluded that presenting this type of nonfactual conjecture to a jury is impermissible. The question itself is not based on evidence but is rhetorical in nature. Answering the question would require a jury to engage in pure speculation about the nature of the charges, diluting the presumption of innocence. There had been no scientific evidence presented to the jury regarding the probability of any particular outcome, although experts in mathematical probabilities are available. The judge determined that this line of argument was improper and in direct conflict with the announced intention of the court. A collection of forty-three suspicious but ambiguous anecdotes does not combine to make a forty-fourth factor that unquestioningly proves guilt.

The court granted the defendants' motion for a new trial. A new prosecutor decided that the case would not be retried, and the charges were dismissed.

Conclusion

Most people view the institutional healthcare setting as one of the least likely places for the crime of murder to be committed. Unfortunately, some healthcare professionals view the healthcare institution as the most inviting place to commit murder. The potential criminality of healthcare colleagues must not be naively ignored.

However, it is important also not to jump to erroneous conclusions based on rumor, innuendo, and casual observations. Conclusions must be based on evidence that has been discovered through painstaking investigation.

Any unexpected death in a hospital must be considered as suspicious. Homicide should not be ruled out until another cause of death has been determined. Systematic studies of healthcare homicide have produced useful information that can be used to detect murderous activities by healthcare personnel.

Key Takeaways

- Follow your instincts if something seems amiss about a patient's death. Don't be deceived by the apparent commitment of your healthcare colleagues. Things aren't always what they seem to be. On the other hand, don't rush to judgment about anything simply because it seems out of the ordinary. There is no "ordinary" in patient care because every patient is unique and every situation is different. The best approach is to objectively gather information that might be useful for others so that they can undertake a systematic investigation later. Record your observations in some sort of paper or electronic ledger. Do not be an alarmist, but also do not be an idealist. Be an objectivist.

- As you reflect on something unusual that has happened in association with a patient's death, consider the research and analysis that have been conducted and published by scholars and practitioners who have shown a professional interest in healthcare homicide. There are useful publications that instruct on how to organize thoughts and what to look for. If you are not looking for relevant factors, then you will likely not see them. Criminals do not announce themselves. Researchers who have studied patterns of healthcare murder have published guidance on what to look for and how to look for what you look for. You can follow their lead rather than developing your own criteria and procedures. An internet search of the literature will provide guidance on how to follow up on suspicions.
- Incorporate all of your concerns into a systematic institutional approach to the evaluation of patient care. There are numerous committees and task forces in the hospital that are charged with the responsibility to review occurrences that raise concerns about the quality of care. The best place to start is with a pharmacy department committee. If your instincts are validated after a review by other members of the pharmacy department, then the data collected by you and your colleagues can be forwarded to a larger hospital committee. Taking the committee approach reduces the possibility that your concerns will be viewed as a witch hunt or as a personal vendetta. This type of investigation is an institutional responsibility and not an individual responsibility. Avoid becoming a private detective who functions outside the system. Let the system to the job.

References

1. Kizer KW, Yorker BC. Health care serial murder: a patient safety orphan. *Jt Comm J Qual Patient Saf.* 2010 Apr;36(4):186–191.

2. Sullivan MK. Serial murder in healthcare. *Nurs Manage.* 2009 Jun;40(6):32–36.

3. McNeil v. Mount Carmel Health System, 643 F.Supp.3d 810 (S.D.Ohio 2022).

4. Menshawey R, Menshawey E. Brave Clarice-healthcare serial killers, patterns, motives, and solutions. *Forensic Sci Med Pathol.* 2023 Sep;19(3):452–463.

5. Roberts v. Sankey, 813 N.E.2d 1195 (Ind. App. 2005).

6. Yardley E, Wilson D. In search of the 'angels of death': Conceptualizing the contemporary nurse healthcare serial killer. *J Invest Psych Offender Profil.* 2014 Jan;13(1):39–55.

7. Jones C. Is a murder charge an occupational hazard of intensive care nursing. *Int Crit Care Nursing*. 1998 Aug;14(4): 208–212.

8. Green PJ, Gill RD, Mackenzie N, Mortera J, Thompson WC. Healthcare serial killer or coincidence? Statistical issues in investigation of suspected medical misconduct. *Royal Statistical Society.* Sept 2022. https://rss.org.uk/RSS/media/File-library/News/2022/Report_Healthcare_serial_killer_or_coincidence_statistical_issues_in_investigation_of_suspected_medical_misconduct_Sept_2022_FINAL.pdf

9. Bowal P, Horvat K. Whatever happened to... the prosecution of Susan Nelles. Legal Resource Center of Alberta. 2011. https://prism.ucalgary.ca/server/api/core/bitstreams/6a7008f1-9a12-4426-81c2-14154f578f27/content

10. Pohlman P. Exclusive: Former ICU doctor struggles with stigma after acquittal on murder charges. Station WKRC. Thu, June 1st, 2023, at 3:23 PM. https://local12.com/news/investigates/exclusive-former-intensive-care-unit-doctor-william-husel-struggle-stigma-death-acquittal-acquitted-murder-charges-mount-carmel-west-hospital-cincinnati-patients-ohio

11. Harrison K. Judge acquits nurse Bolding. *Washington Post.* June 20, 1988. https://www.washingtonpost.com/archive/politics/1988/06/21/judge-acquits-nurse-bolding/b0965636-4228-402a-8f96-45d2b41b3990/

12. United States v Narciso and Perez, 446 F. Supp. 252 (E.D.Mich. 1977); O'Brien T. The V.A. murders. *Litigation.* 1984 Fall;11(4):15–19, 60–62.

Chapter 7

Medication Zone of Danger

Pharmacists have a responsibility to control the supply of medication within a healthcare institution, including various locations outside the pharmacy department where medications are stored and used. This responsibility is challenging. Pharmacists must consider the potential harm to patients within the organized healthcare setting when medications are used unlawfully to harm a patient. The pharmacy department's supervisory responsibility is made even more challenging when one considers that drugs can be removed from a healthcare setting by a hospital employee, and the reality that these drugs can then be used to harm a person outside the healthcare setting.

Danger Zone

The most frequent perpetrators of pharmaceutical homicide within a healthcare setting are nurses. However, outside a healthcare setting, medical doctors and other professionals have just as frequently been implicated as perpetrators of pharmaceutical homicide. Within a healthcare setting, nurses and respiratory therapists have relatively unsupervised access to patients and to pharmaceuticals, so the opportunity to commit crimes arises from the privacy of the situation. Physicians, on the other hand, are often accompanied by other healthcare professionals within a hospital or other organized healthcare setting, so their unsupervised access to patients is limited, as is the opportunity for criminal activity.

Outside the healthcare setting, physicians are often asked to informally provide medical care for family members, friends, and neighbors. The use of medications in the treatment of a patient at a private office or in the home may not be viewed by patients or family members with suspicion. Due to the status and respect afforded to physicians within healthcare institutions, the acquisition and removal of a drug from a particular medical service within the healthcare setting may not arouse suspicions. These illicitly acquired medications may be used in the care of patients outside the formal confines of a healthcare setting.

There is a long history of healthcare professionals removing drugs from healthcare settings and using these drugs to kill persons outside healthcare settings. All healthcare professionals are in a position to commit such a crime, and no healthcare professional is above suspicion when there is an unexpected death involving a patient, a family member, or a friend. Pharmacists have a responsibility not to create an unsupervised "medication danger zone" that invites healthcare professionals to remove drugs from the healthcare setting and use those drugs in the commission of a crimes such as murder.

It is important for pharmacists to participate in the prevention of crimes committed by the intentional use of lethal medications as murder weapons in the healthcare setting. It is also important for pharmacists to avoid developing unreliable medication distributions systems that lack accountability and fail to provide sufficient oversight. A healthcare professional who is tempted to commit crimes with medications may view a pharmacy system with relaxed oversight as an open opportunity to divert potentially lethal drugs.

When pharmaceutical products are diverted from a leaky distribution system and are used as a murder weapon, the criminal is clearly the person who administers the lethal medication and not the person who allowed the criminal to divert the medication for use in a criminal act. Yet it is important to protect potential victims from harmful medications that are intentionally administered as lethal weapons, and the pharmacy department has a significant role to play in restricting access to medications for this purpose.

A pharmacy distribution system that lacks adequate supervision of medication acquisition and fails to monitor unusual requests for medication will not provide documentation for later review to detect problems that may have been caused by the lack of system oversight. A lax system of drug distribution creates a "zone of danger" that puts the public at risk. One significant barrier to creating and implementing a secure system is that a high level of security can project a lack of trust in healthcare colleagues. Trust is an important aspect of any successful healthcare system, but trust can be misplaced.

Trust Barrier

Healthcare professionals are taught "trust bias." This means that the default relationship for those in healthcare is to be trusting of patients and of other health professionals, unless there is good reason, based on confirmed facts, not to be trusting. In a sense, this type of trust is "blind trust" based on professional credentials, licensure, and a shared commitment to common interests for the benefit of the public.

In healthcare, patients and other healthcare professionals do not have to earn each other's trust, because trust is the starting point of a professional relationship. Trust can be lost if circumstances warrant, but it need not be earned, because it is inherent.

Pharmacists trust that other health professionals will use medications safely and effectively for therapeutic purposes. Pharmacists also trust patients to use their medicines as they have been directed to use them for medical treatment. It is a trust-but-verify situation because pharmacists do not merely provide medications to healthcare colleagues and patients. Pharmacists also monitor the use of the medications that they provide, and one important purpose of drug therapy monitoring is verification. Concerns about medication use that arise during the monitoring of drug therapy warrant investigation.

When a suspicious situation suggests that perhaps a healthcare professional no longer deserves to be trusted, then relevant questions must be asked about the person's conduct. Asking such questions can be difficult, because challenging the motives of other healthcare professionals is countercultural in healthcare. It may suggest distrust when trust is assumed to exist.

Trust can be a barrier to the investigation of suspicious situations involving missing drugs and their possible removal from a healthcare setting, because the person with suspicions does not want to wrongly accuse a colleague. There could be major negative consequences for the pharmacist who reports suspected criminal activity by another healthcare professional, even if the pharmacist's concerns are justified.

Safe systems for reporting of suspicions must be developed within healthcare settings both to protect patients from harm and to protect health professionals from unwarranted suspicions. Anonymity of reporting is ill-advised, because it can be abused by people whose intention is to cause problems for another healthcare worker with whom the reporter is having a personal or professional quarrel. The better approach is to require that reports be submitted by reporters who identify themselves for the benefit of the designated recipient of information, within a system that guarantees the confidentiality of the reporter's identity.

Drug-Facilitated Crimes

A special category of pharmaceutical homicide is the drug facilitated crime (DFC). Sometimes when pharmaceutical products are used as weapons in a crime, they are actually used to facilitate the commission of another crime and not as the direct cause of harm to the victim. The United Nations Office on Drugs and Crime has published guidelines for the forensic analysis of drugs facilitating sexual assault and other criminal acts.[1] Drugs are an attractive weapon for the perpetrator of DFC, because they disable the victim, preventing victims from fighting off their attackers. The guidelines discuss the concept of the DFC as an occurrence outside a healthcare institution, using medications that have been acquired within a healthcare setting. According to the guidelines, the source of the drugs used in a DFC is usually a porous pharmaceutical distribution system. The porous system may be either institution-based or community-based, although institution-based leaks are more common.

The UN guidelines report that DFCs have occurred for centuries but that they have significantly increased since the mid-1990s. A common misconception is that a drug must be secretly administered to a victim during a DFC. In reality, most DFCs are committed through voluntary oral ingestion by the victim or with an injection that is agreed to by the victim. It is common for a perpetrator either to take advantage of a victim who has been put off guard by their consumption of alcohol or other drugs or to rely on the misplaced confidence of the victim when the perpetrator appears to have no ill motives toward the victim.

Many DFCs are not reported to law enforcement, and this failure to report is particularly true of attempted murder. The victim's uncertainty about what actually happened, the ambiguous sequence of events, and the uncertainty of knowable facts may delay reporting by a victim. There may be issues with anterograde amnesia suffered by the victim. There is also the possibility of embarrassment that such a seemingly preposterous story could be true. Victims do not want to admit that they allowed themselves to become so vulnerable as to be taken advantage of in the way that the perpetrator committed, or attempted, the crime.

The greater the interval between the occurrence of the crime and a report to law enforcement, the more difficult it becomes for a toxicology lab to identify the incapacitating drug that may have been used in committing or attempting a crime and for a DFC to be identified. For these reasons, the true prevalence of DFCs may never be known. Suspicions that are reported after several days or weeks often cannot be confirmed due to the passing of time.

Drugs Used in DFC

One of the challenges to solving a DFC that has occurred outside a healthcare setting is that there are so many drugs available with which to commit a crime.[2] In a healthcare setting, there are relatively few drugs that are readily available within patient care areas, and toxicology tests can be done to screen for those relatively few drugs. Healthcare institutions have a limited formulary, and the distribution of most drugs is limited to specific services. If there are suspicions about intentionally harmful medication use in the institutional setting, then there are usually only a few drugs that can be considered as the culprit.

When DCF occurs outside the healthcare institution, it is virtually impossible to know from which institutional setting the drugs were obtained. It could have been anywhere. There is no way to narrow down a list of possible drugs based on the place where the drugs were used. All possibilities must be considered.

There have been documented crimes committed with at least fifty medications. These include both prescription-only medications and over-the-counter products. Most of the drugs used in a DCF are fast-acting. They are usually CNS depressants that mimic alcohol intoxication. Victims who feel the initial effects of the drug may mistakenly believe that they have simply had a bit too much alcohol to drink and that the effects will eventually wear off.

The drugs themselves include benzodiazepines (alprazolam, diazepam, lorazepam, oxazepam, temazepam); barbiturates (amobarbital, butalbital, pentobarbital, secobarbital); antidepressants (amitriptyline, desipramine, imipramine, fluoxetine, paroxetine, sertraline); opioids (codeine, hydrocodone, oxycodone, meperidine, methadone, morphine, fentanyl, oxymorphone); and miscellaneous drugs such as carisoprodol, scopolamine, ketamine, and clonidine.

Most of these drugs decrease situational awareness at low doses, and, if not used as the actual murder weapon, they can facilitate the commission of murder with a different weapon. At higher doses, many of these drugs have effects that are similar to anesthetic agents, rendering the victim powerless to avoid being the victim of a crime.

Homicide with Diverted Medications

A DFC is relatively easy for law enforcement to investigate, because the basic crime is a familiar one to those who are trained and experienced in murder investigation. Even though a medication has been used to create a vulnerability of the victim in facilitating the commission of a crime, the crime itself is straightforward for those in law enforcement who are experienced in the investigation of rape or murder or assault.

On the other hand, when a pharmaceutical product is diverted from a healthcare setting and is used as the actual murder weapon, law enforcement is challenged to investigate whether a crime has been committed and to identify the perpetrator if there has been a crime. Pharmaceutical homicides do not produce the evidence that detectives are accustomed to seeing.

When a pharmaceutical homicide is committed within a healthcare setting, staff who are familiar with the toxic effects of drugs and who understand the manner in which drugs are distributed within the healthcare setting may have reasons to suspect that a crime has been committed and that a particular person is likely the perpetrator of the crime. Previous incidents of patient harm under questionable circumstances may allow a healthcare professional to discern a trend in adverse events that could explain the most recent incident in that trend. Outside the institutional setting, even the most experienced and devoted detectives will lack the expertise to appreciate that a pharmaceutical homicide should be considered.

Evidence of a Pharmaceutical Homicide

The most persuasive evidence that a pharmaceutical homicide has been committed is the identification of the drug in the victim's body tissues. Urine is the most useful of specimens because the body concentrates drugs and drug metabolites in the urine for excretion. The general rule is that a urine specimen should be collected within ninety-six hours of the suspected crime and that a specimen of at least 100 mL should be collected. The lab needs a sufficient quantity of urine for the initial test and for retests should they be needed. Specimens should be refrigerated or frozen. There have been suggestions made that the addition of sodium fluoride to a urine specimen will preserve the usefulness of the specimen should there be a delay between collection and testing.

Blood testing is not as useful as urine testing, because drug levels in blood degrade quickly. When possible, a combination of urine samples and blood samples can provide the best opportunity for the laboratory to produce useful evidence. Advances in toxicological analysis have made it possible to use blood samples that were unusable in the recent past.

When a crime has occurred long ago, and there is no longer an opportunity to collect useful urine or blood specimens, it may be necessary to resort to hair analysis. There is significant promise for the future of hair analysis, although there are currently barriers that may stand in the way of using this alternative test.

Because not all drugs have been well studied in hair analysis, there is the possibility of false negative results. Hair analysis is useful as a screen but not as confirmation. Likewise, there is the possibility of false-positive results. Head hair grows at a rate of approximately 1 cm per month. This means that there is a temporal element to hair analysis. Segmental analysis is needed to demonstrate that a drug was ingested on the day of an alleged pharmaceutical homicide.

Forensic Toxicology

Specimens of urine, blood, and hair must be sent to an experienced and qualified laboratory following an alleged pharmaceutical homicide. Frustrated investigators have dealt with the destruction of their evidence by inexperienced laboratory personnel. Laboratory qualifications are subject to challenge at trial, and a case can be lost when qualifications are ruled to be insufficient. Furthermore, when the lab requests an additional sample, because the submitted sample has been completely used up without conclusive results, an investigative case can crumble if no sample remains.

There is a difference between testing for therapeutic levels of a drug and testing for the much smaller trace levels that can support a finding of criminality. There may be a temptation to send a sample to an in-house medical laboratory. This approach would be a mistake. It could use up the existing sample with no possibility of identifying a suspect medication. Medical laboratories may have all the equipment and skills necessary for therapeutic drug level detection, but only a forensic laboratory is sure to have the ability to detect levels that provide evidence of criminality.

Laboratories can enhance the value of their results if the circumstance of sample collection is recorded. The collector of a sample can facilitate success by the laboratory if contextual information is provided to the laboratory. This includes answers to questions such as:

- When and where were the specimens collected?
- What symptoms did the victim exhibit?
- How did witnesses to the alleged crime describe the victim?
- For how long was the victim unconscious or suffering from amnesia?
- Did the victim take alcohol or any other drugs?
- Did the victim urinate, or was the victim incontinent prior to the sample being taken?
- What is known about the suspect with regard to access to pharmaceutical products?
- To what pharmaceutical products did the victim have access prior to the alleged crime?

This background information can assist laboratory personnel in their assessment of the situation and in the analytical decisions they make about specimens submitted for toxicologic analysis.

Laboratory results will be more meaningful and useful if investigators work with the laboratory to identify drugs that should be targeted based on the specifics of the case. There is no need to test for all possible drugs (it is expensive and time-consuming) when a short list of suspected drugs can be made available through investigation. The lab may be able to suggest to investigators the "routine" drugs that are usually detected in a geographic area. There is a distinct possibility that the laboratory is familiar with the concept of pharmaceutical homicide. Identifying the drugs that should be tested for is very much a collaborative effort between the laboratory personnel and the investigative personnel.

Removing Drugs from Healthcare Settings

People who are committed to engaging in criminal activity will develop ingenious ways to remove drugs from a healthcare setting so the drugs can later be used in the commission of crimes. Here are several ways in which this type of criminal activity has occurred in the past (most, but not all, large medical centers are aware of these potential leaks from the system, but some smaller institutions may be unaware of them):

- A healthcare worker stole drugs from a patient care area and stored them in the worker's locker during a shift. At the end of the shift, the worker delayed leaving until everyone else had left, and then removed the stolen drugs from the hospital. After discovering this violation of policy, the hospital developed and enforced a standard that restricted locker access to arrival and departure times, with no access allowed during a shift. The hospital also placed security personnel in the locker area during shift change.
- A hospital worker routinely placed used pharmaceutical products in the trash, and then volunteered to take out the trash, at which time the worker retrieved the (partially) used pharmaceutical products and placed them in her pocket. The hospital developed and enforced a policy of allowing the trash to be removed only by custodial personnel.
- A hospital worker was found to have sewn secret pockets into his uniform top, into which the worker placed pharmaceuticals during a procedure. The worker actually substituted saline for the drugs during the procedure and then removed the real drugs from the hospital. The hospital developed a policy of requiring workers during a procedure to use only hospital-issued uniforms.
- A hospital worker replaced a drug that was provided by the manufacturer in pre-filled syringes with saline and transferred the drug to an empty vial. Then the worker removed the vial with the drug from the hospital. The hospital implemented and enforced a policy that placed pre-filled syringes in locked storage until they were ordered for a specific patient.
- A hospital worker prided himself on always being prepared for any emergency. To meet this responsibility, he carried syringes of various drugs with him as he performed his work. On several occasions, the worker "forgot" that he had the drugs on his person, and he took them home. Later investigation discovered a large stash of

pharmaceuticals that had been removed from the hospital and were stored in the worker's closet at home. The hospital implemented a policy that forbade carrying drugs on one's person unless the drugs had been ordered for immediate administration to a patient.
- A hospital noticed that on multiple occasions sharps waste containers were hidden in areas of the hospital where they did not belong. The hospital conducted video surveillance and discovered that a worker was breaking into the sharps containers, transferring the contents to a lunch box and taking the contents home. The hospital implemented a strict policy for accountability of sharps containers and procured sharps containers that were more difficult to open.

This is not an exhaustive list of ways in which drugs have been removed from healthcare settings. The point of these examples is to show how lax monitoring can lead to removal of drugs by those who have access to them. There is no way to completely prevent the diversion of drugs to criminal use, but diversion can be deterred through identification of the means through which diversion is being accomplished.

Drug Removal and Therapeutic Failure

The most obvious problem with the unauthorized removal of drugs from a patient care setting is the criminal use of the drugs outside the patient care setting, and the harm that can be caused by this criminality. However, another problem arises with injectable drugs when the drugs are removed and are replaced with saline or other nontherapeutic substitutes. Healthcare personnel who use the adulterated vials and syringes think they are administering drugs for the benefit of the patient, but the expected therapeutic effect does not occur. The response may be to increase the dose of the drug, leading to an overdose when a vial of unadulterated product is used.

Lack of an expected patient response to an administered drug can, by itself, be a red flag that the administered product is not what it purports to be. Perhaps an error has been made and the wrong drug has been obtained, or the drug may have been mislabeled. Alternatively, it may be that the drug has been deliberately removed from the healthcare setting and a nontherapeutic substitute has replaced the drug. For this reason, any observation that a patient has not responded to a drug in an expected way should be reported through existing institutional channels, and any syringe or vial other device that has been used in drug administration should be retained for later analysis.

An unexplained lack of expected response is a reportable incident, and it may have significant implications for follow-up patient care. When a patient is not responding to drug therapy as a patient would be expected to respond, a medication error may be the explanation, and the criminal substituting of inactive ingredients for the pharmaceutical entity should also be considered. The crime of pharmaceutical homicide may victimize both the person who is killed with the diverted medication and the patient whose therapy fails because the prescribed drug has been diverted and the administered product contained no active ingredient.

Institutional Risk of Unauthorized Drug Removal

The failure to prevent the removal of drugs from a healthcare setting by a healthcare worker is a significant risk both for the healthcare institution and for healthcare workers within the institution. Harm to the institution includes the loss of the drugs themselves and their lack of availability for patient care. There is also the loss of monetary value to the institution due to the theft.

From a liability perspective, the potential harm from criminal drug removal is enormous. Hospitals are responsible for securing the supply of medications they store for use in patient care. The creation of a "zone of danger" that allows unauthorized access to medications exposes the institution to liability for failing to meet legal expectations for medication security.[3] The risk management department will be very supportive of acquiring resources necessary to secure medications from diversion within a "zone of safety" that the public expects of its healthcare professionals and healthcare institutions.

The healthcare institution may be subject to civil liability if there were indicators that a healthcare worker was removing drugs from the hospital, yet the hospital did not recognize those indicators or recognized them but did nothing in response to them. Individual healthcare workers who had knowledge of these indicators but did not report them could be exposing the institution to civil liability through their inaction.

The appropriate response to indicators of unauthorized drug removal is a comprehensive investigation. Such an investigation requires a commitment of significant internal human resources and the use of forensic expertise that may not exist within the institution. There is also the possibility that the investigation itself will cast the institution in a negative light with those who assume that the investigation is an admission of impropriety. Regardless, this type of investigation is a necessary part of a healthcare system's commitment to responsible patient care. Experts with experience in criminal justice may need to be retained on a consultant basis.

Balanced Approach to Medication Security

While the central pharmacy department is a highly secured area of a healthcare institution where the removal of drugs is closely monitored, there are other areas of every institution that may be less well controlled and where the likelihood of unauthorized drug removal is high. These areas include the emergency department, operating suites, drug carts, automated dispensing units, and other places where procedures are conducted and where pharmaceutical products are stored.

The pharmacy department has full responsibility for all drugs that are used within a hospital or other organized healthcare settings. The goal of the pharmacy department is to both control access to prevent harmful use of drugs and to permit access when drugs are needed in therapy. There is a balance to be found between too much control and too little control.

One of the most effective ways to establish pharmacy control over drugs that should not be removed from a hospital is through a satellite pharmacy program. A satellite pharmacy can dispense limited quantities of drugs on a patient-by-patient basis, instead of using open-access drug carts (which have all but disappeared from modern hospitals) or other leaky drug distribution systems. Satellite pharmacies require staffing, and staffing is expensive. Some hospitals have adopted technological replacements for satellite pharmacies, and this cost-savings approach diminishes pharmacy control over drug distribution.

Healthcare professionals who need medications in the care of their patients can obtain the supply that they need at the start of a shift or at the beginning of an individual procedure, and they must return what they did not use along with documentation of how much was used with each patient. A simple reconciliation step can assure that no drugs are missing. A pharmacist checks for discrepancies, and both parties sign a form to end the transaction.

This process is not perfect. There is still the question of whether the health professional actually used the drugs in patient care and whether what was returned was what was originally dispensed or, instead, was replaced with something else.

One possible check for the first problem is to audit the patient care record and reconcile it with the pharmacy information. A possible check for the second potential problem is to periodically use product testing devices to verify that the returned substance is in fact the expected drug. Testing can be done with a refractometer. In larger institutions that have greater resources, UV spectrometry can be used. Small testing units have recently been developed to facilitate this process.

As is the case with any tracking system, there will be occasional atypical transactions. This is inevitable. It is important to record the results of all transactions in a database and to periodically mine the data to determine whether there is a trend showing that atypical transactions occur on a particular day of the week, a particular time of day, or with a particular healthcare professional. These trends can be investigated to determine whether there is a problem.

Also important is the development of a program called "If You See Something, Then Say Something" (copying unashamedly from the Department of Homeland Security) to create a culture of responsible reporting if things just don't seem quite right.

Accepting the Medication Control Responsibility

As the profession of pharmacy expands into new areas of clinical patient care, the traditional role of product distribution and oversight has become significantly less glamorous. Yet this is a role that continues to be important for pharmacists, for healthcare institutions, and for anyone who might be harmed by a medication that is removed from the hospital without authorization by a person with criminal intent.

The Joint Commission's accreditation standards are quite clear. According to these standards, the pharmacy department is responsible for proper storage, control, and security of medications in all areas of the hospital where medications are located. Compliance with this standard requires that the pharmacy department continually monitor medication control in all areas of an accredited healthcare facility.

A critical component of compliance is the development of policies that specify expectations for medication storage, control, and security within a facility. A next step is the education of personnel involved with medication use, so there is a clear understanding of the expectations.

An effective and standardized audit process is necessary to determine compliance with the policies. Effective auditing must include the development of an audit tool that asks the right questions and produces useful data. In larger institutions, the tool can be loaded onto a handheld device so that the data can be easily uploaded to a central database.

It is usually wise to avoid the perspective that the pharmacy department is the "medication police." This approach will not win many friends among institutional personnel. A preferable approach is that of an educator or colleague, who points out violations of the policies and recommends ways to comply with policies. The security of pharmaceuticals must be sold as a "we are all in this together" program.

DEA's Controlled Substances Model

The epidemic of prescription drug abuse has focused pharmacists' attention on the control of access to DEA-regulated controlled substances, particularly opioid analgesics.[4] Healthcare institutions have increased restrictions on access to these controlled substances to prevent diversion from legitimate medical care to illegal use.

The increased restrictions on controlled substances have also been adopted in many institutions for high-cost drugs that may be diverted to the so-called "gray market" for resale. This expanded control shows that there is no real barrier to applying controlled substance restrictions to yet another category of drugs, including those drugs that are identified as having been used in drug-related crimes.

Using the controlled substance model for control of drugs used in drug-related crimes could mean that all such drugs are received at the hospital by a person other than the one who ordered them, to prevent removal from the hospital of drugs that have been over-ordered. The use of automated dispensing units for all such drugs, and software systems to identify all personnel involved in the handling of the drugs, would also be consistent with the controlled substance model. Supervised disposal of multidose vial waste and reconciliation of returns to the supplier would also fit the model. It may make sense to place all drugs subject to unauthorized use and/or diversion in the same restricted category even if they are pharmacologically dissimilar.

Medication Reconciliation Opportunity

The chain of medication distribution is lengthy and complicated. From start to finish, there are many potential leaks. For this reason, the pharmacy profession has accepted responsibility for an activity often known as "medication reconciliation." Generally performed at the time a patient is discharged from a healthcare facility, medication reconciliation is a process of identifying the most accurate list of all medications that the patient is taking, including name, dosage, frequency, and route. This is done by comparing the medical record to an external list of medications obtained from a patient, hospital, or other provider.

Medication reconciliation gives an overview of a patient's medication use prior to admission, during admission, and after discharge. Because this is such a comprehensive review, it is an opportunity to identify problems that have occurred during a patient's stay in a hospital, including perhaps discrepancies between medications that were provided for the patient and those that were actually used. It is one last chance to reflect on whether there are inconsistencies with the patient's drug therapy showing that some drugs intended for use in the patient's care are missing. There is also the opportunity to educate patients about drug toxicities and the potential danger of inappropriate drug use.

Three legal case studies can facilitate an appreciation for how pharmaceutical products might be diverted from therapeutic use to criminal purposes.

Case Study: "Just Hit Them with a Little Succs"

A nurse and a politician in Nevada were married after having known each other for a relatively long period of time.[5] Following the marriage, the husband's career as a critical care nurse was stagnant. Meanwhile, the wife's political career was meteorically successful. She was elected to a state office. The possibility of her running for Governor was being discussed. The relationship between the two deteriorated. The husband discussed with a nurse colleague how he and his wife were "having marital problems," and that he intended to seek a divorce, but his wife objected due to the damage that could be done to her political aspirations.

The husband and the nursing colleague had a conversation about "a widely publicized case in which a husband killed his wife, shot the judge presiding over the couple's divorce, and fled to Mexico." The husband said to the nurse colleague, "That guy did it wrong. If you want to get rid of someone, you just hit them with a little succs because they can't trace it postmortem." The nurse colleague knew that the husband was referring to succinylcholine. She felt that the comment was "bizarre and scary." But she told nobody about the comment.

At that same time, a pharmacist at the hospital had noticed an unexplained increase in the use of succinylcholine from several crash carts. No other drugs were missing from these crash carts. Despite being concerned about the missing product, the pharmacist told nobody about this unusual observation.

Several days later, while at home, the husband called 911 to report that his wife was unresponsive. Paramedics were able to restore the wife's heartbeat, but she could not breathe on her own. The wife was transported to the hospital. Upon learning of the incident, the nurse colleague informed the wife's

address to the licensing agency. Under close watch by international law enforcement, the nurse was apprehended when he traveled to Mauritania, where extradition to the United States is more easily done. The nurse was returned to the United States, and he was found guilty of first-degree murder. He was sentenced to life in prison.

The victim's family sued the hospital where the nurse had worked and from which the propofol had been diverted. The family alleged that the hospital knew that the nurse had a history of stealing controlled substances and that the hospital should have known that drugs were unaccounted for. The family also alleged that members of the hospital's staff had told hospital administrators that the nurse was stealing drugs and that the hospital's only response was to call a conference with the nurse, after which he resigned, effective two weeks later. It was alleged that during this two-week grace period the propofol that killed the victim was stolen from the hospital by the nurse. The precise circumstances of how the drug was administered by the nurse to the victim are unknown because the nurse took the Fifth Amendment at his trial.

The lower court dismissed the family's lawsuit against the hospital, ruling that the allegations, even if proven to be true, could not support liability of the hospital, because there is no recognized duty by a hospital to prevent murder by one of its employees outside the hospital setting. The lower court ruled that such an abhorrent act is unforeseeable and, therefore, does not violate a hospital's duty of care. From this ruling, the family appealed.

The appellate court noted that the drug used to murder the victim is a "dangerous drug that requires a prescription" and that the hospital was "entrusted with its proper use." The court explained that a common law duty of care is recognized when a person's actions "create a foreseeable zone of risk" posing a general threat of harm to others. The court said that the hospital's failure to ensure the proper use of the stolen drugs created a "zone of risk," because it exposed the general public to a risk that the hospital could have avoided by taking reasonable measures to prevent the drugs' theft and removal without authorization. Dismissal of the family's lawsuit was reversed, and the case was reinstated. The case was apparently settled out of court.

What if hospital administration had shown greater concern for concerns expressed by its own staff regarding the nurse's alleged theft of drugs? What if the nurse had been dismissed immediately after being confronted with the information regarding his theft of drugs? It is impossible to know whether this murder could have been prevented, but it may be possible to prevent similar murders in the future.

Case Study: Physician's Wife Drowns in Bathtub

A Utah physician was convicted of first-degree murder in the death of his wife from drowning while she was under the influence of drugs administered to her by the physician.[7]

Evidence showed that the physician and his wife were experiencing marital difficulties, due in part to the physician's multiple extramarital affairs. He had threatened to kill both himself and the wife several times. The physician's health appeared to be deteriorating. He began limping, walking with a cane, and wearing a surgical boot. He explained to neighbors that he was "having some procedures done," but he told several colleagues at work that he had peripheral neuropathy, while he told other colleagues at work that he had cancer in his big toe.

The physician enlisted an accomplice to unlawfully acquire lethal medication from the hospital where he worked. In March 2007, the physician suggested that the wife have a face lift, to which the wife agreed thinking that it would help her marriage. Following the surgery, the physician requested that the surgeon prescribe injectable diazepam and oxycodone for his wife. The surgeon agreed to do this, as a professional favor for a medical colleague, even though these are drugs that the surgeon did not usually prescribe for his postoperative patients. The order was filled by the hospital pharmacy, and the medication was given to the physician for use by his wife.

Two days after discharge, the wife was found unresponsive, apparently drowned in a bathtub at home. The physician had been with the wife at the time of her bath, and he explained that he had attempted to rescue her but that his physical limitations prevented him from doing so. The death was initially ruled to be due to accidental and natural causes. The couple's children pressed for a toxicology report, which noted the presence of the drugs that the wife allegedly would not have administered to herself. The cause of death was changed to "combined effects of heart disease and drug toxicity."

In August 2012, the physician was charged with his wife's murder. The trial was conducted in October 2013. The prosecution contended that the physician had administered prescribed drugs to the wife so that her death would appear to be from natural causes. There was evidence that the physician had bragged of having committed the perfect crime. The defense claimed that the wife's death was from an accidental fall in the bathtub. The physician was convicted, and he was sentenced to fifteen years to life in prison.

The physician appealed his conviction. He claimed that the evidence of guilt was insufficient. The court disagreed, noting that he had manipulated the wife into a facelift, he requested from the surgeon drugs that deviated from the surgeon's postoperative protocol, and he manufactured an excuse for his own physical inability to lift the wife out of the tub by reporting inconsistent claims of various illnesses to his family, to his neighbors, and to coworkers. The court concluded that "ignoring incriminating evidence does not make it go away." The circumstantial evidence supported "a basis in logic and reasonable human experience" to conclude that the physician wanted the wife out of the way so that he could be with his mistress. The murder conviction was affirmed on appeal.

The most significant "what if" question that this case raises concerns whether the pharmacists could have verified with the surgeon that the ordered drugs were necessary and appropriate. The pharmacists could perhaps have assured that the wife understood the potential adverse effects of the medications. Perhaps pharmacists can find a cautious and respectful way to anticipate that a prescriber has been hoodwinked into ordering unnecessary and potentially lethal medications for a colleague's spouse, and to take necessary step to protect the patient from harm.

System Design to Promote Medication Security

Renowned expert James Thunder suggests steps that can be taken to reduce the incidence of pharmaceutical homicide and to promote detection and resolution of criminal cases after pharmaceutical homicides have occurred.[8] The author is primarily concerned about crimes committed with pharmaceuticals that have been diverted from an institutional setting by a healthcare professional. He is also concerned about crimes that are committed by patients who have been prescribed medications for therapeutic purposes and who then use those medications in the commission of a crime.

The author's advice is primarily directed toward healthcare institutions, yet it has tremendous value for the entire system of medication use (and misuse).

The suggestions offered by James Thunder to prevent pharmaceutical homicide are as follows:

- *Enhance facility security.* Most current security activities are geared toward events that may be immediately harmful to hospital personnel and/or patients. They are to a far lesser degree focused on events that may cause harm in the future. Expanded use of surveillance cameras could document past occurrences that show how medications have been removed from a healthcare facility.
- *Improve background checks.* Rather than trusting a licensed health professional based on the licensure itself, check the history of each

licensed health professional associated with an unexpected death, if there are suspicions of wrongdoing.

- *Improve controls over the dispensing of medicines.* This suggestion is consistent with the idea that systems for limiting access to medications classified as controlled substances by the DEA could be expanded to include other potentially harmful drugs.
- *Require reporting of individual deaths and establish systems to monitor rates, places, and times of death.* Stories of drug-facilitated crimes by health professionals often relate that previous drug-facilitated crimes have been committed by the same person. Any such crimes should be reported to the health professional's licensing agency and should be taken seriously.
- *Treat some death scenes as crime scenes.* Deaths resulting from drug-facilitated crimes often appear to be from natural causes. When there is no obvious cause of death, the possibility of a drug-facilitated crime should be considered.
- *Establish elder death review teams.* This suggestion is the result of an observation made by James Thunder that vulnerable people, such as the elderly and the disabled, die at an unusually high rate as compared with the rest of the population, yet only a small percentage of these deaths are considered as homicides. Thunder speculates that something criminal may be happening that is not being noticed and that formal review could reveal a hidden truth.
- *Establish family profiles.* As difficult as it may be to accept this reality, the spouses and family members of health professionals are at higher risk of drug-facilitated crime than are those who are not related to health professionals. DFC should be considered a risk factor in crime investigations when the victim is a relative of a healthcare professional.
- *Train doctors in certifying death.* There may be a tendency not to suspect a colleague when an unexpected death has occurred. This tendency should be avoided. Nothing should be ruled out as a professional courtesy.
- *Expand medical investigations.* Medical examiners should be required to formally investigate any situation in which there is a suspicion of drug-facilitated crime.
- *Increase autopsy rates and the number of forensic pathologists.* A proper investigation of a drug-facilitated crime depends on the availability of adequate tissue specimens and a competent lab to test them. This expertise should be made available to all investigators.

Most of these suggestions are a matter of institutional policy modification and are not suggestions for changes to be adopted by healthcare practitioners in their day-to-day clinical practice. On the other hand, healthcare practitioners have a role to play in the development of institutional policy, and that role should be taken seriously.

Conclusion

The crime of pharmaceutical homicide may occur outside a formal healthcare setting using drugs that have been acquired within a formal healthcare setting. This is a challenge for institutional pharmacy practice. Pharmacists and other pharmacy personnel have a responsibility to prevent access to pharmaceutical products by those who would use the products as murder weapons. The institutions themselves have a responsibility to create oversight programs that can detect leaks in the pharmaceutical distribution system and to develop processes to plug those leaks.

A body of scholarly literature is available on research works that have studied patterns of pharmaceutical homicide. The results of these studies can facilitate sensible institutional reviews of pharmaceutical distribution systems to prevent the loss of medications that are later used in the crime of pharmaceutical homicide.

Key Takeaways

- Don't contribute to the problem of pharmaceutical homicide. It is important for pharmacists to be aware of the possibility that a healthcare colleague is committing crimes with pharmaceutical products. Detecting, investigating, and reporting these crimes are an essential component of the patient safety activities of any pharmacy department. Unfortunately, these important activities are generally conducted retroactively. They are a reaction to something that has already happened, and the harm that has already been caused cannot be undone. To avoid contributing to diversion of drugs from a healthcare setting, become familiar with the problem of drug leakage from the distribution system (institutional security and loss prevention will already know about this) and proactively plug the leaks before a crime can be committed by an ill-motivated healthcare worker who sees what appears to be an open invitation to divert pharmaceuticals to nefarious uses.
- Include drugs that are associated with pharmaceutical homicide in systematic oversight systems such as those that are established and implemented for controlled substances. The purpose of the controlled substance distribution system is to be able to identify where a drug was diverted from legitimate use and who was responsible for that diversion. The system is not designed to prevent all access to

controlled substances, because they are necessary for patient care. The system limits access to those who have a demonstrated need for a drug, and it records the time and place that the drug was accessed by the person who acquired it. This is not a fool-proof system, as the evidence of opioid use disorder illustrates. There is still controlled substance diversion in institutional and community pharmacy settings. Nevertheless, the diversion is reduced through organized efforts to restrict access, even though it cannot be eliminated. This is a model that could be implemented to prevent drug facilitated crime.

- Prepare yourself to assist with crime scene investigations. It will be tremendously helpful for law enforcement investigating a crime scene to know what drugs might have been available to commit the crime that has occurred and how those drugs are distributed through the distribution system. There might even be a wrapper, or a vial, or another container that can be used as the starting point to investigate what drug was used and where it came from. This will be new information that trained detectives may not be aware of. From that starting point, a pharmacist may be able to reconstruct the chain of custody from the crime scene back to the point at which the drug leaked from an institutional drug distribution system. Don't underestimate your expertise as a consultant to law enforcement. What seems obvious to a pharmacist may not be obvious at all to a person who lacks professional training in pharmacy. Do your part to help the investigation.

References

1. United Nations Office on Drugs and Crime. Guidelines for the Forensic Analysis of Drugs Facilitating Sexual Assault and Other Criminal Acts. 2011. **https://www.unodc.org/documents/scientific/forensic_analys_of_drugs_facilitating_sexual_assault_and_other_criminal_acts.pdf**

2. Volonnino G, et al., Z-Drugs and their use in Drug-Facilitated Crimes: a review of the literature. *Clin Ter.* 2023;174(5):461–468.

3. Grissinger M. Physical environments that promote safe medication use. P T. 2012 Jul;37(7):377–378.

4. United States Department of Justice, Drug Enforcement Administration. Drug-Facilitated Sexual Assault. April 2017. https://www.dea.gov/sites/default/files/2018-07/DFSA_0.PDF

5. Higgs v. State, 222 P.3d 648 (Nev. 2010).

6. Herndon v. Shands Teaching Hospital and Clinics, 23 So.3d 802 (Fla. App. 2009).

7. State v. MacNeill, 397 P.2d (Utah App. (2017); ABC News. Days after death of Utah doctor who killed wife, daughter opens up about decade-long nightmare. April 12, 2017. **https://abcnews.go.com/US/days-death-utah-doctor-killed-wife-daughter-opens/story?id=46730494**

8. Thunder JM. Quiet killings in medical facilities: detection & prevention. *Issues Law Med.* 2003 Spring;18(3):211–237.

Chapter 8

Poisoning as a Cause of Death

In ancient times, all medications were considered poisons, and all poisons were considered medications. It was simply a matter of dosing and intent. The chemical substances that could make a sick person well could also kill a healthy person. This reality was so well established that everyone had a ready supply of antidotes in their home to treat poisoning, regardless of whether the poisons had been intentionally or unintentionally administered. The risk of dying from poisoned food or drink was accepted throughout society. It was similar to the current risk of dying in an automobile crash. Death from poisoning was unlikely to happen, but it was not impossible, and it did occur regularly. Everyone knew, or knew of, someone who had died of poisoning. Death from poisoning was a risk that could not be absolutely prevented, although it could be minimized by taking precautions. When people traveled, they brought their supply of antidotes with them. There was always a concern that wherever a person went, somebody might find a reason to poison them.

Common knowledge of poisoning as a means for committing murder led to consideration of poisoning as the cause of death virtually any time a person died unexpectedly and when no cause of death could be immediately discerned. Tests to detect poisoning were not fact-based, and many people who were found guilty of poisoning another person were innocent. The evidence that led to their conviction was based on observation, intuition, and inference, rather than on science. Those people who were accused of causing another person's death by poisoning had little solid evidence to provide in their defense. Likewise, many people who committed murder by poisoning were not caught. Prosecutors lacked solid evidence that a poisoning had occurred. Early death was accepted as a reality of living in ancient times, and often death by poisoning was attributed to natural causes.

In more recent times, significant progress has been made with instrumentation and analytical processes to enhance the ability of criminal laboratories and law enforcement investigators to detect homicide from poisoning. This improved investigative ability has made poisoning less appealing to perpetrators as a means to commit murder. On the other hand, the vastly expanded availability of pharmaceuticals, and the increased toxicity of them, has provided new opportunities for pharmaceutical homicide. Pharmaceutical products are considered to be relatively difficult to identify as murder weapons, because they are often missed on a toxicology screen, and they may seem innocuous because they are regularly used by many people. From ancient times to the present, the incidence of pharmaceutical poisoning has likely not increased or decreased, but it has changed. The incidence is still high; it is just different. The law enforcement approach to detecting pharmaceutical poisoning has changed also.

Frequency of Pharmaceutical Poisoning

Reported data from poison centers support an assessment that chemical poisonings should be considered as common.[1] This frequency assessment is a matter of perspective. The word "common" is a relative term. For those professionals who are involved day-to-day with the detection and treatment of poisonings, it is no surprise that poisonings would be considered common. For clinicians whose primary focus is on other areas of patient care, the incidence of poisonings may seem less frequent. The data are not very helpful. While there are useful data from a variety of sources that report unintentional poisonings and suicides by poisoning, there are no organized and comprehensive data on homicidal poisonings. No central location or organization serves as a recipient of those reports or aggregates those data in a useful format. The absence of a central repository of information on pharmaceutical homicides hinders the ability to evaluate the scope and nature of the problem and to develop effective solutions.

Anecdotal reports of homicidal poisoning were analyzed in one recent study. The researchers relied on data from the National Mortality Statistics database.[2] The study concluded that the "rate of homicidal poisoning is relatively low as compared with other methods of homicide. However, this rate has been trending upward in recent years." The study also noted that "drugs are the most commonly used poison." Homicidal poisoning of children and the elderly has occurred at a significantly higher rate than with persons in between those age groups, according to the results of the study.

A different study analyzed information that was taken from Centers for Disease Control and Prevention (CDC) data.[3] The investigators acknowledged that the data were far from comprehensive. Nevertheless, the investigators concluded that "Homicidal poisoning, though rarely described in the literature, is an important public health concern in the US. Men, infants, and Blacks were reported to be at higher risk of homicidal poisoning. Drugs were the most commonly used means of homicidal poisoning." The CDC data reviewed by the research team disclosed that about 10,000 suicidal poisoning deaths occur per year and about 150 homicidal poisoning deaths occur each year. These are undoubtedly low numbers that do not represent the true scope of the pharmaceutical suicide or homicide problem. Underreporting presents a challenge for data analysts.

Quantifying the scope of pharmaceutical homicide is a difficult task. Data documenting pharmaceutical homicides will probably never be gathered comprehensively. Information sources such as death certificates are created locally and are maintained in many different ways throughout the country, making it virtually impossible to use that resource to accurately determine the number of pharmaceutical homicides that occur nationally. On the other hand, a problem with pharmaceutical homicide by poisoning clearly exists. The lack of quantification need not stand in the way of those who seek solutions to the challenge presented by the crime of pharmaceutical homicide.

Drugs Used in Pharmaceutical Poisoning: Pre-pharmaceutical Revolution

To help identify deaths due to pharmaceutical homicide, it is important to know the "drugs of choice" that are considered to be most useful by perpetrators of pharmaceutical homicide. Those drugs have changed significantly over time. As one might expect, murderers will use weapons that are available to them. They make their choices from what they can get. As the pharmaceutical business and pharmacy practice have evolved over time, the available drugs have changed and the options for their use as pharmaceutical murder weapons have changed also.

Between 1820 (the founding of the United States Pharmacopeia) and the mid-1900s (the start of massive growth in pharmaceutical technology and innovation), the medications available for pharmaceutical suicide primarily included strychnine, arsenic, cyanide, atropine, digitalis, and thallium. Some of these agents were used for their therapeutic effects. Others were considered as "pharmaceuticals" only in the sense that they were stocked by pharmacies (drugstores), where they could be acquired from a pharmacist (druggist) by prescription or could be purchased without a prescription. Some of these poisonous agents were also available for purchase at non-pharmacy retail outlets. When sold to a purchaser, these products were required to be labeled as a "poison," and records of their sale were required to be kept in a poison register. There are many historic reports of pharmacy malpractice cases in which pharmacists inadvertently substituted one of these poisons for a nonlethal drug that had been prescribed or requested. There are also many reports of homicides in which these drugs were obtained from a pharmacy and were used as lethal weapons.

Strychnine. In times past, strychnine was used as an appetite suppressant, an aphrodisiac, and a purgative. It was often provided as a "tonic" and was prescribed at low doses to speed convalescence from an illness. It is extracted from the seeds of the nux vomica tree. Strychnine was also used to poison rats and other pests. Symptoms of strychnine toxicity begin within five to sixty minutes following ingestion, and they last between 10 and 20 minutes. The toxic dose is in the range of 100 mg. Strychnine toxicity manifests as periodic seizures, with the patient remaining conscious. Coma and death may follow repeated seizures. Respiratory depression is the major life-threatening emergency, caused by spasms of the diaphragm. There is no antidote for strychnine poisoning.

Arsenic. Although rarely used specifically for its medicinal effects, arsenic was included as an adulterant in many medications before standards for product purity were established and routinely enforced. The effects of a medication containing arsenic could easily be detected by the user. Although arsenic is almost tasteless, it can produce a garlicky odor to the breath. Pharmacies were the primary source of arsenic for anyone who needed the chemical for use as a weed killer, pesticide, or rodent poison. Symptoms of arsenic poisoning in humans are largely gastrointestinal (diarrhea, salivation, abdominal pain). Treatment of arsenic poisoning can include bowel irrigation, blood transfusions, and the use of cardiac medications to manage heart failure.

Cyanide. The suicide tablets that are used by spies to avoid divulging information under torture contain cyanide. Cyanide is a rapidly acting, potentially deadly chemical that interferes with the body's ability to use oxygen. There is no medical indication for cyanide. Before modern chemotherapy drugs became readily available, some clinicians promoted the antineoplastic effect of hydrogen cyanide derived from apricot pits. Hydrogen cyanide is converted into cyanide when it is ingested. There is no scientific evidence that this treatment is effective. In fact, it could be harmful. In the early 1970s, cancer patients and their families sued the federal government for the right to use the product laetrile, which was derived from apricot pits. This lawsuit was unsuccessful. There continue to be fringe practitioners who promote this "therapy" for desperate cancer patients. Otherwise, cyanide is criminally used as an adulterant to pharmaceutical dosage forms that converts the therapeutic product to a murder weapon.

Atropine. Also known as "belladonna" (beautiful lady) and extracted from juice of the deadly nightshade bush berries, atropine was, and still is, a staple of anticholinergic pharmacotherapy. It is used as a therapeutic mydriatic and for other medical purposes when administered as ophthalmic drops. It may also be used in its injectable form to treat symptomatic or unstable bradycardia. Potentially fatal effects include ventricular fibrillation and paradoxical bradycardia. Antidotes are physostigmine and pilocarpine. In 2014, atropine poisoning was identified as the causal agent in the death of a man who had been poisoned by his wife and son. The victim was using 1% atropine eye drops, purchasing three 10 ml bottles at a time. Routine toxicology showed the presence of lethal concentrations of atropine in his fluids and hair. The perpetrators had placed the contents of two bottles in the victim's food at mealtime. Both the wife and son were convicted of murder.

Digitalis. Derived from the foxglove plant, digitalis is a familiar cardiac glycoside used in the treatment of congestive heart failure and atrial arrhythmias. Digoxin, the modern form of digitalis, is a narrow therapeutic index drug (the therapeutic level and the toxic level are very close) that has been largely replaced with more effective and less toxic cardiac medications. Nevertheless, there is still a place for digoxin in modern medicine as a third-line therapy. Digoxin overdose can lead to a risk of life-threatening arrhythmias. The antidote for digoxin poisoning is digoxin-specific antibody fragments. A study that was reported in 1983 described ten instances of digitalis poisoning that had been reported as anecdotes in medical literature between 1826 and 1972. The most recent of these, the 1972 report, described how a pharmaceutical chemistry researcher had murdered his foster daughter, foster son, and his mistress, because they were not obeying his instructions to them. He defended these actions by referring to his cultural background, in which the eldest male of the family was permitted to punish other family members for their disobedience. He claimed also that he could not possibly have killed his victims, and that they must have died for some other reason, because he was so familiar with digitalis that he would know how to dose the drug to punish and not kill. He was convicted of murder.

Thallium. The element thallium was discovered in the 1860s and was used to treat venereal disease, ringworm, gout, dysentery, and tuberculosis. Thallium is a cumulative homicidal poison that produces its fatal effects over time. It was used by Saddam Hussain's secret police and is apparently still used by the Russian KGB. Thallium sulfate is water-soluble and tasteless, so it was considered to be desirable as a pharmaceutical agent. These characteristics also make thallium ideal as a poison. It can take several days for toxic symptoms to appear, and the symptoms are often attributed to another illness. By the time thallium poisoning is diagnosed, the poisoner has had ample time to leave the area. Investigations may have difficulty accumulating evidence of what happened and when, prior to the victim's ingestion of thallium.

Liabilities in Dispensing: A SCOTUS Analysis

Of the many historic legal cases implicating pharmacists as negligent providers of poisons used in murder, the most eloquently reasoned is from the Supreme Court of the United States (SCOTUS) in a legal opinion from 1870.[4] Keep in mind that the language used by courts at that time was as outdated for today as the drugs that were then dispensed by pharmacists are outdated for today. The case in question arose from the provision of medication by a pharmacist. The issue presented to the court was whether a pharmacist can be held liable for selling a medication that the pharmacist knows will be used to commit murder. The pharmacist argued that the contractual relationship between the pharmacist and the purchaser of arsenic places the blame for criminal use of the arsenic squarely on the purchaser and not on the pharmacist. The court said:

> The man who sells arsenic to one who, he knows, intends to poison his wife with it, will not be allowed to maintain an action on his contract. The consideration of the contract, in itself good, is there tainted with turpitude which destroys the merits of it. No man ought to furnish another with the means of transgressing the law knowing that he intended to make the use of them.

The court continued:

> Can a man furnish another with the means of committing murder, or any abominable crime, knowing that the purchaser procures them, and intends to use them, for that purpose, and then pretend he is not a participator in the guilt? Can he wrap himself up in his own selfishness and heartless indifference and say "'What business is that of mine? Am I the keeper of another man's conscience?"' No one can hesitate to say that such a man voluntarily aids in the perpetration of the offence, and, morally speaking, is almost, if not quite, as guilty as the principal offender.

The court concluded:

> It is certainly contrary to public policy to give the aid of the courts to a vendor who knew that his goods were purchased for the purpose of being employed in the commission of a criminal act, injurious to society or to any of its members.

The trial court's dismissal of the case against the pharmacist was reversed. There is no further public record of the case or of its resolution. The case establishes the legal principle that a pharmacist can be held liable for selling a poisonous substance that is then used by the purchaser to murder a victim, if the pharmacist knows of the criminal purpose for which the poisonous substance will be used.

Updated Perspective on Poisoning Prevention

A more recent viewpoint, with more contemporary language, was provided by the Court of Appeals of Texas in 1987.[5] In this legal case, the facts showed that a pharmacist received a telephone call from a "regular customer who requested some strychnine for the avowed purpose of killing wolves." The customer advised the pharmacist that he was having problems with wolves attacking his cattle when they were calving. The pharmacist replied that he did not stock strychnine but that he would attempt to find a local pharmacy that did have that product in stock. The customer indicated that he needed the strychnine "immediately" to prevent further loss of livestock. The pharmacist contacted his wholesaler and ordered the strychnine. The customer was instructed to travel directly to the wholesaler to pick up the strychnine, which he did. The strychnine was invoiced to the pharmacy by the wholesaler and was billed to the customer by the pharmacy. The pharmacy never handled the strychnine.

In fact, the customer did not use the strychnine to kill wolves. He used the strychnine to murder his wife. The wife's estate (her surviving family members) sued the pharmacy for negligence. One necessary element of a negligence claim is proximate cause. This element requires that there be foreseeability of harm on the part of the defendant (in this case the pharmacist) to support liability for negligence. The court addressed this foreseeability requirement.

The pharmacist testified:

> At no time during my conversations with the customer, or anyone else, did I ever have any idea that he was going to in some way use the strychnine to harm, injure, or kill his wife. There were no circumstances, inferences, statements, or any other actions by any party that would have in any way led me to believe that the customer would use the strychnine for that reason. No statement, act or conduct in any way suggested that the strychnine would be used for any other purpose than to kill the wolves that were attacking his cattle as he had reported to me in the telephone conversation.

The court concluded:

> The evidence offered by the plaintiffs shows that the pharmacist had no knowledge of any facts even remotely suggesting that the customer had any motive to injure or murder his wife or any other person. In fact, the customer informed him that wolves were killing his cows or newborn calves, and he wanted the strychnine to poison the wolves before more cattle were lost.

The court was willing to overlook the nonstandard way in which the strychnine was acquired, having the pharmacist order it from the wholesaler for pickup by the customer at the wholesaler's place of business. The case against the pharmacist was dismissed because the court ruled that the pharmacist could not have foreseen the murder of the wife based on the information available to the pharmacist at the time the strychnine was provided to the husband.

The major difference between the older case and this more recent case, other than the 100-plus years that separates them, is that the court thought the pharmacist in the older case somehow knew or should have known the criminal purpose to which the purchaser intended to use the product acquired from the pharmacist. The court does not explain how the pharmacist knew this critical piece of information. In the more recent case, the pharmacist was able to offer a credible explanation of why he could not foresee the use of the poison he sold and that was used as a murder weapon.

Case Law: Restricting Lethal Poisons to Sale at Pharmacies

A 1937 case from Indiana summarizes the justification for pharmacy self-regulation, and the exclusion from the pharmacy profession of those businesses that are not licensed by the state board of pharmacy.[6] In this case, legal action was taken by the state board of pharmacy against a "perfumery" that was selling pharmaceutical substances with potentially lethal effects. The substances being sold by the perfumery were listed by a board of pharmacy regulation as being among those potentially lethal substances that could be sold only by a licensed pharmacy. The perfumery challenged the board of pharmacy's legal action that had been taken against the perfumery, contending that the concept of "drug store" and "pharmacy" were so poorly defined that a "perfumery" could not legally be excluded from that classification. The owners of the perfumery also contended that the perfumery's sale of the potentially lethal substances could not be prohibited by the board of pharmacy and that the action taken by the board of pharmacy was based solely on economic protection of pharmacists and not on protection of the public health.

The court began its discussion of the legal arguments by considering whether a "pharmacy" and a "drug store" have a special and identifiable clear meaning from which other businesses can be obviously excluded. The perfumery pointed to the interchangeable use of the terms "druggist" and "apothecary" and "pharmacist" to support its argument that the concepts are so vague that they have no distinct meaning and could apply to anyone. Likewise, the terms "drug store" and "apothecary shop" were undefined in the board of pharmacy regulations; thus, they were arguably without clear meaning. The perfumery argued that if a profession does not define itself, then it cannot exclude anyone from conducting the activities that it claims as its own.

The judge (perhaps an English major prior to attending law school) cited ancient text to begin his analysis (the quoted language below is taken directly from the court's legal opinion):

A drug store or apothecary shop is one of the oldest known places of business. In the 25th verse of Chapter 30 of Exodus, we find the following:

> "'And thou shalt make it an oil of holy ointment, an ointment compounded after the art of the apothecary.'"

The court continued with comments related to the appropriateness of restricting lethal substances to pharmacy sale only. The court quoted Act V, Scene 1 of Shakespeare's *Romeo and Juliet* in which an apothecary shop is described:

> And in his needy shop a tortoise hung,
>
> An alligator stuff'd, and other skins
>
> Of ill-shap'd fishes; and about his shelves
>
> A beggarly account of empty boxes,
>
> Green earthen pots, bladders, and musty seeds,
>
> Remnants of packthread, and old cakes of roses,
>
> Were thinly scatt'd, to make up a show.

And when Romeo requested that the apothecary provide him with specific lethal drugs, the apothecary replied:

> Such mortal drugs I have.
>
> But Mantua's law is "'death to any he who utters them.'

The less literary, but more practical, meaning of this passage is that an apothecary (pharmacist) located in the province of Mantua, Italy, would be convicted of capital murder for selling poisons if they were used to put a person to death rather than to heal an infirmity. The role of the pharmacist was to protect people from death by poisoning. This responsibility was recognized by members of the pharmacy profession and by the public they served. It was so well recognized that it was included in the theater of the day.

Through these interesting citations, the court considering the perfumery's argument noted that the pharmacy profession has existed for centuries, and the court concluded that pharmacies are well-recognized places of business that must be placed under the control of licensed pharmacists. Restricting potentially lethal substances to sale by pharmacies was held by the court to be fully within the prerogative of the state board of pharmacy. The authority of the state board of pharmacy was upheld in this legal case. The challenged regulation had been promulgated and enforced for the purpose of protecting the public from improper use of pharmaceutical substances that could cause death to their user. The perfumery was not allowed to continue its sales of potentially lethal pharmaceuticals.

This case is only one of many cases that reflect a similar theme. Through the late 1800s and the early 1900s, courts consistently rejected challenges brought by general retailers to the authority of the pharmacy profession to restrict the sale of potentially lethal substances to licensed pharmacies. In 1952, that authority was recognized under federal law when the RxOnly category of pharmaceuticals was officially recognized. The pharmacy profession, through its boards of pharmacy, was given clear authority to determine who is qualified to protect the public from the harmful effects of pharmaceuticals that can be deadly if misused.

It is axiomatic that with authority comes responsibility. There may be regulatory consequences for the pharmacist or pharmacy that does not meet the recognized responsibility to protect patients from the lethal effects of dispensed medications. What if a pharmacist's error in dispensing the wrong drug, or dispensing the wrong strength of the right drug, results in the death of a patient? What if a pharmacist's failure to effectively counsel a patient about the method of medication use causes the patient to die? What if a pharmacy is so poorly organized that errors are inevitable and patient deaths result from the failure of management to promote safe pharmacy systems? May these actions result in board of pharmacy disciplinary action? The answer to this question is, "yes."

Having excluded general retailers from the business of distributing harmful pharmaceutical products, the pharmacy profession, through its boards of pharmacy, has a responsibility to implement requirements to assure that consistent, caring, and competent practices are employed by pharmacists in pharmacies that provide pharmacists with the tools necessary to promote successful practices. The means through which these responsibilities are met by the board of pharmacy are licensure and permitting. The consequence of regulatory violations can lead to the loss of a license or permit. State boards of pharmacy have been created to develop standards of practice for the pharmacy profession, and they have been given the responsibility to enforce those standards.

Drugs Used in Pharmaceutical Poisoning: Post-pharmaceutical Revolution

The general rule that murderers will use whatever weapon they can get to commit their crimes continues to be applied today. The pharmaceutical weapons available to murderers are more numerous, and more lethal, than those that were available prior to the pharmaceutical revolution that began immediately following World War II.

Researchers have examined the drugs that have been used as murder weapons in reported prosecutions of pharmaceutical homicide. Based on this research, it is possible to compile a list of drugs that are likely to be used in the commission of pharmaceutical homicide. This is certainly not a complete list of drugs that are actually used in pharmaceutical homicide. Many pharmaceutical homicides are not discovered, and the drug that was used is impossible to know. Some pharmaceutical homicides that are discovered are resolved through a plea bargain or other legal mechanism that does not leave an extensive legal record for researchers to locate and evaluate. Given these caveats, the known drugs that have most frequently been used in pharmaceutical homicide include the following:

- Epinephrine
- Succinylcholine
- Concentrated KCl
- Digoxin
- Insulin
- Lidocaine
- Morphine

This list is not surprising. These drugs are easily acquired, easily used, and are potentially very toxic. None of the drugs is expensive, and only one is a controlled substance. Very little attention is given to missing supplies of these drugs, except for morphine. They are easily leaked from the drug distribution system.

Media reports suggest that three more drugs will likely be added to the list when the next group of researchers conducts a similar investigation. The first of these, and the least surprising, is fentanyl, due to its notoriety and widespread availability. There have been many reports in the media of deaths due to opioids generally and fentanyl specifically. The second, and most disgusting new poison, is misoprostol, secretly given by men to their pregnant partners to terminate a pregnancy. In these cases, the trust that the victim placed in the perpetrator is heartbreaking. The third, and perhaps most unexpected new poison, is tetrahydrozoline (the active ingredient of Visine ophthalmic drops). A quantity of tetrahydrozoline placed in a victim's beverage can cause heart failure in a very short time.

Murder by Digoxin Poisoning

A tablet count of a patient's remaining medication following an alleged overdose death is one of the easiest pieces of evidence to obtain, yet it was omitted in a Missouri murder investigation, and it became a key issue when the alleged murderer appealed her conviction.[7]

An 84-year-old woman was discharged from the hospital after she had been treated for kidney disease and congestive heart failure. She was prescribed a potentially toxic once-daily dosage of 0.25 mg digoxin, and a pharmacist testified that he dispensed a quantity of 100 tablets on the day that the woman left the hospital. The patient was discharged to the care of her neighbor, who took responsibility for the woman's welfare, including the administration of medications, because the woman was unable to administer her medications by herself.

The patient died twelve days after she was moved into the neighbor's house. Cardiac arrest was determined to be the cause of death. The body had already been embalmed by the time of the autopsy, so the blood could not be tested for digoxin levels. An analysis was performed of the vitreous humor that showed a lethal level of digoxin, indicative of digoxin poisoning. The defense contended that the lethal level could have been the result of drug accumulation over time at the prescribed dosage. The prosecution alleged that the lethal level resulted from an acute overdose administered by the neighbor. The neighbor was convicted of first-degree murder, and she was sentenced to prison for life without parole. From this verdict she appealed.

A key issue on appeal was whether the prosecutor had misled the jury in closing arguments. The defense contended that either the elderly patient had committed suicide or that there was no overdose and that the death was from natural causes. The defense attorney told the jury:

> Something we haven't talked about, something that you should be aware of, another small fact, there was testimony about prescriptions being purchased from a pharmacy. They purchased three bottles, a hundred pills in each bottle. If it was such a gigantic dose, where did all the extra pills go? Is there any evidence that there was only one pill left? No, there wasn't any such evidence. I submit to you that all of the pills that were supposed to be there were there, or that you would have heard about it.

In reply the prosecutor told the jury:

> The defendant said where did the extra pills go. I'll tell you where they went. They went right down the deceased's throat. That is where the extra pills went. The person who was in control of that medication is his own client. If the evidence was that there was a bunch of pills left, why didn't he bring it on? Why didn't you hear that evidence, that there were way too many pills left, that there couldn't have been any put down her throat? The pills weren't here. I'll tell you where the pills were. They were in the deceased.

In fact, there was no evidence of how many digoxin tablets remained in the deceased woman's medication supply when she died. The court noted that there was some quantity of digoxin tablets remaining in the patient's medication vial, but that nobody had bothered to count them. Conducting a tablet count in a first-degree murder case seems like an essential piece of investigatory work, but it was not done.

The court admitted that the prosecutor's unsubstantiated assertion that the tablets were in the deceased person's body may have allowed the jury to draw a misleading inference, but the statement made by the prosecutor did not warrant reversal of the conviction. Numerous other questionable actions taken at the trial were challenged on appeal, and the appellate court remanded the case back to the trial court for clarification. There is no further mention of the case in the public record. It is likely that the neighbor's murder conviction was upheld.

The importance of this case is that forensic science can be as simple as basic arithmetic. An elementary approach such as counting tablets is particularly relevant when tissue samples have been contaminated by embalming fluid and the laboratory scientists are unable to provide irrefutable evidence through complex analysis. If a tablet count had been conducted in this case, and if ninety tablets of the original one hundred remained after ten days, then the defense would have been strengthened and the prosecution would have been weakened. The opposite conclusion would have been reached had there been significantly fewer than 90 tablets remaining. When a defendant's conviction for pharmaceutical poisoning by overdose will result in life imprisonment, a tablet count is essential.

Murder by Insulin Poisoning

Insulin can be a very attractive option as a murder weapon outside a healthcare setting. Of all the drugs used in pharmaceutical homicide, insulin is perhaps the drug most frequently chosen by murderers. Insulin warrants special attention both due to its frequency of use and the ready access to it. Insulin serves as an excellent example of how investigative methods can be developed to uncover and prosecute pharmaceutical homicides.

The older types of insulin are available for purchase from a pharmacy without a prescription, and generally with no questions asked and no record made. Even the newer types of insulin that require a prescription are available in many patients' homes due to the high incidence of diabetes in the U.S. population. Anyone who has paid attention to their high school biology class has learned that insulin is a naturally occurring peptide hormone, and a murderer may conclude that it will not necessarily raise suspicions of foul play if a natural substance like insulin is discovered in the tissues of a deceased person.

The notorious murder trials of Claus von Bulow brought attention to the possible use of insulin as a murder weapon. The 1990 movie "Reversal of Fortune" tells the story of how Claus von Bulow was accused of murdering his wife "Sunny" with an injection of insulin. Jeremy Irons won a Best Actor Academy Award for his portrayal of Claus von Bulow. The movie illustrates how the insulin may have been administered to Sunny. It also shows how difficult it can be to convict a person of murder with insulin.

Von Bulow was initially convicted. His conviction was reversed, and he was found not guilty when he was retried. The new evidence presented during the retrial was the testimony of several experts who concluded that Sonny's death was due both to a combination of drugs other than insulin and to her underlying medical condition. The widely publicized Claus von Bulow story and the hugely popular movie version of it provide a clear roadmap for the use of insulin as a murder weapon.

One of the experts who testified for the defense in the second trial was Dr. Vincent Marks, who is the world's leading expert on murder by insulin. In 2009, Marks published the results of a literature review that he had conducted.[8] He described 66 cases of murder by insulin. The included reports were of proven cases of murder, attempted murder, and manslaughter. This is undoubtedly the small tip of a large iceberg, given the challenges of identifying murder by insulin and the difficulties in successfully prosecuting cases of murder by insulin. It is also likely that many successfully prosecuted cases of murder by insulin are not reported in the medical-legal literature, because prosecutors move quickly onto their next case rather than taking a pause in their busy schedule to write an article for publication.

Marks suggests using postmortem toxicological testing with mass spectrometry so that the identification of any insulin analogue is verified. If the substance C-peptide is included in the scope of analysis and if a quantitative method is used, the ratio of insulin to C-peptide can be calculated. High insulin levels accompanied by low C-peptide levels point to exogenous insulin introduced from outside the body's production pathway. Marks cautions that there is no foolproof way to determine murder by insulin solely from laboratory values. Investigation of possible insulin deaths must incorporate many strategies, including thorough scene and postmortem investigations, a comprehensive medical record review, and background checks on each person who may have had the opportunity to inject the victim with insulin.

A Legal Case of Murder by Insulin: Investigation and Prosecution

An actual legal case serves as an illustration of how murder by insulin can be detected and prosecuted. A 68-year-old patient died from an insulin overdose.[9] The patient suffered from several medical conditions, and she was confined to a wheelchair due to partial paralysis. She was not diabetic. The State of Texas charged her home health registered nurse with murder for injecting the patient with a massive dose of insulin. A jury convicted the defendant nurse, and she was sentenced to ninety-nine years in prison. She appealed her conviction based on two grounds: (1) that the trial court abused its discretion in allowing the prosecution to present evidence of extraneous bad acts to which the nurse was linked and (2) that the evidence supporting her conviction was factually insufficient.

The facts presented in the case showed that the patient was living with her daughter and son-in-law. The daughter was a registered nurse. Because of her infirmities, the patient needed domestic support. The daughter contacted a home health agency to obtain assistance for her mother with routine tasks such as feeding and bathing. The agency sent the defendant nurse to provide these services.

The patient did not need help with her medications, which she took on her own. None of her prescribed medications were administered through injection. The patient did like to receive occasional injections of B_{12} that she felt helped her "not feel tired." Because she trusted the home health nurse's credentials as a registered nurse, she asked the defendant to inject her B_{12}.

The son-in-law returned home from work one day and he noticed that the patient was nonresponsive, she was mumbling, and "looking really clammy and dazed." He also noticed that her mobility was restricted because she was struggling to grasp a cup that she ordinarily held easily. He called the patient's daughter at the hospital where she worked, because she "had more knowledge about such things." The daughter had already talked to her mother on the telephone at 3:35 p.m. that day and to the defendant home health nurse at 3:36 p.m. Hospital employment records for the daughter showed that she had

death. Second, she claimed that the evidence against her was all circumstantial and that it was the patient's daughter who had the opportunity and motive to kill the patient. The evidence showed that five years earlier the daughter had inadvertently brought home from work a vial of insulin after having administered a dose to a patient. The evidence also showed that the daughter was a "compulsive gambler" and that she had, in the past, asked her mother to help her pay off her gambling debts.

The defendant nurse claimed that this evidence about the daughter raised a reasonable doubt of her guilt and that she should have been found not guilty. The jury did not agree with the argument and found that the nurse was guilty. The defendant nurse appealed this guilty verdict.

The Appeal: Extraneous Offenses Evidence

The appellate court began its review of the case by focusing on the "extraneous offenses evidence" argument made by the nurse. The defendant nurse contended that the jury had been allowed to hear testimony concerning two prior incidents for which she was not either charged or convicted: (1) the death by insulin overdose of a patient in Oregon and (2) the theft of insulin from the hospital in Texas.

It is a basic principle of law that defendants must only be tried for the crimes of which they have been charged, not for other disconnected crimes. To avoid undue prejudice to defendants, the circumstances under which a court will permit a jury to hear evidence of extraneous offenses are limited. To allow testimony related to other possible offenses, the judge must be convinced that the defendant's involvement in the extraneous offenses was probable beyond a reasonable doubt and that the probative value of the evidence outweighed the unfair prejudice to the defendant.

The appellate court ruled that the evidence of the incident in Oregon was properly presented to the jury because it demonstrated modus operandi, which refers to a defendant's distinctive and idiosyncratic manner of committing criminal acts. Evidence of modus operandi is recognized as an exception to the general rule that precludes extraneous offense evidence.

The modus operandi exception is important because it can implicate the "doctrine of chances." According to this doctrine, the evidence of the repetition of similar unusual events over time demonstrates a decreasing probability that the events occurred merely by chance. The doctrine reflects the principle that evidence of striking similarities between two rather idiosyncratic crimes is evidence that the same perpetrator was responsible for both crimes.

Evidence of the incident in Oregon was appropriately presented to the jury also because the defense strategy was to implicate the patient's daughter as the person who administered a lethal dose of insulin. The Oregon incident was introduced into evidence to show that, even if both the defendant nurse and the daughter had equal access to insulin, only the defendant nurse could be connected to a modus operandi. This particular modus operandi was to murder elderly patients with an insulin overdose and steal from them.

Similarly, the court ruled that evidence of the defendant nurse's access to insulin at the Texas hospital was properly presented to the jury. The defense had argued to the jury that the defendant nurse lacked access to insulin at the time of the alleged crime. To rebut this argument, the prosecution showed that the defendant nurse had access to insulin at her previous place of employment. Thus, the evidence of access to insulin at the Texas hospital was not extraneous to the case.

The Appeal: Sufficiency of the Evidence

The defendant nurse had been convicted on the basis of circumstantial evidence. She argued that her conviction should be overturned because there was no direct evidence of her guilt. Nobody saw her inject the patient with insulin. There were no vials or syringes found that implicated the defendant nurse as having administered insulin to the patient. In short, the defendant nurse argued that circumstantial evidence alone cannot support guilt beyond a reasonable doubt.

The court disagreed:

> In this case, we believe the cumulative evidence—even if it is primarily circumstantial—is overwhelmingly against [the defendant] because the inferences which the jury was required to draw about her motive and opportunity were reasonably supported by the facts adduced at trial. For example, a jury could have made a reasonable inference about [the defendant's] motive to murder [the patient]. In its closing argument, the prosecution told the jury that its theory of motive in this case was that [the defendant] was stealing from [the patient] and that she wanted to cover up these thefts because she was about to get caught. A reasonable jury could have heard the evidence and inferred that [the defendant] was systematically stealing from [the patient], feared being caught, and had the motive to kill her.
>
> Moreover, while it is true that there is some evidence in the record that conflicts with the jury's verdict, it is hardly enough to describe the guilty verdict as being against the great weight of the evidence. To

> begin, we recognize that the cause of death in this case is indefinite because no autopsy was performed, but the logic of this point is limited. After all, no autopsy was performed because the revelations about the C-peptide test emerged only after the cremation had already been performed. At that point, while an autopsy would have been helpful, it was not necessary because multiple medical experts examined the C-peptide test results and agreed on the cause of death. The doctors were, in fact, so convinced that [the patient] had died of an insulin overdose that they changed her death certificate to reflect this finding.

The court affirmed the verdict, denying the defendant nurse's appeal.

Significance of the Case

Contrary to the assertions of the defendant in this case, circumstantial evidence can be used to convict a person of committing pharmaceutical homicide. Evidence from previous incidents that happened at other times and in other places can be used to establish a perpetrator's modus operandi. Evidence brought to the attention of medical staff can change conclusions as to the cause of death when the evidence supports the use of pharmaceuticals in the commission of a crime.

The challenges faced by a prosecutor in a case of this kind are obvious. There is no "smoking gun" that can be shown to a jury as direct evidence tying the defendant to the crime. The employment record of the suspect must be examined, and interesting leads must be pursued. The pharmacological issues are complex, and they must be thoroughly evaluated.

An investigation of a potential pharmaceutical crime requires significant time and significant financial resources. Many of the suspicious cases of suspected pharmaceutical homicide that are presented to prosecutors are not pursued. Prosecutors want clear-cut cases. They can't justify expending public resources on difficult prosecutions that are likely to fail. This is the main reason why relatively few successfully prosecuted insulin murder cases can be found through a literature review. Despite these challenges, or perhaps because of them, forensic pharmacists must be alert to the possibility of murder by insulin.

Conclusion

It is often difficult to solve crimes caused by poisoning. Several factors contribute to this confusion:

- The symptoms displayed by the victim may be confused with the symptoms of a disease, delaying treatment of the poisoning.
- Even if poisoning is initially suspected, there are often very few clues as to the poison that has been used.
- Many poisons act slowly, giving the poisoner time to create an alibi to avoid suspicion.
- Poisoning by healthcare professionals is often done using professional knowledge of how to commit a crime without being detected.

All of these factors provide an incentive for those who are interested in forensic pharmacy to become more knowledgeable of the means through which crimes by poisoning are committed. Pharmacists must be more attentive to the possibility of poisonings as they perform their professional services, and they can participate actively in the investigation of potential poisonings. The frequency of poisonings through the use of drugs and other toxic substances as murder weapons creates an opportunity for pharmacists to become essentially involved in the analysis of an unexpected death.

Key Takeaways

- Consider the toxic doses of the medications that you dispense and monitor. Recognize the possibility that an overdose of medication may have caused the death of a patient whose death is otherwise unexplained. Many pharmaceutical murders are copycat murders. The perpetrators read about a crime that has been committed by another murderer, and they learn from the media how to use a particular medication, at a particular dose, and using a particular route of administration, to kill an unsuspecting victim. Be aware of the medications that have been used in the past to commit pharmaceutical homicide and be prepared to recognize the use of them by a copycat murderer.
- Think like a criminal. The pharmaceutical distribution system is set up to provide medications for those who need them. Pharmacists are medication providers; they are not medication deniers. From a therapeutic perspective, the pharmacist's goal is to develop systems that improve the distribution of medications. Criminals will appreciate that the system of drug distribution has specific openings to provide access to therapies that are necessary for patient care. These openings in the system can be exploited as leaks from the system by criminals who have dark motives. As you examine the system you use to distribute medications, particularly those medications that have been associated with past pharmaceutical homicides, ask yourself how a criminal might obtain a medication from the system to use as a

murder weapon. Then adopt system changes that reduce the probability of a criminal obtaining medication to use in the commission of a crime.

- Think like a jury member. Direct evidence is rarely found at the scene of a pharmaceutical homicide. Forensic ballistic testing can't be used on bullet fragments following a pharmaceutical homicide because there is no bullet. Likewise, there is no shell casing to test for DNA. There is no blood left behind by the perpetrator after a fight with the victim. Successful prosecutions of pharmaceutical homicide are based on circumstantial evidence. How much circumstantial evidence is enough? Where is the "tipping point" where the circumstantial evidence becomes convincing rather than simply suggestive? To answer these questions, put yourself in the position of a jury member who is considering whether there is a reasonable doubt as to the defendant's guilt. Don't stop gathering evidence until what you have gathered is sufficient to overcome a reasonable doubt in your mind if you were on a jury. Prosecutors want to spend their time on cases that can be successfully prosecuted. Do your best to provide the volume of evidence that a prosecutor would need to convince a jury of the perpetrator's guilt beyond a reasonable doubt.

References

1. Gummin DD, Mowry JB, Beuhler MC, Spyker DA, Rivers LJ, Feldman R, Brown K, Pham NPT, Bronstein AC, DesLauriers C. 2022 Annual Report of the National Poison Data System® (NPDS) from America's Poison Centers®: 40th Annual Report. *Clin Toxicol (Phila)*. 2023 Oct;61(10):717–939.

2. Shepherd G, Ferslew BC. Homicidal poisoning deaths in the United States 1999–2005. *Clin Toxicol (Phila).* 2009 Apr;47(4):342–347.

3. Muazzam S, Swahn MH, Alamgir H, Nasrullah M. Differences in poisoning mortality in the United States, 2003–2007: epidemiology of poisoning deaths classified as unintentional, suicide or homicide. *West J Emerg Med.* 2012 Aug;13(3):230–238.

4. Hanauer v. Doane, 79 U.S. 342 (1870).

5. January v. Peace, 738 S.W.2d 355 (Tex.App. 1987).

6. Carroll v. State, 7 N.E.2d 970 (Ind. 1937).

7. State v. Baldridge, 857 S.W.2d 243 (Mo.App. 1993)

8. Marks V. Murder by insulin: suspected, purported and proven-a review. *Drug Test Anal.* 2009 Apr;1(4):162–176.

9. Hannah v. State, 2008 WL 5689958 (Texas App. 2008).

Chapter 9

Family, Friends, and Betrayed Trust

There have been many recent media reports of horrifying random murders in public locations such as schools, movie theaters, nightclubs, concert venues, and other gathering places where victims have been gunned down by a person they did not know. The reality is that stranger homicide is very rare. Most victims are murdered by someone known to them. The initial investigation of most murders begins with a focus by detectives on the people who are, or have been, close to the victim. Until these "persons of interest" are eliminated as suspects, through a firm alibi, by forensic testing, or by other solid evidence, they are the focal point of investigative attention. The types of homicide that are committed within a family are classified by law enforcement and by academic scholars, using terms that are of Latin derivation.

Categorizing Familial Murder

Mariticide is a category of homicide that refers to the murder of one's spouse or of one's romantic partner. A subcategory of mariticide is uxoricide, which refers to the killing of a wife by a husband. Although some people limit their use of the word "mariticide" specifically to the act of a wife killing a husband, that term and concept technically apply to spouse either as the murderer or as the victim. There is technically no separate word that specifically describes the killing of a husband by a wife. Despite the lack of formal terminology to specifically describe a wife's murder of her husband, or a female murder of her male romantic partner, the slang phrase "Black Widow" has often been used by law enforcement with regard to a woman who kills her husband. A 1987 Hollywood movie called "Black Widow" tells the story of a woman who places penicillin in her husband's toothpaste, knowing of his penicillin allergy, and planning that the husband would have an acute hypersensitivity reaction from which he would die. After this movie came out, the US Food and Drug Administration (FDA) was concerned that copycat murderers might learn from the movie's plot how they could commit a murder using adulterated toothpaste. Toothpaste is one of only a few over-the-counter (OTC) products for which tamper-evident packaging is not required. In most circumstances, access to a person's toothpaste is limited to family members. There is no evidence that any copycat murders actually occurred.

It is important to distinguish the term "mariticide" from the very similar technical term, "matricide," which refers to the crime of murdering one's mother. To avoid confusing "mariticide" with "matricide," consider the difference in meaning between the English word "marital" (Latin form "maritalis") and the English word "mother" (Latin form "mater"). The crime of murdering one's father is referred to as "patricide." The crime of murdering a parent, or both parents, is referred to as "parricide." Aggregated data on murders of family members suggest that parricide is often a crime of passion committed on the spur of the moment. The weapon of choice is a firearm, or a sharp blade, or a blunt instrument, and not a medication. Pharmaceuticals are used much more frequently in the commission of mariticide than in the commission of matricide.

A Focus on Mariticide

Law enforcement authorities have become acutely aware of mariticide as a crime that can be prevented. Many preventable cases of mariticide were not thwarted in the past, due to a reluctance by law enforcement officers to interfere in what has historically been viewed as a family disagreement. Activist groups in the area of domestic violence prevention have successfully lobbied for changes in legislation, and changes in standard approaches to policing, that provide greater protection for those individuals who have been abused by a person to whom they are married or with whom they are in a romantic relationship. In many jurisdictions, there is no longer a requirement that a battered spouse press charges against the perpetrator as a requirement for the police to make an arrest. In these jurisdictions, police do not exercise discretion in the decision of whether to arrest an abusive spouse or a domestic partner. Any evidence of abuse, either physical or testimonial, will automatically result in the arrest of a suspected abuser or at least will result in a requirement that the abuser leave the abused partner alone for a period of time. Separating the parties who have participated in a violent dispute can de-escalate a confrontation that might otherwise result in a murder.

One of the most frequently used weapons in mariticide is a medication. People who have, or have had, strong passionate feelings for another person will often prefer to avoid using a murder weapon that causes obvious harm when that person is their murder victim. Even if love has been lost in a relationship, a level of respect or concern may linger, and a weapon that avoids bloodshed, physical disfigurement, and any other visible trauma may be easier for a murderer to justify using. A peaceful killing through a method where the victim "just goes to sleep," may result in less remorse for the killer than a violent approach that produces observable suffering. Killers may also believe that they have a greater chance of getting away with murder when they use pharmaceuticals to kill their partners, as opposed to firearms or knives or other murder weapons that are easier to detect. This explanation for the use of pharmaceuticals as murder weapons may seem irrational because victims of pharmaceutical homicides are no less dead than victims of other homicides, but there is nothing rational about murder.

Multiple Mariticides

Mariticide is usually not a serial crime. Although there are a small number of known cases in which a spouse has murdered multiple partners over a period of time, it is far more likely that mariticide is a one-time event. For this reason, it is difficult to prevent. Even pharmacists who are aware of the forensic nature of their responsibilities, and who make every effort in their practice to prevent pharmaceutical homicide, may face a huge challenge in the recognition and prevention of mariticide. Unlike the serial killers who regularly prey on vulnerable persons, and who leave a trail of murderous activity that can be tracked, leading to their discovery, one-time murderers are not trackable. A separate factor is the human tendency to stay away from other people's intrafamily matters and to keep out of other people's personal business. Despite having discovered evidence that a spouse may be intending to harm their partner with a medication, very few people will look forward to the experience of taking sides in a disagreement between spouses.

One striking example of mariticide as a serial crime is the case of William Archerd, who was accused in 1967 of murdering three of his wives, as well as the ex-husband of another wife, a nephew, and a friend.[1] According to the Supreme Court of California, in its affirmance of Archerd's conviction, each of the wives seemed to have deeply loved him, and the nephew and friend seemed to have trusted him. Each of the victims became an unwanted burden to Archerd, and each murder brought a financial gain for Archerd.

Archerd was charged with the murder of his three wives, and evidence of the other uncharged murders was provided to the jury to show a common plan or scheme. The murder weapon in each case was insulin, and all six victims died from hypoglycemia. Archerd had been employed many years earlier as an attendant on the insulin shock ward of a state mental hospital. Although insulin shock is now considered barbaric, it was used extensively in the 1940s through the early 1960s, when it was replaced by pharmacotherapy. The ward shock team on which Archerd served was comprised of two physicians, two registered nurses, and four attendants. The attendants were trained to administer injections of insulin, to observe danger signals while the patient was experiencing insulin shock, and to administer glucose to terminate the insulin shock.

Archerd's prosecution is the first known case of murder by insulin poisoning in the United States. To say that the science of insulin poisoning was in its infancy would be an understatement. The trial judge allowed fifteen experts to testify, including "treating physicians, autopsy surgeons, and experts in the fields of diabetes, hypoglycemia, pathology, insulin research, and insulin shock therapy." The trial judge was apparently overwhelmed with the complexity of the medical and scientific evidence.

Archerd was convicted on all three counts of first-degree murder. On each count, he received the death penalty. This penalty was later reduced to life in prison based on a ruling from the Supreme Court of the United States.

One of Archerd's key points in his appeal was based on interactions between the trial judge and "many men of the medical profession" with whom the judge had attended a social affair during the trial. Through conversations at this event, the judge was amazed to learn "how many men had been consulted by one side or the other." Although the judge insisted that he had learned nothing new from his casual conversations with these medical and scientific experts, the defense challenged the legitimacy of the guilty verdict, because defense lawyers had not been given the opportunity to interview or examine the judge or the attendees at the social function to determine the content of the interactions they may have had.

The Supreme Court of California "disapproved of the action by the trial judge in consulting experts outside of court," but the court did not find that this error in judgment by the trial judge was sufficient to overcome the huge weight of evidence supporting the conviction. The court noted that the "interviewing of potential witnesses anywhere but on the witness stand should be avoided." The conviction was affirmed, and Archerd died in prison seven years later. Subsequent review of the evidence presented against Archerd, using more refined and updated understanding of analytical techniques, suggests that the evidence may not have been as strong as it was thought to be at the time.[2] Being the first to be prosecuted for a particular type of pharmaceutical homicide brings with it the strong possibility that the scientific evidence will be misunderstood or misapplied.

Pharmacist's Traditional Gatekeeper Role

Pharmacists who accept the challenge to address mariticide prevention will face a daunting task. Yet pharmacists are in a position to rise to this challenge. Pharmaceutical homicides committed by a person with a healthcare background often rely on the superior knowledge of the perpetrator as opposed to the victim. There is a professional opportunity for pharmacists to alter the imbalance of information that exists between people who are trained in healthcare and those who lack healthcare training. The responsibility to protect innocent and trustful potential victims of poisoning is inherent in the pharmacy profession.

As gatekeepers of the nation's drug supply, pharmacists have traditionally served as a barrier to the acquisition of potentially lethal substances by those who would use them to harm other persons. The “poison log” that was maintained by pharmacists from colonial times through the 1950s served as evidence of who had acquired what poisonous substance, much as the record of methamphetamine precursors, is kept by pharmacists today. Most poison logs recorded the name and quantity of the poison that was purchased, the identity of the purchaser, and the purchaser’s intended use of the poison. The requirement for entry of purchases in a poison log did not apply to medications dispensed pursuant to a prescription, because the prescription retained on file at the pharmacy was deemed sufficient to serve as a record of a poison’s distribution. If suspicions arose about the use of poison as a murder weapon, then the police could visit area pharmacies to find out who had recently purchased the suspected poison. Purchasers who requested that pharmacists evade the regulatory requirements for the sale of poisons were rejected by pharmacists. The possibility of discovery through pharmacy poison log review served as a deterrent to the purchaser’s commission of a crime by means of poisoning.

Pharmacists also served the public as a source of information about the benefits and risks of medications. Prior to 1952, most nonnarcotic medications could be acquired either with a prescription or directly from a pharmacist without a prescription. From colonial times through the early 1900s, people might hear by word-of-mouth that a particular remedy had been used successfully by a friend or acquaintance for a particular condition. These people would consult a pharmacist about the utility for them of what they had heard through a friendly conversation. If a person consulting a pharmacist seemed overly interested in the toxic effects of a medication, then suspicions were aroused, and acquisition of the medication was denied.

Intentional Poisoning and Contemporary Pharmacy Practice

Many pharmacists have accepted a professional role in the management of poisoning, through a position on the staff of a poison control center. The primary objective of contemporary pharmacy practice is the effective treatment of poisoning to restore a patient’s health. Pharmacists are administratively responsible for poison centers in many areas, and the clinical advice they provide can facilitate the treatment of suspected poisoning. The aggregated data recorded and published by poison centers can establish trends in poisonings either locally or regionally, and from knowledge of these trends, poison prevention programs can be developed.

Pharmacist responsibilities have expanded far beyond the traditional role as custodian and guardian of poisonous substances to prevent their harmful use. Pharmacists today are in a position not only to control access to beneficial, yet potentially poisonous drugs. Pharmacists can also anticipate unauthorized and harmful misuse of drugs by those who have unlawful motives. Pharmacists continue to be the gatekeepers who protect patients from toxic drug effects.

The opportunities to cause harm to others from criminal drug use increase as the expanding complexity of drug therapy brings into the healthcare system new molecular entities with strict limitations on their use. These opportunities for harm justify requirements for extensive monitoring to promote effective and safe therapy. This is a pharmacy role. Pharmacists "own" the professional turf of medication safety.

Many adverse drug events are well recognized and cannot be prevented. They are sometimes viewed as simply an unfortunate, yet unavoidable by-product of effective drug therapy, based on the "no risk; no reward" philosophy. Criminals are in a position to exploit this view of inevitable harm by using medications to intentionally cause harm to others. Traditional poisons continue to be used in criminal activity, while a new generation of beneficial, yet also poisonous, pharmaceutical products has provided new weapons that must be monitored and restricted by vigilant pharmacists.

The Office of Justice Programs within the US Department of Justice conducted a study of homicidal poisonings and concluded that those at highest risk for being victims of poisoning are the terminally ill and mentally incapacitated, drug addicts, the elderly, and the very young.[3] The study also concluded that spouses or lovers with whom a murderer has become emotionally separated compose another high-risk group. According to the study, the murderers are often employed in the medical or caregiving fields. Finally, the study suggests some factors that indicate homicidal poisoning. These factors include sudden and unexpected death, the close connection of a victim with a caregiver who has been treating the victim for an illness, and the victim receiving medical treatment and being "nursed" back to health by the perpetrator but dying soon thereafter. Other factors include caregiver access to pharmaceuticals and isolation of the victim.

Legal case studies illustrate how the murder of family and friends with medications can occur within contemporary healthcare and pharmacy. Pharmacists who practice in a community setting are likely to understand the circumstances of their patients' lives and the extent of access to pharmaceutical products within their patients' homes. Based on this information, pharmacists can be in a unique position to understand the risks of pharmaceutical homicide within their community. Keep in mind that means, motive, and opportunity are the foundational keys to understanding a crime such as pharmaceutical homicide. In many cases of pharmaceutical homicide, the courage of one person to speak up about something peculiar that they saw or heard has facilitated an investigation that otherwise would have grown stagnant. The application of forensic principles to clinical expertise within a specific context can support the prevention, investigation, and prosecution of pharmaceutical homicide.

Money as Motive

Tami Duvall, a certified nurse's aide, was convicted of murdering her estranged husband.[4] She was sentenced to over sixty years in prison. She appealed her conviction. The basis of her appeal was the admission into evidence of testimony regarding a missing bottle of oral liquid morphine from the care facility where she worked. Duvall contended that the allegation of her having stolen the morphine was "tenuous at best," because the morphine had been documented by the facility as having been spilled, and the facility could not prove where it went.

Duvall placed a 9-1-1 call and told the dispatcher that she had found her estranged husband dead in the back yard. According to Duvall, the husband had come over to her house the prior evening to work on a malfunctioning air conditioner, he then became overheated, and he went outside, where he slept overnight.

It was initially believed that the husband, who had a blood alcohol level of 0.436%, had died of alcohol poisoning. However, toxicology reports revealed that the husband's blood had a morphine concentration of 6,590 ng/mL (approximately 100 times the therapeutic level) and a cyclobenzaprine concentration of 2,229 ng/mL (approximately eight times the therapeutic level). A pathologist concluded that the cause of death was an overdose of morphine.

An investigation revealed that the couple, who had been separated for several months, had significant financial problems. A short time before the husband's death, Duvall had encourage him to obtain a US$100,000 life insurance policy naming her as the beneficiary. The husband agreed to do this because he thought it was mortgage insurance and he expected to reconcile with Duvall and move back home. The policy was issued by an insurance agent with whom Duvall was having an affair.

A charge nurse testified at trial that he had been working with Duvall several months prior to the husband's death, when he had absent-mindedly left a nearly full bottle of liquid morphine on a hospice patient's bedside table. When he went to retrieve the bottle shortly thereafter, Duvall was the only staff member present, and the bottle was missing. When questioned by the charge nurse, Duvall responded that she had not seen the bottle but that the patient's daughter had been in the room. According to the charge nurse, he "kind of knew better" because the daughter was a teacher, and she never visited her mother during the daytime. The prosecution used this testimony as evidence that Duvall had access to the murder weapon. In her appeal, Duvall challenged this testimony as speculative and inadmissible.

The appellate court concluded: "The value of evidence that Duvall had access to the murder weapon, a rare form of morphine typically used for palliative care for dying patients, was high. Moreover, the access had been in recent proximity to the husband's death. The admission of such evidence was not unfairly prejudicial." The conviction was affirmed.

This case illustrates the importance of demonstrating access by an alleged perpetrator to the medication that was used as a murder weapon. Any sort of recollection regarding the availability of a medication to an alleged perpetrator, within a logical time frame, may be considered as relevant in a murder prosecution.

Broken Relationship as Motive

Nurse Stephanie Stephens was convicted of murdering her surgeon husband.[5] She was sentenced to life in prison. She appealed, contending that the trial court should have granted her motion to dismiss the case due to the prosecution's failure to prove all of the essential elements of the crime charged beyond a reasonable doubt. She argued that sufficient credible evidence existed to prove that her husband, who suffered from end-stage liver disease, had committed suicide.

Shortly after Stephens and her husband were married, the husband suffered a stroke that resulted in his partial loss of eyesight. He was no longer able to perform surgery. He was also diagnosed with diabetes. He began to draw disability benefits, and he was given a part-time work at the hospital where he had previously been a prominent heart surgeon. His monthly income dropped from US$50,000 to US$6,000.

Stephens reportedly awoke one morning to find her husband lifeless in bed. The initial conclusion was that the husband had died from natural causes related to his end-stage liver disease. The coroner saw no indication of foul play other than the possibility that the husband's insulin pump had malfunctioned. The coroner drew two vials of blood from the husband's body and sent them to the crime lab. The lab report revealed that the blood sample contained etomidate and a metabolite of the paralytic drug atracurium. The cause of death was determined to be an overdose of these drugs. Based on this information, Stephens was arrested.

During the trial, one of Stephens' friends testified that Stephens admitted to her that the husband wanted to die and that he had requested Stephens's help. Stephens told the witness that she had injected the husband with "two sedatives and a heart medication." Stephens argued on appeal that this testimony did not prove that she had murdered her husband.

The appellate court noted that when a defendant confesses to a crime, the confession itself is not sufficient to support a felony conviction unless it is corroborated by independent evidence. The court then noted that there had been sufficient independent evidentiary proof offered at trial. The evidence revealed that Stephens had the opportunity, ability, knowledge, and motive to commit murder. She was alone with the husband in a locked bedroom when he died.

The crime lab report revealed the presence of drugs that are intended to induce anesthesia and to which Stephens had access during her previous employment as a nurse. She possessed knowledge of the drugs as well as the workings of her husband's insulin pump.

There was also evidence that the husband had a deferred compensation account valued at US$732,000 and that he was planning to leave Stephens.

In her defense, Stephens offered the testimony of a forensic psychiatrist who had reviewed the husband's medical, personal, and work history. The forensic psychiatrist concluded that, due to the husband's personal history and health problems, he was "definitely a candidate for suicide." The prosecutor presented contrary evidence from members of the husband's family that he was upbeat before his death and that he anticipated receiving a liver transplant.

The appellate court concluded that the prosecution had adequately established the crime of murder. The murder conviction was affirmed. The presence outside a healthcare setting, of drugs that would never legally be found other than in a healthcare setting, and to which the alleged perpetrator had access, was seen as critical to the conviction.

Burden as Motive

Katherine Dendel, an insulin-dependent diabetic, was convicted of second-degree murder for injecting her live-in partner with a lethal dose of insulin.[6] Dendel and her partner were in a long-term relationship. The partner had been taking numerous medications for serious illnesses, including HIV, herpes, hepatitis B and C, epilepsy, ataxia, neuropathy, chronic obstructive pulmonary disease, severely impaired vision, dementia, lymphoma, and throat cancer. He was not diabetic.

The partner was a challenging person to care for, and Dendel was solely responsible for making sure that he used his medications appropriately and for tending to his everyday needs. One week before the partner's death, feeling frustrated with the partner's demands, Dendel told the partner's sister, "I can't take this," and "I feel like giving him a shot of insulin."

Dendel also expressed her frustration to a person employed by a family support agency. That employee told Dendel that she should have her partner evaluated at a mental health facility or have him placed in respite or hospice care. Dendel then requested help from the local agency on aging, but the request was denied because both she and her partner were under sixty years old.

On the day before the partner's death, a visiting nurse who had been helping Dendel care for her partner terminated her services because the partner had been uncooperative. Dendel told the nurse that she did not know how long she could continue caring for the partner by herself.

At 3:00 am on the day of the partner's death, Dendel called 9-1-1 to report that the partner had been hallucinating and running around with a knife. Dendel asked the police to take the partner to a mental institution, as had been recommended to her by the family support agency employee. When the police arrived, the partner was sitting calmly in a chair. He told the officers that he was fine and that there was no problem. The police determined that the partner was not a threat to himself or others, so they left and took no further action.

Later that day, Dendel said that she discovered the partner slumped over on a couch and unresponsive. Dendel called a friend who called the police. While the police and emergency personnel were removing the partner's body from the house, the partner's sister telephoned Dendel, who quickly ended the conversation without telling the sister that her brother had just died.

Dendel requested that the partner's body be cremated without an autopsy, but an autopsy was performed despite her wishes. When a detective incorrectly told Dendel that the medical examiner had detected insulin in the partner's tissues, Dendel called him a liar and explained to him that insulin cannot be detected in the human body after death because it breaks down and depletes naturally.

After she was arrested, Dendel told detectives that her partner had injected himself with insulin and that he had talked about suicide for many years. At trial, Dendel instructed her defense attorney to pursue the suicide theory. The prosecution presented expert testimony that, despite the lab results showing the partner's insulin and C-peptide levels were normal, the complete lack of glucose in the samples taken from the partner confirmed that the death was due to hypoglycemic shock from an overdose of exogenous insulin. The defense attorney did not retain an expert to refute this testimony, because, under the suicide theory, the issue was not what had caused the partner's death but who had caused it.

In appealing the jury's verdict of second-degree murder, Dendel argued that it was a reversible error for her attorney not to have retained an expert witness on her behalf. The court of appeals agreed and reversed the conviction. From this ruling the prosecution appealed to the state supreme court, where the ruling by the court of appeals was reversed and the conviction was reinstated.

The state supreme court noted that the primary evidence in the case had been circumstantial and that this considerable circumstantial evidence was sufficient to support the conviction. Any expert testimony that might have been offered by the defense attorney to refute the testimony that exogenous insulin was the cause of the partner's death would have been irrelevant, because an insulin overdose was consistent with the defense of suicide on which Dendel had insisted her attorney rely.

The story was not over. Dendel filed a writ of habeas corpus in federal court. Once again, she argued that her attorney had provided her with an ineffective defense by failing to fully investigate the cause of her partner's death, through expert analysis of evidence and trial testimony. Eight years after her conviction was affirmed by the state supreme court, and after Dendel had fully served her prison sentence, a federal court of appeals granted her petition for a writ of habeas corpus, setting the stage for a new trial.[7] Because Dendel had completed her term in prison, the prosecutor saw no point in conducting a new trial.

Revenge as Motive

Vicki Jensen appealed her fixed life sentence (no possibility of parole) that was imposed following her plea of guilty to first-degree murder.[8] She contended that the sentence was unreasonably harsh and that the district court had abused its discretion by imposing such a harsh sentence.

The facts of the case revealed that Jensen's husband had left her and had moved into an apartment with another woman. Jensen was distraught, and she was obsessed with winning her husband back. Using her knowledge and experience as a registered nurse, Jensen devised a plan to kill the woman by injecting her with a lethal dose of insulin. She enlisted the help of her niece and her niece's boyfriend to carry out the plan.

Jensen and her accomplices entered the victim's apartment after the husband had left for work. While one of her accomplices restrained the victim, Jensen injected a lethal dose of insulin into the victim's arm. To make it appear as though the victim died of a drug overdose, Jensen also injected the victim with methamphetamine, and she placed methamphetamine in the victim's purse. The court noted that "as a registered nurse, Jensen knew that injecting the victim with insulin when the victim did not need it would be fatal and virtually undetectable."

After several months of investigation, Jensen was arrested and was charged with first-degree murder. The state filed a notice of intent to seek the death penalty. Pursuant to a plea agreement, Jensen pled guilty to first-degree murder, and the state withdrew its notice of intent to seek the death penalty. The imposition of the determinate life sentence was then imposed, and Jensen's appeal followed.

On appeal, the court first considered factors related to Jensen and her actions. The evidence showed that two years prior to the murder for which she had been convicted, Jensen had threatened to kill her husband's first wife by injecting her with insulin.

Other evidence showed that after killing the woman for whom her husband had left her, Jensen had stalked her husband and another female friend of the husband, threatening to harm them. Although a neuropsychological examination determined that Jensen was unlikely to reoffend, the court concluded that the egregious nature of Jensen's crime, coupled with her conduct before and after the murder, justified a determinate life sentence.

The court also considered the need for the protection of the public as justification for the harsh sentence. The court noted that the gravity of the offense, as shown by the circumstances, was sufficient to justify a significant measure of retribution and deterrence. The court concluded that "given Jensen's escalating pattern of violence, society must be protected from her." The district court's indeterminate sentence of life imprisonment without possibility of parole was affirmed on appeal.

Addressing Pharmaceutical Homicide in the Community Setting

Proof of motive is an essential element in the prosecution of a single event of pharmaceutical homicide that has allegedly occurred outside an institutional healthcare setting. When multiple murders have occurred within a healthcare institution, the facts are often so incriminating that the need to determine a motive is secondary to the development of scientific and circumstantial evidence that a crime has been committed and by whom the crime was committed. Pharmacists can play an integral role in healthcare institution investigations.

It is more difficult to know the extent to which pharmacists can perform professional functions to facilitate the prevention, investigation, and prosecution of pharmaceutical homicide in the community setting. The extent of the problem is unknown, and solutions are elusive in the absence of problem definition. A continued commitment to promoting positive outcomes from drug therapy is a fundamental role for pharmacists, and this commitment can contribute to the reduction of incidents of pharmaceutical homicide.

The acquisition of medication is a privilege, and not a right. Under most circumstances, patients have the right to refuse medications, but they do not have the right to demand medications. If a prescriber or a pharmacist is concerned about potential harm to a patient, or to another person who could be harmed by a medication, then the standard of care will support refusal to prescribe and/or dispense the medication. At the very least, a prescriber or a pharmacist will insist that the patient should listen to important information about a medication and agree to use the medication as it has been prescribed.

The reporting of adverse drug effects (ADEs) is an important means through which pharmacists can contribute to the body of knowledge concerning possible pharmaceutical homicide in the community setting. The formal program for communication about ADEs from pharmacists to the FDA is called MedWatch. Pharmacists are not required to participate in MedWatch. They voluntarily submit reports out of a sense of professional responsibility. Among healthcare professionals, pharmacists are the most frequent reporters of ADEs through the MedWatch system. The agency assigns pharmacy staff to review MedWatch reports and to detect potentially problematic trends from the data submitted. MedWatch is a system run by pharmacists to promote patient safety.

The intentional poisoning of a person with a drug is clearly a reportable ADE. It should be reported to the FDA through MedWatch and to the product sponsor (manufacturer) for inclusion in an Alert Report made to the FDA by the sponsor.

Patient confidentiality should not stand in the way of reporting suspicious activities. Pharmacists and other health professionals are understandably respectful of patient privacy, and this respect is codified in a very familiar federal law, the Health Insurance Portability and Accountability Act (commonly referred to as HIPAA). The general rule under the HIPAA is that protected health information (PHI) must be maintained as confidential. The HIPAA rules designate how and with whom PHI may be shared by covered entities that maintain PHI on record.

Recognizing that there may be a need to share PHI with law enforcement, the HIPAA rules specifically allow reporting to a law enforcement official any PHI that the covered entity believes is necessary to alert law enforcement to the death of a covered individual when there is a suspicion that death resulted from criminal conduct. Reports of PHI to law enforcement are allowed under the HIPAA to prevent or lessen a serious and an imminent threat to the health or safety of an individual or the public. The HIPAA confidentiality requirements do not stand in the way of contacting law enforcement when a pharmacist or other health professional has a reason to believe that a pharmaceutical homicide is being planned or has already occurred.

Discerning Patterns of Homicide

Circumstantial evidence is key to the investigation and prosecution of pharmaceutical homicide. Scientific evidence is necessary, but it may not be sufficient. The possibility of recognizing trends in criminal behavior, by looking for situational anomalies and considering the implications of them, can lead to knowledge that otherwise might not be discovered. Those who seek information may find it. Those who choose not to look will not see it.

Official court reports and media coverage of pharmaceutical homicide in the community setting can provide background information that pharmacists and other healthcare professionals may find useful in recognizing incongruities with what one might expect in the use of medications. The similarities in these stories suggest that homicidal patterns may exist, and the trends may be worthy of recognition. A review of several such potential trends can provide a framework for the evaluation of homicidal patterns.

Pharmaceutical Product Tampering Homicides

A pharmaceutical product may serve as the vehicle through which a homicide is committed by removing the therapeutic contents of the product and replacing the contents with a lethal poison. The Chicago Tylenol tampering murders were widely publicized when they occurred in 1982. Seven victims died from ingesting Extra Strength Tylenol capsules that had been adulterated with cyanide and had then been returned to retail store shelving from which they were selected and purchased by customers who were unaware of the potentially fatal nature of the adulterated product's content. The murderer was never caught. In response to this tragedy, the FDA promulgates rules that require most OTC products to be packaged in containers with tamper-resistant or tamper-evident features.[9] Federal law now provides that any person who tampers with a consumer product and places another person in danger of death or bodily injury shall be fined or imprisoned for any term of years or for life, or both, if the death of an individual results.[10] The imposition of new packaging requirements and the threat of severe penalties have not prevented homicides from pharmaceutical product tampering.

Joseph Meling, of Olympia Washington, took out several hundred thousand dollars in life insurance on his wife, and he stood to collect US$700,000 if his wife happened to die an accidental death.[11] The day after the coverage became effective, he fed his wife a capsule of Sudafed 12-hour cold capsules that was laced with cyanide. The wife recovered but Meling worried that he might be suspected of the poisoning. He laced five packages of the Sudafed product with cyanide and planted them on pharmacy shelves, killing two people before the manufacturer could institute a national recall of the product. Meling's goal was to divert attention from himself as the poisoner. He contended that his wife had purchased cyanide-laced Sudafed from the pharmacy.

Meling soon became the central focus of the Federal Bureau of Investigation (FBI) investigation of the two deaths. He was convicted of six counts of product tampering, one count of causing serious bodily damage to his wife, two counts of causing the deaths, and three counts of planting packages of Sudafed that were recovered unopened. He was sentenced to life in prison. Meling appealed his conviction, challenging the evidence and contending that the punishment was too harsh.

In affirming the conviction, the appellate court said, "Meling knowingly killed two people. Callously disregarding the suffering he might inflict, Meling had the basest of motives: He wanted to divert attention from his heinous attempt to kill his wife for profit. Acting without compassion, Meling calculated that a few random deaths would throw the FBI off his trail. To this end, he laced five packages of Sudafed with poison, intending that they be ingested by unsuspecting victims, and knowing that these victims would die horrible deaths. The only detail missing from Meling's calculus was the identity of the people he would kill. That he was unaware of the victims' identities, however, does not make his conduct any less culpable. Meling was aware to a practical certainty that someone—perhaps as many as five people—would die to help save his skin. Nor does the victims' anonymity make his crime any less gruesome. If anything, the randomness of the act only renders it more cruel." The conviction was affirmed.

Perhaps not so coincidentally, Meling's modus operandi had been utilized seven years before by Stella Nickell, from the nearby city of Seattle.[12] Nickell was accused of killing her husband by putting cyanide in an Excedrin capsule that the husband later took for a headache. The husband died, but the cause of death was listed as emphysema and not as cyanide poisoning. This determination caused a problem for Nickell, because her life insurance payout would be reduced by US$100,000 if the husband's death was not ruled an accident.

Nickell then adulterated five additional bottles of Excedrin and she placed them on store shelves in the Seattle area. Six days later, a woman took one of the poisonous capsules and she died. Nickell notified police that she thought her husband had also been poisoned by Excedrin that was contaminated with cyanide. Although the police were suspicious of this claim, they lacked solid evidence that Nickell had killed her husband as well as the second victim. The case was widely publicized in the media, and a reward was offered for any information leading to a conviction of the murderer. At this point, Nickell's daughter contacted the police and told them that her mother had been planning to murder her husband and that she had remarked about how the Tylenol murders demonstrated an effective method for murder.

Nickell was convicted of five counts of tampering with an OTC product and two counts of product tampering that resulted in deaths. She was sentenced to serve two 90-year terms in prison for the deaths of her husband and the woman who died from using the adulterated Excedrin.

There have been many reports of copycat murders that followed the plan of the unknown Chicago Tylenol murderer.[13] A lawsuit in New York challenged the adequacy of measures taken by a retailer and a manufacturer following the death in 1986 of a woman due to her ingesting cyanide-laced Tylenol capsules that were purchased for her by a friend. The capsules were packaged in conformance with federal tamper-resistant standards. The lawsuit alleged that compliance with these federal standards was insufficient to meet legal responsibilities.

The legal representative of the victim's estate contended that the retailer should be held liable for negligence because the retailer should have recognized the danger of placing the product on open shelving and should have instead required that the product be placed in a "behind the counter" area where it could be safeguarded from contamination. The court disagreed. The court said, "Short of eliminating over-the-counter shopping, no practical, feasible, affordable way of ensuring against this kind of tampering has been suggested by the parties or imagined by the court." The court ruled that to hold that a retailer has a duty in this regard is "illogical, undermines sound notions of public policy, and contorts all principles of justice."

The lawsuit also alleged that the manufacturer should be held legally liable for continuing to formulate the product in gelatin capsules as opposed to tablets or caplets. The court disagreed with this allegation. The court first noted an FDA statement that tablets and caplets are less susceptible to tampering, but they are not tamper-proof, and that known methods of tampering are simply more difficult to apply. The court concluded that the plaintiff could not demonstrate that had the manufacturer eliminated gelatin capsules the criminals would not be able to commit crimes with poisoned tablets or caplets.

The case against the retailer and the manufacturer was dismissed.

Pharmaceutical product tampering homicides do not all follow the formula of the Chicago Tylenol tampering tragedy.

Former Ohio physician Yazeed Essa was convicted of one count of aggravated murder in the death of his wife from cyanide poisoning.[14] His wife took a calcium capsule laced with cyanide, given to her by the Essa just before she left the house to run an errand. Shortly thereafter she was involved in an automobile accident. She had been observed driving erratically. She was pronounced dead at the hospital, although there were no signs of trauma.

An autopsy was conducted, and the initial toxicology report did not reveal any unusual substances in the wife's tissues.

Based on evidence that the wife had been given a calcium capsule by Essa, a search was conducted of the house, and the search revealed cyanide contamination in the wife's medications. A more elaborate test for cyanide was conducted on the wife's tissues, and a determination was made that the wife had died of acute cyanide intoxication.

Essa was an expert on cyanide poisoning and had "given courses at a hospital addressing the subject." He also had access to cyanide through his well-documented connections to the jewelry industry. There was evidence that Essa was having an affair and that his wife had recently confronted him about it.

Essa was sentenced to life in prison with parole eligibility after twenty years. From his conviction and sentencing, Essa appealed. On appeal, the court concluded that the state had presented "competent, credible evidence" that the defendant had "purposely, and with prior calculation and design," caused the death of his wife. Essa's conviction was affirmed.

Fetal Homicides

Regardless of one's perspective on the legality or morality of elective abortions, it is both heartbreaking and maddening that pharmaceuticals would be used criminally by one person to involuntarily end another person's pregnancy. The legality and availability of abortifacient drugs creates an opportunity for these drugs to be used unlawfully. The most common type of pharmaceutical abortion uses the drugs mifepristone and misoprostol sequentially. There is also a misoprostol-only regimen that is less frequently used. In a 9-0 unanimous ruling, the Supreme Court of the United States rejected a challenge to the FDA's determination that mifepristone is a safe and highly effective means of pregnancy termination.[15] As is the case with every other drug, pharmacists and pharmacies have a responsibility to provide access to abortifacient drugs only when the intended use of the drug is lawful.

A lawsuit in Texas challenged the decision by a hospital pharmacist to honor a resident physician's prescription for dinoprostone (a pharmaceutical cousin of misoprostol).[16] The lawsuit was initiated by the resident's former girlfriend, to whom the resident had secretly administered the drug, resulting in an unwanted abortion. The facts showed that the resident contacted a pharmacist at the hospital's inpatient pharmacy, asking about the availability of the drug. The pharmacist indicated that the drug was in stock. Shortly thereafter, the resident went to the pharmacy and wrote a prescription for the drug, without writing a patient's name on the prescription. The pharmacist called this omission to the resident's attention, and the resident said to use his own name as that of the patient.

The trial court dismissed the woman's case against the hospital because the hospital was a subdivision of the State of Texas. The lower court ruled that the hospital was shielded from litigation by sovereign governmental immunity under the Texas Tort Claims Act. The appellate court disagreed, noting that the law acknowledges an exception from governmental immunity for injuries caused by the use of tangible personal property. The court concluded that "the dispensing of a drug by a hospital pharmacy is a use of tangible personal property and falls within the waiver provision of the statute." This ruling permitted the woman's negligence lawsuit against the hospital to proceed.

The appellate court also ruled that the injury to the former girlfriend was foreseeable to the hospital pharmacist. The court relied on an explanation by the hospital's medical residency director who testified that a resident physician is not allowed to write prescriptions for anyone outside the hospital, including family members. The residency director testified that "anyone working in the pharmacy would be aware of this restriction, and the pharmacy department advises residents of this restriction during their portion of the orientation."

Moreover, the court reasoned that the pharmacist should have foreseen that an injury such as the injury alleged in this case could occur, because the resident was a male prescribing a female hormone either for himself or for an undisclosed person. Yet the pharmacist did not inquire whether the drug was for a hospitalized patient and did not ask why the resident needed it.

The dismissal of the woman's lawsuit was reversed, and the case against the hospital was reinstated. There is no public record of its resolution, likely meaning that it was settled out of court. There is no public record of any criminal prosecution of the resident physician.

John Andrew Weldon of Tampa, Florida, was sentenced to thirteen years and eight months in prison for tampering with a consumer product, resulting in the termination of his then girlfriend's pregnancy.[17] In a lawsuit filed by the girlfriend, the allegations stated that Weldon had stolen a prescription blank from his father's medical practice and had forged a prescription for misoprostol, which was filled for him at a community pharmacy. A technician allegedly agreed to omit the name of the drug from the label, and Weldon later labeled the medication as amoxicillin. The girlfriend used the misoprostol, believing it to be amoxicillin. As a consequence of using the misoprostol, the girlfriend miscarried. The outcome of the girlfriend's lawsuit is unknown, although the court ruled that the pharmacy's premises liability insurance company had a duty to defend the lawsuit.[18]

Mason Herring of Houston, Texas, entered a plea of guilty to causing injury to a child and assault on a pregnant person.[19] Evidence showed that Herring had mixed misoprostol in his wife's drink. Hidden cameras in the couple's home showed Herring mixing a substance into one of the wife's beverages. Herring was sentenced to 180 days in jail and ten years in prison. The wife filed for divorce. Their child was ten weeks premature with developmental delays. The wife's brother was a state senator in Louisiana, and his experience with this crime committed by Herring led the state senator to introduce a bill intended to classify mifepristone and misoprostol as Schedule IV controlled substances in Louisiana.[20] The bill was passed and has become law.

Scott Bollig of WaKeeney, Kansas, was found guilty of conspiring to commit intentional first-degree murder as a principal in a plot to terminate his then girlfriend's pregnancy by secretly causing her to ingest mifepristone and misoprostol.[21] He was sentenced to just under ten years in prison. Bollig told investigators that he had purchased the medication on the Internet pursuant to advice from a nurse with whom he had a "romantic involvement" and that he laced pancakes with the drugs, which he then served to his victim. At trial, Bollig changed his story, and he testified that the girlfriend wanted to end the pregnancy, so she put the drugs in the pancakes herself and voluntarily ate the pancakes. On appeal of his conviction, the court was incredulous, asking "Why would Bollig's girlfriend opt for a medication abortion after she had adamantly rejected that idea when she and Bollig weighed terminating the pregnancy? Why would she have had Bollig obtain drugs for the medication abortion rather than asking her physician? Why wouldn't she simply take the medications with a sip of water rather than going through some odd ritual with the pancakes?" The conviction was affirmed.

Manishkumar Patel of Appleton, Wisconsin, was convicted of attempted first-degree homicide of an unborn child.[22] Patel placed mifepristone in his girlfriend's smoothie, resulting in two miscarriages. He was sentenced to twenty-one years in prison. The trial judge characterized Patel's actions as despicable and noted that the lengthy sentence was based on the seriousness of the offenses rather than on the protection of the public. Patel appealed the sentence as overly harsh. The appellate court determined that the lengthy sentence was rationally justified by the trial judge and that it was based on relevant sentencing factors. The appeal was denied.

Eye Drops Homicides

As attractive as pharmaceutical products may be for criminals with murderous intent, the delivery of an overdose is a challenge with most dosage forms. Solid oral dosage forms are difficult to administer to a victim without the victim knowing, because it requires some sort of subterfuge that can raise suspicions for the victim. Rectal and vaginal suppositories raise even greater challenges. Injections require expertise, and they leave evidence that is easily detected in an autopsy. Oral liquids are designed to be therapeutic in normal quantities and can reach toxic levels only when suspicious volumes are ingested. The search for the perfect dosage form for homicide may be trending toward ophthalmic drops that contain concentrated strengths of drugs. Ophthalmic drops permit the addition of a high oral dosage of a drug to a liquid beverage that can be offered to a victim without raising concerns.

The use of atropine eye drops as a murder weapon has been reported.[23] The possibility of atropine eye drops being the murderer's long-sought "perfect weapon" has been suggested.[24] A major problem with atropine eye drops as a murder weapon is that they require a prescription, and a prescription leaves a trail of evidence from a pharmacy to a perpetrator. Using an OTC eye drop has significant advantages for pharmaceutical homicide, because no evidence of acquisition is available.

Tetrahydrozoline (THZ) is the active ingredient in several OTC ophthalmic products. The cardiotoxic effects of THZ from oral ingestion have been understood for many years.[25] Yet the criminal use of THZ as a murder weapon

A nurse who had worked with the defendant nurse at an Oregon rehabilitation hospital testified about an incident that occurred when she arrived at 6:30 a.m. one morning as the defendant nurse was completing her night shift. The defendant nurse had instructed the testifying nurse "in an unusually adamant fashion" not to enter an elderly patient's room to check on her because the patient "had had a rough night." The testifying nurse found this instruction odd, and she ignored it. The defendant nurse followed the testifying nurse into the patient's room and insisted that the testifying nurse "verify the insulin amount that she had administered to the patient." The testifying nurse found this also to be odd behavior.

The nursing supervisor at the Oregon hospital testified that at 9:00 a.m. on that day, she found the patient unconscious and with a very low blood sugar level of 13. She testified that just two hours before the patient's blood sugar level had been measured at 100. The patient died later that day.

This patient appeared to have signed a DNR order, but an expert in forensic document examination testified he did not believe the order had been signed by the patient. Rather, he indicated it was likely that the defendant nurse had signed the patient's name to the order.

The patient's daughter testified that after her mother's death, a diamond ring was missing from her finger. Nurses and others who had cared for the patient remembered the ring but did not know what happened to it. The nursing supervisor announced that she would be launching an investigation into the missing ring. Two days later, the ring was placed in the supervisor's office mailbox. It had been left anonymously in an envelope. No charges were filed over this incident.

Shortly after the Oregon incident occurred, the defendant nurse moved to Texas. She was initially employed at a hospital. The hospital director testified that the defendant nurse had "access to the hospital's insulin cache" while she worked there and that over 70% of the hospital's patients received regular insulin injections. The hospital director testified that the insulin was stored in a locked refrigerator and that the defendant nurse had a key to the refrigerator. There was no accounting system for the insulin in the refrigerator, and if someone stole insulin then it would be impossible to know.

The defendant nurse left the hospital due to a work-related injury and immediately began working for the home health agency that assigned her to care for the patient whom she was alleged to have murdered.

The defendant nurse pursued two defense strategies at trial. First, she questioned whether an insulin overdose was the actual cause of the patient's clocked out of work at 3:23 p.m. to go on a shopping errand and had returned to work at 4:20 p.m.

The call from the son-in-law to the daughter was made at 5:43 p.m. The daughter rushed home and sat with her mother for about forty minutes. She grew concerned that her mother's condition was deteriorating, and she called for an ambulance at 6:26 pm. The ambulance crew conducted blood draws and determined that the patient was suffering from unusually low blood glucose levels. At the hospital, the patient's glucose levels fluctuated for the next twenty-four hours, and the medical personnel could not determine the cause of the instability. The patient died the following evening. The attending physician listed secondary adrenal insufficiency as the cause of death.

After the patient died, the daughter reviewed her mother's bank accounts, and she discovered that the defendant nurse had stolen thousands of dollars from the patient. The daughter testified that her suspicions were "overwhelming" at this point. She asked a physician colleague at the hospital to examine the results of a C-peptide test that had been conducted at the hospital. The results of this test had not been reported by the laboratory until after the patient's funeral. The physician indicated to the daughter that the patient had a massive excess of insulin in her body when she was admitted to the hospital. The C-peptide test conclusively ruled out both pancreatic cancer and endogenous hyperinsulinism. The physician told the daughter, and later testified in court, that although he could not determine how much or what type of insulin had been injected, it was clear that the amount was vastly greater than would be necessary to treat any patient, even a patient with diabetes.

These opinions were echoed by an endocrinologist who examined the patient's insulin levels before her death and observed that the patient had an insulin level of 400, well above the normal level of around 27. The attending physician then amended the patient's death certificate, listing the cause of death as "exogenous insulin overdose."

The daughter notified local police. By this time, the patient had been cremated. Based on circumstantial evidence, the defendant nurse was arrested and indicted for murder.

The Trial

At her trial, certain aspects of the nurse's work history were entered into evidence, despite the objections of her attorney, who claimed that this historical evidence was irrelevant to the recent death of the patient. The evidence showed that the nurse had changed jobs frequently and that she had used different names at different jobs.

pharmacist had reported the unusual succinylcholine crash cart replacements to a pharmacy supervisor? What if the two supervisors had met to discuss the two reports that were made to them, and at the meeting they had concluded that the husband's conduct should be closely examined? Might the wife's life have been saved? This is an impossible question to answer, yet it is a question that can provide incentives for hospital personnel to think critically when something unusual happens and to consult with others at the hospital to consider whether a problematic situation may exist.

Case Study: Spurned Suiter Commits Murder

A Florida nurse killed a woman who resisted his affections.[6] The murder weapon was the anesthetic drug propofol that had been stolen by the nurse, along with midazolam and etomidate, from the hospital where the nurse worked. The nurse almost committed the perfect crime. His victim was found deceased in her apartment with no obvious indication of foul play. She had been dead for two days. The medical examiner discovered a tiny injury on the victim's arm. The injury looked like it could have been caused by a drug injection, if a trained person had administered the drug.

Interviews of the victim's friends disclosed that the nurse was infatuated with the victim, despite the victim having recently announced her engagement to another person. There was evidence that the nurse had overheard the victim refer to him as "an annoying little man." Telephone records indicated that the nurse had called the victim several times each day for nine days prior to her death, but the calls ended on the day of the victim's death.

The crime scene investigators noticed that a trashcan in the victim's apartment was clean and empty. They went out to the apartment complex dumpster, but it had just been emptied by a trash truck. An investigator noticed that some material was stuck to the bottom of the otherwise empty dumpster, and that material turned out to be some mail belonging to the victim, along with two empty medication vials labeled as propofol, and an injection needle cap. Later investigation disclosed that the nurse had procured two vials of propofol from a hospital automated dispensing unit, with no accounting of their use in the hospital. The nurse's DNA was found on the needle cap. The investigators theorized that the victim, who suffered from migraines, had trusted the nurse to inject her with what she thought would be an effective treatment for migraines.

A first-degree murder warrant was issued for the nurse, but the nurse had fled to Ireland. Extradition from Ireland to the United States is very complicated, if not impossible, when a capital crime has been charged. The nurse was difficult to locate in Ireland until he applied for a nursing license there and gave his attending physician of her previous bizarre and scary conversation with the husband. The nurse colleague told the wife's attending physician to order a succinylcholine level. The hospital staff obtained a urine sample. The wife died shortly after.

The antemortem urine sample was positive for both succinylcholine and succinylmonocholine, a metabolite of succinylcholine. Postmortem tissue samples tested negative. Hospital personnel had not used any succinylcholine in their treatment of the wife.

The evidence offered by the prosecution at the husband's trial focused on the positive laboratory test for succinylcholine and the nurse colleague's testimony about her conversation with the husband. Testimony by a representative of the pharmacy department confirmed the husband's access to succinylcholine in the hospital, and he explained how the shortage of succinylcholine had occurred in crash carts located in areas of the hospital where the husband worked.

It was never determined how the husband had injected the wife with succinylcholine. A forensic pathologist was not able to determine whether a tissue sample that appeared to be a puncture wound was the site of a succinylcholine injection. The pathologist testified that an experienced nurse could administer an injection without "a resulting bruise or large bloody track underneath the skin." The absence of any discernable injection site led to speculation that the wife was too trusting of the husband's ability to provide her with safe medications that would be of benefit to her. If a struggle had occurred during the injection, then evidence of the struggle would be apparent at the injection site during an autopsy.

The husband was convicted of first-degree murder. His conviction was affirmed on appeal.

The court in this case did not criticize anything that was done or not done by the nurse colleague who had the "bizarre and scary" conversation with the husband, and there was no criticism of the pharmacist who noticed the unusual removal of succinylcholine from crash carts. Hindsight is always 20–20. There is simply no realistic way that either of these people could have foreseen, at the time they noticed something odd, such a hideous murder being committed. Yet this case review does offer an opportunity to consider alternative actions that might be appropriate should circumstances similar to this arise in the future.

A series of "what if" questions can guide an after-the-fact analysis of this case, with a focus on reasonable preventive measures that might be appropriately adopted moving forward. What if the nurse colleague had reported the bizarre and scary conversation with the husband to a nursing supervisor? What if the has been recognized only recently due to a significant number of reported murders caused by THZ overdosage.[26] As a clear, colorless, and tasteless liquid, THZ drops have become a drug of choice for pharmaceutical homicide.

The first criminal defendant to be charged with using THZ as a weapon was Byron Shull from a suburb of Cleveland.[27] Shull and his girlfriend moved to Ohio from Florida to live with his parents, and there was a conflict between the generations. Shull told detectives that he stole two bottles of Visine from a pharmacy and poured them in his father's milk to give him diarrhea. Apparently Shull had seen this done on television as a prank. The father was hospitalized with a dangerously low heart rate, and he was not discharged for several weeks. The father survived, but he suffered permanent injuries. Shull's girlfriend went to the police and told them of the intentional poisoning. Shull entered a plea of guilty to felonious assault, domestic violence, and contaminating a substance for human consumption. He was sentenced to five years in prison.

Lana Sue Clayton, a nurse from South Carolina, was charged with murder in the death of her husband from doses of THZ that Clayton had allegedly placed in the husband's water over a period of three days.[28] Shortly after her trial began, Clayton entered a plea of guilty to voluntary manslaughter and tampering with a food or drug causing death. She was sentenced to twenty-five years in prison. Although her husband suffered from numerous medical conditions, and the initial investigations concluded that he had died from natural causes, Clayton was charged with murder based on toxicological evidence. Law enforcement authorities were aware that a very similar alleged THZ murder occurred in a North Carolina town just 12 miles away from where Clayton lived.[29] In that case, a paramedic is accused of poisoning his wife with THZ. The possibility of a copycat murder has been considered, but it has not been resolved.

Jessy Kurczewski has been sentenced to forty years in prison, following her conviction of first-degree intentional homicide.[30] A jury found that Kurczewski, of Waukesha County, Wisconsin, had poisoned a friend with six bottles of THZ that were added to the victim's water bottle. The victim was found dead in her condo surrounded by prescription bottles and with crushed medication on her chest. The prosecution alleged that Kurczewski had staged the scene to look like a suicide. Evidence showed that for a period of time Kurczewski had been stealing money from the victim to the total of almost US$300,000.

Although it is very difficult, if not impossible, to prevent pharmaceutical homicide with THZ ophthalmic products, there is a significant role for pharmacists and other health professionals in the detection of this crime through collaboration with law enforcement. Expert witness testimony at trial can validate the ease with this the product can be both acquired and used in the commission of pharmaceutical homicide. Jurors need to know that simply because a medication can be acquired at a convenience store without a prescription, this does not mean that the product is safe under all circumstances of use. The successful prosecution of THZ murderers can make the crime seem less "perfect" and can serve as a deterrent to similar crimes in the future.

Conclusion

It may seem counterintuitive to consider family members and close friends as likely murder suspects when a homicide is investigated. One might assume that caring and nurturing personal relationships (either past or present) would make it less likely that a murderer would have a special family or friendship connection with the victim. It is a false assumption. Anecdotal evidence and limited data suggest that this is exactly what one must consider when investigating the cause of a homicide. When the suspected murder weapon is a pharmaceutical product, then the investigation should consider whether there is anyone with a healthcare background who has a family or friendship connection with the victim. No seemingly unusual circumstances should be disregarded as insignificant, regardless of how bizarre they may seem. Standard approaches to the prevention of adverse drug events can help protect patients and others from being victimized by a homicidal family member or friend.

Key Takeaways

- Counsel patients on both the expected therapeutic effect and the possible adverse effects of all "high-alert medications" (as defined by the Institute for Safe Medication Practices). Do not wait for the patient to ask for counseling. Do not explain precisely what a toxic dose is or how to administer the medication to produce a toxic dose. Avoid teaching the patient how to commit a crime. The message for patients should stress the need for appropriate therapeutic use, and not teach any method for toxic use. Emphasize that the instructions provided by the prescriber, and included on the product label, are the only acceptable way to use the medication. All medications should be kept in a safe place where they cannot be accessed by anyone other than the person for whom they have been prescribed. They should be discarded when they are no longer needed. They should not be stockpiled for later use. Never use any other person's medication. Never allow anyone to administer medication unless it is done as authorized by a prescriber. This is all a matter of patient safety, for the protection of the patient and for the protection of the public.
- Be alert for any requests for "rule bending" with regard to drugs that may have lethal effects. Make sure that patients have authorized

pickup of their medication by anyone who requests the medication at the will-call area. Consult with the prescriber when any refill patterns seem to suggest medication use outside the instructions that have been provided to the patient. Be particularly cautious if a healthcare professional asks for medication to be provided without the usual safeguards to assure accurate recordkeeping and oversight of medication use. Do not allow any prescriptions to be issued without a patient's name, or with a pseudonym, particularly if the prescriber has explained that she/he will be taking the medication to the patient. Do not allow informal "borrowing" of medication by prescribers or other healthcare professionals. All transfers of medication between licensed facilities must be conducted pursuant to recordkeeping requirements that assure product integrity.

- Offer your expertise to law enforcement if you learn that one of your patients has died under suspicious circumstances. In a murder investigation, no information is too small or insignificant. Everything matters. Let the law enforcement investigators decide whether what you have to offer is of value to them. Investigators may not know what to look for until they are told of medications that have been dispensed to a deceased patient. Answer questions carefully when an investigator interviews you. Do not share any unfounded suspicions. But do not withhold any information that could possibly be relevant. Just state the facts as you know them.

References

1. People v. Archerd, 477 P.2d 421 (Cal. 1970).

2. Marks V, Richmond C. William Archerd: A serial matrimonialist killer. *J R Soc Med.* 2008 Feb;101(2):63–66.

3. Steck-Flynn K. Just a pinch of cyanide: The basics of homicidal poisoning investigations. *Law Enf Tech.* 2007 Oct;34(10):118, 120, 126.

4. Duvall v. State, 978 N.E.2d 417 (Ind.App. 2012).

5. Stephens v. State, 911 So.2d 424 (Miss. 2005).

6. People v. Dendel, 748 N.W.2d 859 (Mich. 2008).

7. Dendel v. Washington, 647 Fed.Appx. 612 (6th Cir. 2016).

8. State v. Jensen, 46 P. 3d 536 (Ida. 2002).

9. 21 CFR § 211.132, Tamper-evident packaging requirements for over-the-counter (OTC) human drug products.

10. 18 U.S. Code § 1365, Tampering with consumer products.

11. United States v. Meling, 47 F.3d 1546 (9th Cir. 1995).

12. United States v. Nickell, 883 F.2d 824 (9th Cir. 1989).

13. Elsroth v. Johnson & Johnson, 700 F.Supp. (S.D.N.Y. 1988).

14. State v. Essa, 955 N.E.2d 429 (Ohio App. 2011).

15. Food and Drug Administration v. Alliance for Hippocratic Medicine, 144 S. Ct. 1540 (2024).

16. Quinn v. Memorial Medical Center, 764 S.W.2d 915 (Tex.App. 1989).

17. United States Attorney's Office, Middle District of Florida, Press Release, Tampa Bay man sentenced to more than 13 years in federal prison for product tampering, causing the death of an unborn child. January 27, 2014. **https://www.justice.gov/usao-mdfl/pr/tampa-bay-man-sentenced-more-13-years-federal-prison-product-tampering-causing-death#:~:text=Lazzara%20today%20sentenced%20John%20Andrew,conspiracy%20to%20commit%20mail%20fraud**

18. Alicea Enterprises v. Nationwide Insurance Company, 252 So. 2d 799 (Fla.App. 2018).

19. *AP News.* Texas man sentenced to 180 days in jail for drugging wife's drinks to induce an abortion. February 8, 2024. **https://apnews.com/article/abortion-texas-guilty-plea-sentence-c5e6a1b71ddf8cfdcf0258fb5b7bff23**

20. *AP News*. Louisiana Legislature approves bill classifying abortion pills as controlled dangerous substances. May 23, 2024. **https://apnews.com/article/abortion-pills-louisiana-legislature-controlled-substance-06ea3e8df86b72b473efe8fc71054ddf**

21. State v. Bollig, 523 P.3d 1 (Kan.App. 2023).

22. People v. Patel, 2022 Westlaw 17420572 (Wisc.App. 2022).

23. Carlier J, Escard E, Péoc'h M, Boyer B, Romeuf L, Faict T, Guitton J, Gaillard Y. Atropine eye drops: An unusual homicidal poisoning. *J Forensic Sci.* 2014 May;59(3):859–864.

24. Di Fazio V, Vanhaebost J, Wille Sarah MR, Samyn N, Schmit G, Bonbled F. Poisoning with atropine-based eye drops: An almost perfect murder? *Tox Analy et Clin.* 2022 Sept;34(3):S46.

25. Spiller H, Griffith J. Prolonged cardiovascular effects after unintentional ingestion of tetrahydrozoline. *Clin Toxicol* (Phila). 2008 Feb;46(2):171–172.

26. Menshawey E, Menshawey R. More than meets the eye: A scoping review on the non-medical uses of THZ eye drops. *Forensic Sci Med Pathol.* 2023 Jul 28.

27. Staff. Cuyahoga County judge sentences man to 5 years in prison for poisoning father with eyedrops. *Cleveland Plain Dealer* (June 15, 2012). https://www.cleveland.com/metro/2012/06/eyedrops_story_shell.html

28. Miller R. Woman who poisoned husband with eye drops gets 25 years in prison. *USA Today* (January 17, 2020). https://www.usatoday.com/story/news/nation/2020/01/17/south-carolina-woman-who-poisoned-husband-eye-drops-25-years/4498134002/

29. Roppolo M. Former paramedic, accused of killing wife, faces arson charges. *CBS News* (April 1, 2021). https://www.aol.com/former-paramedic-accused-killing-wife-173510824.html

30. Griffin A. Wisconsin woman convicted of fatally poisoning friend with eye drops, stealing $300K. *New York Post* (November 15, 2023). https://nypost.com/2023/11/15/news/wisconsin-woman-jessy-kurczewski-convicted-of-fatally-poisoning-friend-with-eye-drops-stealing-300k/

Chapter 10

Opioid-Related Mortality

The abuse of opioids is killing people. Media headlines tell the clear story with sensational phrases like "Killer Opioids," "Drug Deaths Skyrocket," "Prescription for Death," and "Narcotic Fatalities." There is unquestionably a public health problem with opioid-related deaths. Most of these tragic deaths occur in the community setting. Many of those who have died were using products originally acquired from a pharmacy. Some people who became addicted to products that were dispensed by a pharmacy have died from the lethal effects of street drugs because pharmaceutical opioids were no longer available. As the guardians of the nation's drug supply, pharmacists have been heavily involved in efforts to reduce opioid-related deaths. Pharmacists have been criticized for dispensing opioids under suspicious, or outright unlawful, circumstances. Some pharmacists have been convicted of crimes for their incautious provision of opioids. Unintended death from opioid abuse is a problem that a very few pharmacists have caused and that every pharmacist can address.

Opioids and the Pharmacist's Responsibility

Pharmacists find themselves in a challenging position. As health professionals, they are responsible for providing necessary medications to many patients with chronic pain who need opioids and who use them therapeutically to live better lives. Yet, having been conscripted into the nation's so-called "War on Drugs," pharmacists are responsible for reducing the incidence of prescription drug abuse by denying opioids to people who do not need them. The choice of who should receive opioids and who should not receive them is not a comfortable decision for pharmacists to make, but it is unavoidable in the current climate of epidemic proportions. A pharmacist's decision to deny opioids for those who need them can be as problematic as providing opioids to those who do not need them. Making good decisions about access to opioids is a significant challenge for pharmacists.

The focus of law enforcement and public health officials on reducing deaths from opioid abuse is unsurprising. The abuse of opioids is lurid and dramatic. Medications prescribed by physicians and dispensed by pharmacists are supposed to be helpful rather than harmful. There is a keenly felt sense of treachery and disloyalty when medications are diverted to harmful nonmedical use. As the last link in the distribution chain of pharmaceutical products, pharmacists are charged with the responsibility to review decisions made "upstream" from them and to press the "stop button" when criminal activity may be occurring. The failure to meet this expectation is often seen as a betrayal of public trust.

Risk of Denying Necessary Medication

Pharmacists have the authority to refuse dispensing of controlled substance medications to any patient when circumstances suggest that the medications will be abused or diverted to illicit use. This responsibility for denial of medication can be misapplied through knee-jerk deference to simplistic rules that fail to recognize the complexities of the disease of opioid use disorder and the debilitating nature of the disease of chronic pain. Refusing medication because a patient "looks like an abuser" or because "this just does not feel right" is an inappropriate play of the "trump card" that pharmacists hold. Subjective feelings must be supported by objective facts to validate a refusal to honor a prescription. A pharmacist's uncomfortable feelings can be a starting point, but should not be an endpoint, of a decision to fill or not to fill an opioid prescription.

Decision assistance algorithms and other evidence-based programs have been developed to support pharmacists as they make dispensing choices by considering objective factors related to the risks of opioid diversion. The dispensing of medication to an abuser or a diverter is obviously a huge error that can lead to misery and death. The refusal to dispense medication to a patient with appropriately diagnosed chronic pain is an error that can lead to continued suffering by the patient. Denying necessary medication for a patient with chronic pain can also lead to loss of respect for a pharmacist's clinical judgment and diminished collegiality with the prescriber. A pharmacist's exercise of the power of prescription refusal must be done with care and for valid reasons.

Pharmacist Legal Responsibility for Opioid Monitoring

A classic legal case of liability for opioid overdose encapsulates the concerns that may arise in pharmacy practice when accusations are made that a pharmacist has not adequately monitored a patient's use of opioids and/or other controlled substance medications, resulting in a patient's death.[1]

This case is from 2015. The Court of Appeals of Florida reviewed the dismissal of a lawsuit filed by the estate of a deceased patient against the pharmacy that dispensed opioids and other controlled substances to the patient in an allegedly negligent manner. The owner of the pharmacy was named as a defendant along with the pharmacists who had dispensed the medications.

The trial court granted what is called "summary judgment" for the defendant pharmacy and for pharmacists, essentially ruling that there was no possible liability under the facts as they had been alleged in the plaintiff's lawsuit.

The patient's estate (the plaintiffs) appealed the dismissal of the case, arguing that the trial court misunderstood the important duties of pharmacists in the screening of controlled substance prescriptions and in the monitoring of controlled substance use by patients. The facts of the case tell a familiar story that has appeared in various forms in many pharmacy malpractice lawsuits.

In May 2009, a patient began treatment from a physician who diagnosed him with "stress syndrome." The physician prescribed alprazolam, hydrocodone/acetaminophen, and oxycodone/acetaminophen. It was alleged that, over the next two years, the physician repeatedly prescribed these drugs before the patient should have depleted the preceding prescriptions. The plaintiff alleged that the pharmacy filled at least thirty of these prescriptions without question, "even though the prescriptions were issued too closely in time and days before the patient should have exhausted the preceding prescription." In March 2011, the patient died due to "combined drug intoxication of alprazolam and hydrocodone."

The plaintiff sued the pharmacy for negligence, alleging that the pharmacists at the pharmacy owed the patient a duty to: (1) use due and proper care in filling and dispensing all prescriptions; (2) exercise the level of care and skill recognized by reasonably prudent and similar pharmacy professionals; (3) not dispense or fill prescriptions that were unreasonable on their face or in light of the circumstances; (4) warn the patient of the risk of using the medications; (5) comply with relevant policies and procedures; (6) comply with relevant statutory and regulatory provisions; and (7) not subject the patient to an unreasonable risk of harm from their foreseeable conduct.

The pharmacy filed a motion to dismiss the case, arguing that based on a prior Florida legal case, there was no duty owed by the pharmacy to the patient other than properly filling his valid and lawful prescriptions. The trial court granted the motion to dismiss the case. The pharmacists claimed that they had never filled an illegal prescription for the deceased patient and that all prescriptions had been filled in accord with the prescriber's directions. From this dismissal, the plaintiffs appealed.

The appellate court ruled that the trial court erred in dismissing the negligence claims against the pharmacy.

The court said:

> A pharmacist owes a patient a duty of reasonable care. Pharmacists are required to exercise that degree of care than an ordinarily prudent pharmacist would exercise under the same or similar circumstances. We hold that a pharmacist's duty to use due and proper care in filling a prescription extends beyond simply following the prescribing physician's directions. In the instant case, the pharmacy filled, without question, numerous prescriptions that were so close together that the pharmacists should have been put on notice that the patient was getting too many pills within a too short period. We refuse to interpret a pharmacist's duty to use "due and proper care in filling the prescription" as being satisfied by "robotic compliance" with the instructions of the prescribing physician.

The appellate court continued:

Pharmacists are specifically charged with knowledge of prescription medication and the risks presented by taking particular prescription drugs, such that they should be able to evaluate and explain the operative risks of taking a medication or series of medications. In essence, a strong policy basis already exists supporting a pharmacist's duty to warn customers of the inherent risks in filling repeated and unreasonable prescriptions with potentially fatal consequences.

The trial court's ruling that dismissed the case against the pharmacists and pharmacy was reversed and sent back to the trial court for further proceedings. The case was eventually settled out of court. The take-home message of the case is that pharmacists can be held legally liable for the death of a patient that results from foreseeable overuse of opioids. The legality of controlled substance prescriptions and a pharmacist's accuracy in order processing does not completely protect pharmacists from liability when controlled substance prescriptions are filled "too early" resulting in the death of a patient.

Focus on Opioid Quantity and Acquisition Timing

As the ruling and discussion in this case demonstrate, one of the most challenging issues for pharmacists is the "too early" controlled substance prescription. The problem the court described of prescriptions being "so close together that the pharmacist should have been put on notice" can mean either a too early refill of a C-III through C-V medication or a too early new supply of a C-II medication. Faced with this interpretation of pharmacist responsibility for controlled substance monitoring, pharmacists may legitimately ask: "How early is too early?" In many situations, early acquisition of a new supply of medication is a good thing. Patients with pain are very concerned about maintaining an available supply of pain medication. They don't want to run out, just as people don't want to run out of cleaning supplies, or food, or gasoline, or paper products, or any other item that makes life more comfortable. For many patients with chronic pain, running out of medication can lead to withdrawal symptoms and/or the need to modify an ongoing therapeutic plan and completely start over with a different drug or a different dose of the same drug. Pain management physicians and patients with chronic pain prefer not to interrupt analgesic therapy that is working. Patients with chronic pain are instructed by pain management experts not to run out of their medication.

Responsible patients with chronic pain plan ahead. They acquire an additional supply of medication before they run out of their existing supply. "Early" is good. "Too early" is not good. The goal for pharmacists is to define what "too early" means. Some pharmacies have adopted a policy of "20% early" as being too early. In pharmacies with such a policy, a 30-day supply should not need to be replenished until 24 days have elapsed. Insurance companies may have their own criteria for a "too early" resupply of medication. If a patient requests an additional supply earlier than this, there must be a valid justification for the request. Some explanations by the patient can be considered acceptable, as long as they do not become routine ("I am going on vacation," "I don't have transportation to get here next week," etc.). At other times, it may be necessary to consult the prescriber ("The doctor increased my dosage," "Somebody stole my medication," etc.). Any explanation that seems out of the ordinary should be investigated. The process of the investigation (who was contacted) and the results of the investigation (what was decided and why) should be documented.

Focus on the Prescriber

The regulatory challenge for pharmacists in meeting their responsibility to screen controlled substance prescriptions has led some pharmacies to blacklist physicians whose prescriptions will no longer be filled at the pharmacy regardless of who the patient may be. The blacklisting of these physicians is often based on opioid volume and on physical surveillance of the physician's clinic or office. Blacklisting of physicians is a very blunt instrument that is certain to eliminate many invalid orders, but it has the additional consequence of potentially eliminating some valid orders. Drug diverters may patronize blacklisted prescribers, but legitimate patients may also go to these physicians because their primary care provider has a "no opioids" policy for fear of regulatory investigation. Rejecting all of a physician's prescriptions necessarily means that some needy patients will not receive their medication. In addition, this approach ignores the reality that many nonlisted physicians are likely being duped by abusers and diverters. Since these implicitly cleared physicians are not on the list, pharmacists may decide to fill their prescriptions with a level of confidence that is not warranted. Abusers and diverters won't just stop when a blacklisted physician can no longer provide what they need. They will just take their illegal business elsewhere. A preferable approach is to focus on problematic prescriptions, regardless of the prescriber.

On the other hand, a small number of prescribers have succumbed to the temptation to provide opioids to persons who obviously do not need them. Alert pharmacists have brought these prescribers to the attention of law enforcement authorities. In some cases, the prescribers have been found guilty of homicide. It is important to examine the facts and rationale of the physician convictions that were based on the issuance of prescriptions that were honored by pharmacists.

Physician Found Guilty of Felony Murder

Physicians have been charged with murder for the inappropriate prescribing of opioids leading to the death of their patients. Most of these murder charges were later reduced to a lesser charge, and the physician was found guilty of that lesser charge, or the physician agreed to a plea bargain based on a lesser charge than on a murder. One of several notable exceptions to this result was Georgia physician Noel Chua who was found guilty of felony murder for overprescribing opioids to one of his patients.[2] Felony murder occurs when a perpetrator kills a person during the commission of a separate felony, even if the killing was unintended.

In most cases when felony murder is charged by a prosecutor, the perpetrator has killed a victim during a robbery of the victim. Kidnapping, rape, and arson are other examples of felonies that can elevate the murder charge if a victim dies during the commission of that felony. The result of being found guilty of felony murder is that the crime is punished as first-degree murder, which is a capital offense in many jurisdictions. A charge of felony murder raises the stakes considerably for a perpetrator, and it will lead to a much more substantial sentence if the perpetrator is found guilty. For a charge of felony murder to be successfully prosecuted, the prosecution must prove that the death of the victim was a "foreseeable result" of the underlying felony.

The jury in this Georgia case found the physician guilty of "multiple counts of distributing controlled substances by prescribing them in a manner that was not in the usual course of his professional practice and was not for a legitimate medical purpose." This drug distribution charge, based on prescriptions for methadone and oxycodone issued to a single patient, was the underlying felony that led to additional charges of felony murder against the physician when the patient died.

By referencing language contained in the federal Controlled Substances Act, prosecutors have consistently argued, with considerable success, that when a prescriber issues a controlled substance prescription outside the usual course of professional practice, or not for a legitimate medical purpose, then the prescriber is acting as a street drug distributor and not as a healthcare professional. This argument has been successfully used for pharmacists and for prescribers. In the Georgia case, the patient's death was alleged to have been the "probable consequence" of the crime of unlawful drug distribution.

The facts of the Georgia case showed that the patient died from a fatal ingestion of controlled substances prescribed for him by the defendant physician. He was found in his bedroom surrounded by "numerous pills bottles, loose pills, syringes, and drug patches." The medications had been prescribed for the patient by the defendant physician.

The physician's defense was that he had not operated a "pill mill." There was no evidence that he had overprescribed opioids for any other patients. There was no evidence that he was selling prescriptions without any medical examination. There was no evidence that there were long lines of drug-seekers waiting to see him outside his office. This was not the typical "death by opioid overdose case" that has frequently been alleged against a physician who ran a huge practice devoted almost entirely to the prescribing of opioids for persons who the physician knew were abusing them or were diverting them.

Testimony by a pharmacist indicated that the physician was practicing outside the usual course of professional practice with regard to this one patient. All it takes is one patient to violate the Controlled Substances Act. According to the pharmacist, on one occasion, the physician took the unusual step of visiting the pharmacy to write a prescription for drugs for the patient. This was something that the physician had never done before and that rarely occurred with any other physicians. At another time, the patient presented to the pharmacist a prescription that was written "for two opioids on the same prescription," and the pharmacist consulted by telephone with the physician regarding the excessive dosage. A record of this consultation was made by the pharmacist on the prescription, noting the physician's authorization to dispense both medications despite the pharmacist's concerns. On another occasion, the pharmacist documented his concerns that the patient "had been prescribed six different pain medications in the last twenty days." The physician explained to the pharmacist that the previous medications were not working and that the patient had destroyed them. The court offered no criticism of the pharmacist's efforts on behalf of the patient. The documentation produced by the pharmacist was vital to the prosecution of the physician and to the exculpation of the pharmacist.

There was also expert testimony that the patient "exhibited signs of drug abuse that should have been recognized by a treating physician" and that the physician's prescriptions constituted "providing drugs" rather than patient care. The physician argued that the evidence demonstrated "nothing more than poor performance by a physician in treatment and record keeping." The court disagreed, noting that the physician was aware of the patient's drug problem, but he "nonetheless provided him with drugs that were dangerous to such a person." The physician claimed that the patient "did not take as directed the drugs that caused his death," but the court noted expert testimony that "a drug addict may not take medication as prescribed, and that is one reason that providing controlled substances to one who may be an addict is dangerous."

The court concluded that since the physician knew the patient's medical condition and history, the felony of illegally providing controlled substances through prescriptions was a dangerous felony and the patient's death was "a foreseeable result within the meaning of the felony murder statute." The physician's conviction of felony murder was affirmed on appeal.

Pain Specialist Convicted of Second-Degree Manslaughter

A board-certified anesthesiologist and pain management specialist from New York was accused of running a "pill mill" at his pain management clinic.[3] Dr. Stan Xuhui Li was convicted of two counts of manslaughter in the second degree. The prosecutors presented evidence that Li prescribed medically unnecessary high doses of opioids, alprazolam, and other controlled substances "as a first resort." The evidence showed that Li did not verify the source of the pain complained of by the patients. He did not order diagnostic tests for objective confirmation of pain, and he did not consider pain management treatment options other than opioids. He conducted little or no physical examinations. Li often prescribed high doses of whatever medication the patients requested. He required payment in cash, and he scaled the required payment based on the dose of opioids prescribed.

Two of Li's former patients testified at trial that they were opioid addicts. They testified that they used the drugs that Li prescribed to get high, rather than for legitimate pain management. Li had been advised by other healthcare professionals and patients' family members that several patients were addicted to opioids and were at risk of dying from opioid abuse.

Two of Li's patients allegedly died of overdoses caused by a combination of oxycodone and alprazolam. In addition to his conviction on two counts of manslaughter, Li was convicted of three counts of reckless endangerment and 170 counts of criminal sale of a prescription. Li appealed his conviction, arguing that the law contains no provision by which a prescriber of medication can be convicted of any homicide offense that results in an overdose of the prescribed medication.

The appellate court noted that to convict a defendant of second-degree manslaughter requires proof beyond a reasonable doubt that the alleged perpetrator recklessly caused the death of the victims. The court concluded that the evidence was sufficient to support the jury's finding that Li had acted recklessly. The court explained that a rational juror could have concluded, based on a valid line of reasoning and permissible inferences, that Li was aware of and consciously disregarded the risk that his patients would take drugs more rapidly than instructed and would die by overdosage. Particularly given that Li was a medical doctor, with specialty expertise in anesthesiology and pain management, his conduct "constituted a gross deviation from the standard of conduct that a reasonable person would observe in the situation."

The conviction was affirmed.

Drastic Changes in the Approach to Medical Practice

California Internist Dr. Hsiu Ying "Lisa" Tseng was convicted of three counts of second-degree murder.[4] The facts showed that Tseng joined a general medical practice in 2007. According to the court, when Li began at the clinic, "the patients were mostly from the local Hispanic and Asian communities, the wait time for each patient was 15 to 20 minutes, and 90 percent of the patients paid for treatment through their insurance." One year later, the practice and the clientele had changed. Most of Tseng's patients "were now white males in their 20s and 30s who came from outside the community seeking pain and anxiety medications."

By 2010, the clinic had developed a reputation as a place where patients could easily obtain prescriptions for controlled substances, including opioids, sedatives, muscle relaxants, and drugs used to treat drug addiction. In addition, fees had doubled and nearly all patients paid cash. The court quoted one visitor to the clinic who said that it "looked like a parole office" with "drug dealing." The wait time had increased to about six hours with twenty to thirty patients inside the waiting room or outside the clinic at any one time. When the clinic's receptionist expressed concern about the number of patients waiting and the level of anxiety and agitation they expressed in the waiting room, Tseng allegedly told her that they were "druggies" and that they could wait.

The court stated that "Beginning in 2008, pharmacists began to refuse to fill prescriptions written by Tseng because the prescriptions raised red flags, and the patient's profiles, conduct, and the combination of substances and quantities that Tseng prescribed indicated no legitimate medical purpose for writing the prescriptions. When Tseng learned of this, she referred her patients to 'mom and pop' pharmacies that continued to fill her prescriptions."

Law enforcement investigators, including investigators from the coroner's office, began calling Tseng to discuss the deaths of several of her patients and to apprise her that the patients had died of suspected drug overdoses shortly after obtaining prescriptions from her. Nevertheless, Tseng continued her prescribing practices until she was arrested in 2012. At trial, the prosecution presented evidence that nine of Tseng's patients died shortly after receiving prescriptions from Tseng for controlled substances.

In appealing her convictions, Tseng contended that although she acted with negligence sufficient to support convictions for involuntary manslaughter, there was no evidence that she acted with conscious disregard for her patients' lives and that the conviction for second-degree murder was a misapplication of the law. Specifically, she asserted that because coroner and police investigators never informed her that she was responsible for her patients' deaths, her continued practice of prescribing high doses and large quantities of opioids and other controlled substances did not show the necessary reckless mindset to support a finding of implied malice.

The appellate court responded that, as a licensed physician, Tseng had expert knowledge of the life-threatening risks posed by her prescribing practices. She knew that the drugs she prescribed were dangerous and that the combination of the prescribed drugs, often with increasing doses, posed a significant risk of death. Tseng's experience and medical training regarding opioids and other controlled substances provided her with special knowledge of those dangers. During the investigation of her practice, Tseng admitted to undercover the Drug Enforcement Administration (DEA) agents that she understood that the drugs she was prescribing were addictive and typically would only be prescribed to treat pain from cancer or bone fractures. She knew that she was prescribing those drugs in high doses and in dangerous combinations to patients who did not suffer from those conditions.

The court also described how Tseng took actions that showed her awareness of the danger of her prescribing practices. After large national pharmacies contacted Tseng to raise questions about the lack of medical justification for her prescriptions, and ultimately refused to fill those prescriptions, Tseng sent her patients to smaller local pharmacies that she knew would continue to fill her prescriptions. Moreover, although she knew that some patients were also obtaining similar prescriptions from other physicians and were taking the drugs in lethal combinations, she did not contact those other physicians to determine which other drugs they were prescribing or in what doses.

The appellate court concluded that the evidence supported a finding of implied malice with respect to each of the murders. The second-degree murder convictions were affirmed.

Pharmacist's Corresponding Responsibility

The convictions of physicians for homicide following the deaths of their patients illustrate how the prescriber has the primary responsibility for lawfully issuing a controlled substance prescription. Under federal regulations, pharmacists have a significant corresponding responsibility to that of the prescriber. Federal law clearly defines the pharmacist's role in the screening of opioid prescriptions. Pharmacists have a responsibility that corresponds with that of the prescriber to avoid knowingly honoring unlawful controlled substance prescriptions. Many prescribers are surprised to learn that federal law imposes this requirement on pharmacists. When a pharmacist has unresolved concerns about the legality of a controlled substance prescription, consultation by a pharmacist with the prescriber is not optional—it is mandated by federal law. Here is the language of the federal law:

> A prescription for a controlled substance to be effective must be issued for a legitimate medical purpose by an individual practitioner acting in the usual course of his professional practice. The responsibility for the proper prescribing and dispensing of controlled substances is upon the prescribing practitioner, but a corresponding responsibility rests with the pharmacist who fills the prescription. An order purporting to be a prescription issued not in the usual course of professional treatment or in legitimate and authorized research is not a prescription within the meaning and intent of [the Controlled Substance Act] and the person knowingly filling such a purported prescription, as well as the person issuing it, shall be subject to the penalties provided for violations of the provisions of law relating to controlled substances.[5]

The language of this federal law leaves pharmacists with no choice. Pharmacists have a responsibility to evaluate the legitimacy of any prescription that appears to have been issued inconsistent with this rule. Pharmacists have discretion to decide how they will exercise that responsibility. The language of the federal law is difficult to interpret. There is no definition of the words and phrases used in the federal law, leaving it to pharmacists to figure out how to apply the words and phrases to relevant circumstances in pharmacy practice.

"Legitimate Medical Purpose"

Federal law requires that a controlled substance prescription is not be issued for anything other than a "legitimate medical purpose." This is a curious phrase, because it is difficult to imagine a medical purpose that is not legitimate. Medicine is an inherently legitimate profession. One way to understand the phrase is that the words "legitimate" and "medical" are redundant and that what the law requires is the issuance of a prescription for a medical purpose. This interpretation would mean that under DEA regulations a pharmacist is not required to screen prescriptions for their therapeutic appropriateness. A pharmacist is required to determine a prescription's legal validity, and what matters is whether the prescription is intended for use in therapy rather than for its euphoric effect.

The companion phrase "usual course of professional practice" is also somewhat challenging. The "course" of a medical practice is not the same as the "scope" of medical practice. Course of practice refers to the process of taking a history, conducting an assessment, developing a treatment plan, and prescribing consistent with the treatment plan. Scope of practice, on the other hand, refers to the training and licensure of the practitioner.

Pharmacists usually cannot know whether a prescriber was acting in the usual course of professional practice unless someone explains the process used by the prescriber (i.e., selling prescriptions for cash and conducting no physical examination) and the pharmacist recognizes that nonmedical process as being outside the usual course of professional practice.

"Knowingly"

A pharmacist who knowingly dispenses medication pursuant to what the DEA refers to as a "purported prescription" has violated the federal law. "Purported prescription" is an important phrase since the similar phrase "invalid prescription" has little meaning. If an order is a prescription, then it is valid. A prescription cannot be invalid because validity is an element of a prescription.

According to the DEA regulation, a pharmacist who honors a purported prescription, but does not do so "knowingly," has not violated the law. As the DEA has interpreted this word, the concept of "knowingly" means both what is actually known and what should be known by the exercise of judgment based on the facts available to the pharmacist. "Knowingly" incorporates what a pharmacist knew and what a pharmacist had "reason to know." The pharmacist must investigate if there are problematic red flags associated with a prescription.

Pharmacists usually won't avoid legal responsibilities by using the "naïve pharmacist" defense ("Sorry, I just didn't recognize any sort of problem at all."). This is sometimes also called the "ostrich defense" because it is based on burying one's head in the sand. It never works.

The concept of "knowingly" applies an objective standard. When they are presented with a suspicious controlled substance prescription, pharmacists must follow up on clues that a reasonable pharmacist would identify. Having done that due diligence, and having received reasonable explanations, the pharmacist can fill the order without having knowingly filling a purported prescription.

Identifying and Managing "Red Flags"

The phrase "red flags" is applied generally to any situation in which anyone who is doing anything needs to slow down, examine the evidence, consider the circumstances, and move forward only when the "coast is clear." A red flag attached to a long or wide load on a vehicle that is traveling on a street conveys the need to be cautious and not the need to stop or to drive in a completely different direction. Similarly, a "red flag" that signifies a reason to know that a prescription has not been issued for a legitimate medical purpose or in the usual course of professional practice means that a pharmacist should examine the situation closely and not that a pharmacist should automatically decline the prescription. Red flags can be resolved.

The DEA does not provide a formal list of what the agency considers to be red flags. Only by examining the enforcement actions pursued by the agency is it possible to develop an understanding of what situations may be considered as reasons to know of prescription illegitimacy. Here is a list of several red flags that have been identified by the DEA during legal proceedings against pharmacists.[6] This is not a complete list of all "red flags."

- Patient has traveled from a "long distance."
- Multiple prescriptions for different patients issued by the same prescriber for the same drug, in the same quantity, on the same day.
- Multiple patients with the same address have the same prescription for the same drug and same strength.
- Patients are issued prescriptions for the same drug in different strengths, such as an immediate release as well as a higher strength sustained release dosage form of the same drug.
- Patients are issued prescriptions for what the DEA refers to as a "drug cocktail," which is usually an opioid along with a benzodiazepine.
- Patients pay cash when other red flags are present.

- Patient is issued a new prescription for a supply of opioid before they should have finished the previous supply.
- Price gouging/black market pricing substantially higher than the market price at other nearby pharmacies.

Each one of these "red flags" could be applicable to a patient with chronic pain. None of these "red flags" is unique to drug diverters or drug abusers. Every one of these "red flags" could be resolved through consultation with the prescriber and/or conversation with the patient. If a "red flag" exists, then the responsibility of the pharmacist is to identify the "red flag." Having identified "red flags," it is the responsibility of the pharmacist to resolve them prior to honoring the prescription. When "red flags" cannot be resolved, then the prescriptions must be declined.

Conducting the Inquiry

Most patients with chronic pain have been treated with such a high level of suspicion by prescribers, pharmacists, and others that they are accustomed to answering probing questions about their opioid use. As long as a pharmacist conducts a polite inquiry (not an inquisition), patients with chronic pain will understand this questioning to be a necessary part of the solution to the problem of prescription drug abuse.

If done with care and with professional tact, a pharmacist inquiry can legitimize patients with chronic pain by recognizing that they have a medical need for the opioids that abusers use recreationally. This legitimization of patients with chronic pain validates them, and it usually provides very welcome support. For those persons who are offended by pharmacist inquiries to address red flags, and who opt to take their prescriptions elsewhere to avoid pharmacist questioning, the choice they make is a choice that pharmacists simply must accept.

The best approach to the inquiry is to begin by explaining that there are risks to the patient, risks to the pharmacy, risks to the prescriber, and risks to the public from the distribution and use of opioids. The goal of the pharmacist's questions is to reduce all those risks. This is not just some pointless government rule. It is a matter of public and patient safety. Questions must be asked of patients by their pharmacist to provide answers for those who will eventually ask similar questions of the pharmacist.

Discomfort of Taking a Balanced Approach

Balance is the cornerstone of effective healthcare regulation, and it is also often the cornerstone of effective healthcare practice. Balance is not an unfamiliar concept. Most people balance themselves physically as they walk so that they don't fall down. People balance their work and personal lives. People balance their physical and emotional well-being.

The dark side of balance is that there are always two sides of the balance, and the more one emphasizes one side, the more one neglects the other. In pharmacy, for example, emphasizing caution sacrifices speed. Emphasizing speed sacrifices accuracy. Missing the balance point can cause frustration and can lead to errors.

Consider the pharmacist who says: "I will always be so cautious with opioid prescription screening that I will never fill a purported prescription." That goal can be achieved, but only at the expense of refusing many valid prescriptions. Distinguishing between the two is just too difficult.

Alternatively, there may be a pharmacist who says: "These are medications that chronic pain patients need, and I am never going to deny medication to a patient whose quality of life I can improve." This pharmacist will fill many illegal prescriptions.

The problem with balance, and the dirty little secret that goes with it, is that in a balanced practice there inevitably will be some illegal prescriptions that get filled and there will be some valid prescriptions that are denied. Pharmacists know this. Pharmacists don't like it, but there is no avoiding it. Despite this reality, balance is a better approach than either of the two extreme positions.

Judicial Affirmation of Balanced Policy in Practice

Federal judges have a responsibility to justify the sentences they impose on convicted criminals. Although sentencing guidelines exist, judges may opt for non-guideline sentences if the nature and circumstances of the offense warrant. In 2011, Senior United States District Judge Jack Weinstein, of the Eastern District of New York, issued a written legal opinion explaining his reasons for a non-guideline sentence, and in doing, so he made some interesting observations about the challenges pharmacists face when dispensing opioid analgesics and monitoring their use.[7]

Judge Weinstein explained that the criminal defendant was the youngest son of "hard-working parents who were married and lived together in one home. There was apparently no physical, emotional, or substance abuse in that home." When the defendant was 18 years old, he was in a serious automobile accident and injured his back. He sought medical treatment from a pain specialist who prescribed oxycodone. The defendant soon began to receive oxycodone from multiple physicians, without telling any of the physicians about the others. The defendant claimed that none of the physicians warned him of the addictive qualities of oxycodone, nor was he told of this danger by pharmacists who dispensed his medications, although written information he received from the pharmacies included this warning.

According to Judge Weinstein, "The drug took control of his life. Predictably it began to unravel." The defendant dropped out of college and began to support his expensive addiction by selling oxycodone tablets, and this conduct led to his arrest, guilty plea, and criminal conviction.

Although the guidelines for this offense call for a range of imprisonment between 57 and 71 months, Judge Weinstein sentenced the defendant only to five years of probation. Judge Weinstein focused on the importance of cooperation between healthcare professionals and law enforcement. Referencing opioid analgesics used for chronic pain, he said:

"Physicians' and pharmacists' combined ethical and legal obligations in regard to distributing such pharmaceuticals can provide substantial protection against their abuse. Nevertheless, the physicians and pharmacists may themselves contribute to abuse, necessitating intervention by law enforcement. Although complicated, a working relationship between the medical community and law enforcement is essential to realizing the potential benefit that these substances hold for patients suffering from severe or chronic pain while avoiding their deleterious effects on society from rampant abuse and addiction."

Rather than blaming pharmacists for drug diversion, Judge Weinstein described the burdens placed on pharmacists when dispensing controlled substances. "When considering whether to fill a prescription for an opioid painkiller, pharmacists find themselves subject to pressures similar to those placed on physicians when initially deciding to issue the prescription. The pharmacists' constraints derive from their legal and ethical obligations."

Noting that "fear of investigation by federal or state authorities has proven to be a significant disincentive to pharmacists in filling prescriptions for opioid painkillers," Judge Weinstein acknowledged that "pharmacists act as gatekeepers." He recognized a responsibility of pharmacists to "assure that patients who need pain medications get them" and that "this force acts as a counterbalance to the pressures of intense scrutiny from government agencies."

Citing the American Pharmacists Association (APhA) Code of Ethics for the Profession of Pharmacy, Judge Weinstein concluded that pharmacists are ethically obligated "to consider the impact of filling a particular prescription not only on the individual but on society at large." The relevant section of the APhA

Code of Ethics states, "The primary obligation of a pharmacist is to individual patients. However, the obligations of a pharmacist may at times extend beyond the individual to the community and society. In these situations, the pharmacist recognizes the responsibilities that accompany these obligations and acts accordingly."

The compassionate approach taken by Judge Weinstein is typical of many judges who consider substance abuse disorder to be a medical condition that requires treatment, rather than a crime that must be punished. Judges resolve specific controversies with awareness of the broader public policy considerations that the controversies may raise. Chronic pain is primarily an individual patient problem, while substance abuse disorder is primarily a public health matter. Yet in many ways chronic pain raises public health issues, and substance abuse disorder is critically important for specific patients. It is impossible to say that under all circumstances one factor is more important than any other. A balancing of all considerations is essential to meeting professional responsibilities.

Challenges in the Application of a Balanced Approach

Pharmacists don't always get it right. Compassion for the needs of patients may get in the way of a pharmacist's responsibility to prevent opioid diversion and abuse. On the other hand, suspicions of ill motives by honest patients with unusual behaviors can interfere with a pharmacist's commitment to effective patient care.

Numerous legal cases have addressed the pharmacist's standard of care in evaluating opioid prescriptions. In many of these cases, the unfortunate result has been the death of a patient or another person who has used medication dispensed by a pharmacist for a patient under circumstances that allegedly should have been considered as suspicions. It may not be sufficient for a pharmacist to assure that an opioid prescription has been issued legally. It may also be necessary for a pharmacist to anticipate that appropriately prescribed opioids will be used inappropriately.

Pharmacist as a Gatekeeper

Courts are understandably reluctant to impose on pharmacists any onerous responsibilities for controlled substance prescription screening that could lead to denial of medications to patients with legitimate medical needs. On the other hand, there are circumstances in which courts cannot ignore the gatekeeper role of pharmacists when patients may be acquiring unnecessary controlled substance medications that could be put to unlawful use.

The judicial record in a New Mexico case revealed that a patient died from multiple drug toxicity.[8] The autopsy report identified oxycodone, oxymorphone, and alprazolam in her tissues. The patient's estate sued both the prescribing physician and the dispensing pharmacy. The undisputed facts showed that over a four-month period, the patient had, on at least seven occasions, been dispensed oxycodone by the pharmacy between two and twenty-three days "early." The patient's medications were covered by Medicaid, yet "on a few occasions" she had "paid a substantial amount of cash to purchase oxycodone from the pharmacy." On one occasion, she paid US$1,107 for oxycodone, although the prescription would have been covered by Medicaid several days later.

An expert witness for the defendant pharmacy testified that if a pharmacist "does not dispense medication in accordance with the medical doctor's prescription, that pharmacist risks interfering with the doctor/patient relationship and may be inappropriately practicing medicine without a license." In contrast, the plaintiff's expert testified that a pattern of "early" requests for medication "is highly suspicious of abuse and/or diversion and would preclude the pharmacist from filling the prescriptions."

The trial court dismissed the pharmacy from the case, ruling that the plaintiff's expert had not refuted the contentions of the defendant's expert. The plaintiff appealed the dismissal of the pharmacy from the case.

In its review, the Court of Appeals noted that the pharmacy's expert advocated "what amounts to a clerical-accuracy standard, requiring only that a retail pharmacist fill a prescription accurately, unless the prescription is facially invalid, or the pharmacist has personal knowledge that filling the prescription would harm a specific customer." The court referenced New Mexico statutes and regulations requiring that pharmacists identify potential problems with drug therapy, such as clinical abuse/misuse, prior to dispensing prescribed medication to a patient, and take appropriate steps to avoid or resolve these potential problems. The court cited a requirement that a pharmacist requests a prescription drug monitoring program (PDMP) report under a variety of circumstances including a patient "paying cash when the patient has prescription insurance."

The court recognized the existence of policy concerns associated with pharmacists "intruding into the doctor–patient relationship or practicing medicine without a license." However, the court noted that "a standard of care that requires nothing more of pharmacists than that they accurately fill an apparently valid prescription raises other policy concerns related to the potential harm to patients and to the public at large."

Applying policy concerns to the facts of the case, the court stated that "the circumstances presented here involve repeated early fills of opioid medications prescribed in combination with benzodiazepines, and at least one instance in which the patient paid a substantial amount of cash to purchase OxyContin from the pharmacy, although her prescriptions were paid with insurance on other occasions." Based on this analysis, the Court of Appeals reversed dismissal of the case against the pharmacy.

The court did not say that "too early" dispensing requests are necessarily problematic. What the court said is that consistent "too early" requests combined with large cash payments for medications covered by a program such as Medicaid should be cautiously evaluated before they are honored. A pharmacist who fails to resolve questions raised by such "too early" requests for medication cannot escape liability by using what the court disdainfully referred to as the "clerical accuracy standard."

Long-Term Liabilities for Short-Term Opioid Use

Many opioid-related legal cases are currently being pursued against pharmacies, alleging that a patient's brief period of opioid use years earlier caused the patient to become addicted to opioids and that the dispensing pharmacy should be held legally liable for causing the patient's overdose death years later. An Ohio appellate court explained why this theory of liability could be legally maintainable.[9]

A high school football player injured his shoulder during a football game, and he required surgery. His physician prescribed opioid medication one time prior to the surgery and four times following the surgery, all within a period of less than two months in late 2009. The court indicated that the pharmacy dispensed "260 opioids" to the patient during this two-month time frame. The patient allegedly "became addicted to drugs based on the initial opioid pills." The patient "entered rehabilitation five times to treat his drug addiction." However, despite periods of sobriety, he overdosed on fentanyl and oxycodone and died in the fall of 2017.

The patient's estate sued the pharmacy, contending that the "overdispensing of medication to the decedent caused him to become addicted to opioids and to ultimately overdose." A physician expert witness, who was qualified as a pain and an addiction specialist, testified that "there was a causal connection between the prescribed opioids in 2009, the decedent's diagnosis of opioid use disorder, and untimely death in 2017."

The trial court concluded that the estate "could not demonstrate that the pharmacy's actions were the proximate cause of the decedent's death." The trial court ruled that the expert's opinion was "speculative, and based on assumptions, not facts in the record." The case against the pharmacy was dismissed, and the patient's estate appealed.

The appellate court reviewed evidence presented by the pharmacy concerning the pharmacy's 2009 policy for pharmacist review of duplicate controlled substance prescriptions. The policy indicated that overprescribing of opioids would be flagged by the pharmacy computer, bringing the problem to the attention of the dispensing pharmacist. However, the court noted that there was "no testimony that demonstrated the pharmacy's policy of flagging a duplicate prescription occurred even if it was designed to do so." The pharmacy's electronic recordkeeping system had been purged of any records from 2009, so there was no way for the pharmacy to prove compliance at that time with the existing policy.

The appellate court also noted that the patient's opioid prescriptions maintained on file did not show that any telephone calls were made by a pharmacist to the prescriber. The court acknowledged that "the period between the dispensing of the drugs and the decedent's overdose is significant." However, the court concluded that "addiction is a long-term, chronic, and relapsing disease that is complex to evaluate in this context." The dismissal of the case against the pharmacy was reversed. The case was remanded back to the trial court for further proceedings against the pharmacy. The outcome of the case is not available in the public record. The plausibility of the estate's legal argument has been judicially recognized.

This judicial ruling is significant for several reasons. First, an allegation that five opioid prescriptions dispensed over a two-month period may be the legal cause of a patient's death eight years later can be legally pursued, despite how far-fetched it may seem. Second, simply because a pharmacy's policy from years ago required that a particular action be taken by a pharmacist does not support a legal conclusion that the action was taken at that time. If there is no written notation on an opioid prescription, then an expert witness may be allowed to speculate that the prescriber was not contacted by a pharmacist. Lastly, although concerns for the effects of opioid abuse disorder have expanded over time, judicial rulings may reflect perspectives of today rather than perspectives from the time care was provided. Current recognition of a crisis with opioid use disorder was not anticipated when these prescriptions were processed in 2009.

These observations suggest that effective pharmacy risk management programs must anticipate judgments that will be made years in the future. Pharmacies must create enduring records that will support future judicial evaluations of decisions made today.

Identifying a Patient with Opioid Use Disorder

A New Jersey case addressed a novel approach to pharmacist liability.[10] Rather than alleging that the defendant pharmacies were liable for causing a patient to become addicted to dispensed opioids, this case contended that the defendants' pharmacists knew, or should have known, that a patient was already addicted to opioids and that their negligent dispensing of opioids exacerbated the patient's preexisting condition.

The plaintiff was the estate of a deceased patient. The estate sued four pharmacies that had dispensed oxycodone to the patient, sometimes in combination with alprazolam. The patient allegedly died as the result of the defendants' negligence. The prescriber of the controlled substances was also sued, but that lawsuit was separated from the pharmacy litigation.

The lawsuit against the defendant pharmacies alleged that pharmacists honored prescriptions for the patient "that they knew or should have known were negligently, carelessly, and or recklessly prescribed, given their amount and frequency." The lawsuit alleged that the pharmacists "engaged in professional malpractice by not noticing that the amount and frequency of the prescriptions were for addictive medications outside reasonable practice, and by not refusing to fill those prescriptions."

The pharmacies moved to dismiss the lawsuit based on what is known as the "learned intermediary" doctrine, contending that it is the physician as a learned intermediary, and not the pharmacist as a dispenser, who has a duty to warn the patient. The pharmacies also contended that the lawsuit did not properly allege proximate cause, because it was the patient's underlying condition that caused her death, and not any action or inaction by the pharmacists. The trial court granted the pharmacies motion to dismiss the lawsuit, and the plaintiff appealed.

On appeal, the court first considered the defendants' defense based on the learned intermediary doctrine. The court recognized that the doctrine appropriately applies absolve pharmacists of a duty to warn when they accurately process prescriptions a a e ee "issued in amounts and at frequencies within reasonable medical standards." According to the doctrine, it is the prescriber, and not the pharmacist, who is the learned intermediary and who has the duty to warn the patient of medication-related risks. However, the plaintiff's lawsuit did not allege the breach of a duty to warn the patient of risks. The lawsuit alleged the breach of a duty to refuse the improperly issued prescriptions. Therefore, the learned intermediary doctrine was ruled to be inapplicable. The learned intermediary doctrine does not pertain to duty to refuse cases; the doctrine applies only to duty to warn cases. The doctrine cannot absolve pharmacists of liability when the allegation is that they should have refused opioid prescriptions.

The appellate court also disagreed with applicability of the defendants' proximate causation defense. The court noted that a plaintiff need not allege that a defendant's conduct was the only cause of the plaintiff's injury. Rather, "a plaintiff may recover if he establishes that professional negligence increased the risk of harm posed by a preexisting condition and the increased risk was a substantial factor in producing the harm." The dismissal of the plaintiff's lawsuit was reversed on appeal, and the case was remanded to the trial court for further proceedings against the pharmacies.

This case illustrates a variation of the legal principle known as the "eggshell plaintiff" doctrine. Under that doctrine, an allegedly negligent defendant must accept the plaintiff's condition as it existed when the plaintiff was presented to the defendant, even if that condition is as fragile or as delicate as an eggshell. The defendant cannot escape liability by arguing that the action taken by the defendant toward the plaintiff would have been harmless if the plaintiff had not been so susceptible to the harm.

The significance of this case is that pharmacists may have a legal duty to know a patient's underlying condition and to refuse pharmaceutical products or services that exacerbate the underlying condition. Pharmacists can know of an underlying condition based on a patient's medication history or information contained in the medication record. Suspicions about a patient's underlying condition that arise due to a pattern of medication use can be investigated by consulting with the patient or with the prescriber.

Patient with Inherited Chronic Pain

New patients who present an opioid prescription at a pharmacy raise particularly challenging concerns for the application of a balanced approach to prescription assessment. A pharmacist who receives a prescription from a new patient for a thirty-day supply of an opioid with a dose exceeding 60 mg oral morphine equivalent daily must face the reality that this is likely to be an inherited patient. For some reason, the patient has chosen to change pharmacies. While this change in pharmacies is perfectly within the rights of the patient, it is the pharmacist's right to know why the change is being made. Was the previous pharmacy biased against patients with pain? Was that pharmacy shorted on their order for the prescribed drug? Did the patient violate pharmacy rules, resulting in a decision by that pharmacy to no longer provide opioid medications to the patient? What does the previous pharmacy know, if anything, that the new pharmacy needs to know?

There will be some investigation necessary to find the answers to these basic questions, and the investigation may include contacting the former pharmacy or the prescriber of the opioids. It is not a violation of the Health Insurance Portability and Accountability Act for one pharmacy to contact another pharmacy, or the prescriber, to discuss issues of patient safety related to opioid prescriptions. Care must be taken not to make disparaging remarks when these conversations are held.

Under all circumstances, inherited patients need to be told the rules of the new pharmacy. The state PDMP must be consulted the first time an inherited patient presents an opioid prescription for filling. Inherited patients can be welcome additions, or they can spell big trouble.

Patient Education/Attestation

Just as patients to whom pseudoephedrine is being sold must attest that they will not cook the drug to manufacture methamphetamine, patients receiving opioids should verify that they understand their responsibilities as patients with pain. They need to take responsibility for (1) using the medication only as directed, (2) not sharing the medication with anyone, (3) not using alcohol or illicit drugs while using the medication, (4) storing the medication in a discreet and secure place, (5) disposing of the medication safely when it is no longer needed, and (6) not driving or using heavy machinery if the medication causes the patient to be drowsy.

This is an attestation process that can be conducted in the same way that patient attestation is used for the purchase of methamphetamine precursors. Perhaps the same hardware and software can be used. It need not be computerized, but it needs to be done. The main message is that opioid medications must be used only by the person for whom they have been prescribed, and they must be used as directed by the prescriber. The consequences of ignoring this important advice can be deadly.

Patients who attest to responsible use, and who later betray that trust, may forfeit their privilege of access to medications, and they need to be told of this possible consequence. Patients do not have a right to medication simply because they have a prescription. Pharmacists have a responsibility to meet their standard of care, and that standard may include the responsibility to decline an opioid prescription.

Patient's Responsibility

The conservative approach taken by most pharmacists to the screening of opioid prescriptions is completely understandable given the challenges that pharmacists have faced in litigation alleging liability for harm caused by opioids. In a West Virginia case, twenty-nine individuals sued various pharmacies, physicians, and clinics, alleging that the defendants caused the plaintiffs to become addicted to opioids.[11] These assertions were made despite the evidence that the plaintiffs had deliberately lied to pharmacists, duping the pharmacies into supplying unnecessary opioids to the plaintiffs.

All of the opioid abusers admitted to engaging in most, if not all, of the following illegal activities: criminal possession of pain medications; criminal distribution, purchase, and receipt of pain medications; criminally acquiring and obtaining opioids through misrepresentation, fraud, forgery, deception, and subterfuge (not advising doctors of addiction or receipt of opioids from other doctors); criminally obtaining opioids from multiple doctors concurrently; and abusing and/or misusing pain medication by ingesting greater amounts than prescribed and snorting or injecting the medications to enhance their effects.

The pharmacies sought to invoke the "wrongful conduct rule" as it had been adopted in other jurisdictions. The "wrongful conduct rule" takes the position that a plaintiff may not "profit" from wrongdoing when his or her unlawful conduct or immoral act caused or contributed to the injuries. The goal of the rule is to deter people from engaging in self-destructive behaviors because they know they can hold someone else legally liable for their own misconduct.

The West Virginia court was skeptical about the applicability of the "wrongful conduct rule" to this case. First, the suggestion that the absence of such a rule allows a plaintiff to "profit" from his wrongdoing is misguided, said the court. If a plaintiff is injured as the result of someone's negligence, merely obtaining compensation for his loss does not constitute a "profit." An award of compensatory damages for a person who has become addicted to drugs due to the negligence of another person is not a "profit."

Second, the idea that precluding personal injury suits by those who engage in criminal conduct serves as a deterrent to such conduct lacks credulity, said the court. Refusing to allow a patient to sue a pharmacist when the patient has become addicted to a drug dispensed by the pharmacist will not prevent the patient from becoming addicted. The disease of substance use disorder is more complicated than that.

The court concluded: "We find that in cases where a plaintiff has engaged in allegedly immoral or criminal acts, the jury must consider the nature of those actions, the cause of those actions, and the extent to which such acts contributed to their injuries, for purposes of assessment of comparative fault. In the instant case, there is an obvious threshold factual question which perfectly illustrates the potential inequity in applying a wrongful conduct bar: did the respondents suffer from preexisting addiction and abuse of controlled substances which was merely enabled by the petitioners, or was their addiction and abuse a result of the petitioners conduct? We hold that a plaintiff's immoral or wrongful conduct does not serve as a bar to his or her recovery for injuries."

Other states have ruled to the contrary and have adopted the wrongful conduct rule in cases filed against pharmacies by opioid abusers and diverters. The significance of this West Virginia case is that when a pharmacist provides opioids to a person who does not need them, and who is not telling the truth, then the pharmacist may be open to a lawsuit by the deceptive patient.

Pharmacists are targeted by fakers and liars who take advantage of pharmacists' trusting nature. As this case suggests, it can be difficult, if not impossible to tell the difference between a legitimate patient with chronic pain and a drug diverter or an abuser. Using a systematic approach to prescription screening can help, but it can't replace common sense. When an organized group of criminals decides to target a pharmacy, the pharmacist's instincts and street smarts must override any sympathy for patients.

In Pari Delicto

When a medication has caused harm, everyone involved with the distribution and use of that medication is potentially accountable for the harm, and this includes any person who abused the medication resulting in that person's death. A case from Pennsylvania applied the legal doctrine of *in pari delicto* (in equal fault) to absolve a pharmacy from liability following the death of a person who fraudulently acquired an opioid medication from the pharmacy.[12]

A lawsuit against the pharmacy was filed by the estate of a deceased college student. The decedent's mother suffered from multiple myeloma. She had on file at the defendant pharmacy a prescription for fentanyl patches that could be dispensed at her request. A friend of the decedent called the pharmacy pretending to be representing the decedent's mother, and the friend requested that the fentanyl patches be dispensed pursuant to the prescription. The decedent drove the friend to the pharmacy, and the friend picked up the fentanyl patches. The friend and the decedent each ingested the contents of a fentanyl patch. The decedent fell asleep and could not be awakened. He was pronounced dead after being transported to a hospital.

The lawsuit against the pharmacy alleged negligence by the pharmacy in allowing a person who was not a family member to acquire the medication with no questions asked. The pharmacy moved the court for dismissal of the lawsuit based on the *in pari delicto*. The pharmacy's motion was granted, and the estate appealed.

The appellate court first noted that the *in pari delicto* defense applies "when the plaintiff is an active, voluntary participant in the wrongful conduct or transaction for which he seeks redress and bears substantially equal or greater responsibility for the underlying illegality as compared to the defendant." The plaintiff contended that the doctrine was inapplicable in this case "because the decedent did not engage in anything that was immoral or illegal." Rather, it was the decedent's friend who had engaged in immoral and illegal conduct. The friend was named as a codefendant in the lawsuit, but only the pharmacy moved for dismissal of the case.

The appellate court disagreed with the plaintiff's contention. The court concluded that "by participating in the scheme to obtain fentanyl and by illegally possessing the fentanyl at the friend's house, the decedent was an active, voluntary participant in the wrongful conduct for which the plaintiff seeks redress and bears substantially equal or greater responsibility for the underlying illegality as compared to the pharmacy." The court affirmed the dismissal of the case against the pharmacy.

This case illustrates that pharmacists have a responsibility to provide medications to those who need them for medical treatment and also to prevent acquisition of medications by those who would divert and/or abuse them. It is not uncommon for a person other than the patient to pick up a controlled substance medication at a pharmacy. This is particularly true when the patient has a cancer diagnosis. If pharmacists routinely refused controlled substances under these circumstances, then many patients who need medications would not get them.

On the other hand, the DEA has advised that it can be considered a "red flag" when "a patient presents prescriptions written in the names of other people." A cancer diagnosis does not, by itself, justify ignoring indicators of controlled substance diversion. The plaintiff in the Pennsylvania case argued that the defendant pharmacy could have called the patient to verify her request for the fentanyl, and the medication would not have been dispensed if that call had been made. The court in this case engaged in a balancing of illegality, as courts often do. The court held that the decedent's illegal conduct tipped the balance away from liability of the pharmacy.

Using Cautious Language When Prescriptions Are Declined

Pharmacists are frequently put in a position where they cannot honor a controlled substance prescription. The inability to honor a prescription could be the result of factors that simply do not provide the pharmacist with the confidence necessary to conclude that the prescription has been issued for a legitimate medical purpose and in the usual course of professional practice. Communication to the patient of a pharmacist's inability to honor a prescription must be done with tact. The failure to use cautious language may result in a lawsuit for defamation being filed by the prescriber against the pharmacy. Patients will understandably want to know why their opioid prescription cannot be honored. Both pharmacists and the pharmacy technicians they supervise must refrain from untruthful and/or disparaging comments about the prescriber when the explanation is provided.

Allegedly incautious comments at a pharmacy led to litigation based on a physician's claim that a pharmacy's employees uttered false and defamatory statements to his patients, causing him to suffer embarrassment, damage to himself and his practice, and loss of clients from his pain management practice.[13] The pharmacy disputed that its employees made any actionable defamatory statements and contended that if the employees did make defamatory statements, then they were protected by a qualified privilege.

The physician contended that when the pharmacy declined his opioid prescriptions, the pharmacy, through its employees, defamed him with the following statements:

- "His license has been suspended or revoked."
- "He has been arrested, and if he hasn't been, he soon will be, therefore find a new doctor."
- "We no longer fill prescriptions for him because he has been to jail and is a bad doctor."
- "He is under DEA investigation."
- "We don't fill his prescriptions or prescriptions for any other pill mills."

The pharmacy contended that the statements were protected by what is known in the law as a "qualified privilege." A professional person is granted a qualified privilege to speak about matters that the law either allows or requires the professional person to speak about. In this case, the pharmacy asserted that the law requires a pharmacist to counsel a patient about the risks of medications that have been prescribed for the patient, and therefore any pharmacist who made the alleged comments did so under a qualified privilege while being engaged in legally mandatory patient counseling.

In response, the physician contended that the pharmacy's argument failed because the law that the pharmacy relied on applies only to licensed pharmacists. The physician contended that qualified immunity should not be applied because the pharmacy's employees who used this language were not pharmacists, but rather, they were pharmacy technicians. The physician argued that pharmacy technicians do not have the same duties and responsibilities as pharmacists and are not entitled to the protections of qualified privilege.

The court agreed with the physician that qualified privilege does not apply to pharmacy technicians. Pharmacy technicians are prohibited from providing advice or consultation to patients and from performing any activity required by law to be performed only by a pharmacist. In addition, the statements at issue were particularly disparaging and went beyond the scope of the purposes for which qualified privilege exists.

The result of this case, to put it bluntly, is that when a patient is told that a prescription cannot be honored, pharmacy personnel need to shut up about the prescriber. No editorializing about the quality or legality of the prescriber's practice should be offered. Period. Pharmacists can comment about the risks of drug therapy, but not about the qualifications or activities of the prescriber. A conversation of drug risks is likely protected by qualified privilege. Technicians must say nothing. Neither pharmacists nor technicians should say anything critical of the patient or of the drug. The prescription simply cannot be honored. It is a matter of patient safety and professional responsibility.

Conclusion

Pharmacists must accept responsibility for the death of people from the abuse of opioids that have been dispensed by pharmacists under questionable circumstances. Federal laws restrict access to controlled substances so that only those who need them may acquire them. Pharmacists implement those restrictions based on what they see and what they know when opioid prescriptions are presented for filling. A "trust but verify" approach must be used when questions about opioid prescriptions arise.

Key Takeaways

- Don't be responsible for opioid deaths due to your own inadvertence. Most opioid prescriptions are legitimate, but this reality should not lead pharmacists to relax their concerns about opioids when questionable circumstances arise. Patients are dying from the abuse of opioids. People who are not pharmacy patients are also dying from the abuse of opioids that have been diverted from use by patients to whom they have been dispensed. Vigilance by pharmacists in the evaluation of opioid prescriptions can save lives and can reduce pharmacist exposure to potential legal liability for the death of a patient.

- Take a balanced approach to opioid prescription screening. There are many patients who need opioid analgesics for the treatment of acute and chronic pain. These drugs continue to be approved by the US Food and Drug Administration (FDA) as safe and effective. Although some opioid critics contend that opioids should be removed from the market by the FDA, that drastic step has not been taken and likely will not be. In a balanced approach to opioid prescription screening, and to the monitoring of ongoing opioid use, pharmacists must not usurp the authority of the FDA regarding the safety and efficacy of opioids. The drugs are safe and effective when they are prescribed appropriately and when they are used consistent with the prescriber's instructions for use. It is the pharmacist's responsibility to review opioid prescriptions to ascertain potential problems with the prescriber's issuance of the prescriptions, and it is the pharmacist's responsibility to monitor a patient's use of opioids to ascertain whether the patient is using them safely as prescribed.
- Use a "tough love" approach toward your patients with chronic pain. Many chronic pain patients are accustomed to being treated disrespectfully by prescribers and by pharmacists. They have been told over and over again that the opioids they receive can lead to abuse and addiction if they are used for their euphoric effect rather than for their medicinal effect. Patients with chronic pain will appreciate respectful treatment by pharmacists who accept that chronic pain is a disease that warrants treatment rather than condemnation. Respect and responsibility go hand in hand. It is perfectly acceptable, in fact it is necessary, to impress on patients with chronic pain the responsibilities they have to safeguard their medication. In exchange for the privilege of receiving their opioid analgesic medications, patients must use the medication only as directed, not share the medication with anyone, avoid alcohol or illicit drugs while using the medication, store the medication in a discreet and secure place, dispose of the medication safely when it is no longer needed, and not drive or use heavy machinery if the medication causes the patient to be drowsy. Violation of these stipulations may result in loss of the privilege to receive opioid analgesics.

References

1. Oleckna v. Daytona Discount Pharmacy, 162 So.3d 178 (Fla.App. 2015).

2. Chua v. State, 710 S.E.2d 540 (Ga. 2011).

3. People v. Xuhui Li, 140 N.E.2d 965 (N.Y. 2019).

4. People v. Tseng, 241 Cal.Rpt.3d 194 (Cal.App. 2018).

5. 21 C.F.R. §1306.04. Purpose of issue of Prescription.

6. Pharmacy Doctors Enterprises d/b/a Zion Clinic Pharmacy, Federal Register. Vol. 83, No. 49, Pages 10876-10903 (March 13, 2018).

7. United States v. Ilayayev, 800 F.Supp. 417 (E.D.N.Y. 2011).

8. Oakey v. May Maple Pharmacy, 399 P.3d 939 (N.M.App. 2017).

9. Estate of Mehrer v. Walgreens Specialty Pharmacy, 218 N.E.3d 301 (OhioApp. 2013).

10. Shamey v. Gamao, 2013 Westlaw 6939135 (N.J.App. 2013).

11. Tug Valley Pharmacy v. All Plaintiffs Below, 773 S.E.2d 627 (W.V. 2015).

12. Albert v. Sheeley's Drug Store, 265 A.3d 442 (Penn. 2012).

13. Goulmamine v. CVS Pharmacy, 138 F.Supp.3d 652 (E.D.Va. 2015).

Chapter 11

Lethal, But Lawful Pharmaceuticals

Pharmaceutical manufacturers may be held liable for the lethal effects of a product that they distribute, if the product is defective and unreasonably dangerous. However, product liability cases can be difficult for a plaintiff to prove. Pharmaceutical products are legally considered to be unavoidably unsafe. The concept of "safety" is a relative concept when it comes to pharmaceutical products. Simply because a pharmaceutical product has caused harm to a patient does not mean that there will be product liability due to any harm that has occurred. All pharmaceuticals cause adverse effects in some patients. Some pharmaceuticals cause adverse effects in many patients. It would be illogical to hold manufacturers liable for all harm caused by their product, when harm to a patient is a risk that must be accepted in order to provide a therapeutic effect. The only way to completely avoid adverse drug effects is to remove all pharmaceuticals from the market. Obviously, this unbalanced solution would not only eliminate drug risks, but it would also eliminate beneficial drug therapy, to the detriment of patients and the public. To achieve balance between the benefits and risks of pharmaceutical products, drug product liability law has recognized necessary limitations on liability.

Drug Product Liability

Pharmaceutical manufacturers are not exposed to product liability for unpreventable adverse effects caused by their products. Unlimited exposure to liability could lead to withdrawal from the market of useful, but inherently risky drugs. Pharmaceutical manufacturers are exposed to product liability only when their products are deemed to have been marketed in a defective and an unreasonably dangerous condition. For any specific drug, what is reasonable and what is not reasonable depend, in large part, on the risk versus benefit calculation for the drug. The more beneficial a drug is for a patient, the more reasonable it is to risk harm to a patient from the use of the drug by a patient. This is true even if there is a risk that harm from the drug could be fatal.

Drug product liability is an important area of forensic pharmacy. If a death results from medication use, then the evidence may show that the death was caused by an aspect of the drug product itself rather than by a person who prescribed, dispensed, or otherwise directed the use of the drug product. Recognition of "thing responsibility" as opposed to "agent responsibility" can lead an investigation in a useful direction. Things do not have moral responsibility, while agents do have moral responsibility. Assigning blame to an inanimate object such as a drug (thing responsibility) can relieve a person (agent responsibility) of legal liability. A thorough understanding of drug product liability will facilitate the legal analysis of medication-related deaths.

A Legal Case Study of an Alleged Fatality Due to Pharmaceutical Product Defect

Legal case analysis can clarify how a pharmaceutical product that causes the death of a patient may be the focus of product liability litigation and perhaps excuse from liability healthcare professionals or others who were associated with a patient's use of the drug. A classic case from Indiana is as an excellent illustration of how product liability and professional liability can overlap.[1] The case resulted from the death of a 4-year-old child following the administration to the child of allegedly superpotent promethazine syrup (plain). The child was seen at a hospital emergency room with symptoms of coughing, choking, and diarrhea. A physician at the hospital gave the child's mother a prescription for promethazine syrup, and the physician instructed the mother to also administer Kaopectate to the child.

The mother had the prescription dispensed by a local pharmacy, where she received a generic version of the drug. That evening, the mother administered a first dose of promethazine, after which the child became extremely drowsy. The mother called the hospital, and a nurse told the mother that drowsiness is an expected side effect of promethazine. The mother checked the child a few hours later and discovered that the child was not breathing. The child was transported to the hospital where the child was pronounced dead on arrival. The parents sued the hospital, they sued the pharmacy, and they sued the pharmaceutical manufacturer based on a legal theory of product liability. All defendants moved the court for summary judgment, arguing that the facts could not support liability and that the case should be dismissed.

Toxicology testing showed lethal levels of promethazine in the child's postmortem tissues. Testing of the contents of the medication bottle showed that the product was superpotent. The attending physician concluded that the child "died of acute diarrheal enteritis" and that "promethazine intoxication" was a significant factor contributing to her death.

Pharmacy records did not include any notation as to the lot number of the stock bottle from which the syrup used in processing the prescription had been removed. Nevertheless, the manufacturer's end testing data indicated that each lot of recently manufactured promethazine syrup had been tested prior to its distribution, and each lot had met all the US Food and Drug Administration (FDA) strength requirements. Based on sale and distribution patterns for their product, representatives of the manufacturer contended that the product used by the pharmacy in filling the child's prescription must have been taken from one of the compliant lots of the product. There was evidence, however, that "for an earlier formulation of promethazine syrup, the concentration of promethazine was more likely to be defective." The court concluded that this earlier defective lot of promethazine syrup could have been used by the pharmacy to fill the child's prescription. If the pharmacy filled the prescription with promethazine syrup from an outdated or recalled stock bottle, then that could explain the overdose.

The trial court granted summary judgment in favor of the pharmacy and dismissed the case. From the dismissal of their case, the parents appealed. The appellate court noted that, in a product liability case, there is a presumption that a product is not defective. The plaintiffs must rebut that presumption. The appellate court ruled that the trial court had improperly dismissed the case before contested facts could be considered by a jury. Perhaps the laboratory testing was flawed, and the product was not superpotent. Perhaps the mother had administered an overdose of medication. Alternatively, the product might have been superpotent despite the manufacturer's testing data, even if the mother administered the appropriate dose. The pharmacy might have dispensed outdated and defective promethazine syrup. These are fact questions that must be considered by a jury. Because these important questions had not been resolved, the case was not in an appropriate posture for dismissal through summary judgment. The appellate court reinstated the case against the defendants because the facts were in dispute. The case was later settled out of court.

This case is important because it raises a variety of issues relevant to allegations of pharmaceutical product defects. Postmortem laboratory testing is important, but it is not foolproof. Circumstantial evidence is necessary to facilitate a complete understanding of how a patient has died and who may be responsible. The inability of a pharmacy to identify the manufacturer's lot number of a dispensed product may expose the pharmacy to product liability. Facts are rarely clear in cases like this, and it is up to a jury to decide what version of the facts to believe based on the evidence presented.

Product Liability and Pharmacy

Because the provision of pharmacy professional services is closely tied with the distribution of pharmaceutical products, lawsuits against pharmacists for malpractice sometimes resemble product liability lawsuits against manufacturers. Product liability lawsuits against pharmacies and/or pharmacists often arise when a patient has not been told of a potential adverse effect of a prescribed medication, and the patient sues both the pharmacy and the manufacturer without knowing who (if anyone) failed to inform whom of the adverse effect. One possibility is that the manufacturer warned the pharmacist through product labeling, and the pharmacist did not pass on that warning to the patient. This could be a case of pharmacy malpractice. Another possibility is that the manufacturer did not adequately warn the pharmacist. This could be a case of drug product liability as opposed to pharmacy malpractice. The product-focused allegation of warning defect (a product liability case) is often not clearly distinguished from the practice-focused allegation of failure to warn (a professional malpractice case). The difference between professional malpractice and product liability is an important distinction that courts must make in addressing the allegations within a lawsuit, because pharmacists and manufacturers fulfill very different roles in drug distribution and in drug therapy.

With the notable exception of extemporaneous compounding cases, pharmacists are rarely sued for a patient's death or for other harm caused by a defective pharmaceutical product. There may be litigation against a pharmacy if it is unclear whose responsibility it was for an alleged product defect. For example, in one case, a patient alleged that a pharmacist dispensed an antibiotic to her and that when the patient opened the vial she noticed "a foul odor" that alarmed her.[2] The patient called the pharmacist, and the pharmacist told the patient that this was to be expected and that she should take the medication despite the foul odor. The patient alleged that after taking the medication she "experienced nausea, vomiting of blood, upper abdominal pain, and epigastric burning." Her lawsuit against both the pharmacy and the manufacturer contended that either the medication had been improperly manufactured or the pharmacy had contaminated the medication after receiving it from the manufacturer. A judgment was entered in favor of both defendants because the patient was unable to prove who was responsible for the defect in the product or that there was even any defect at all. The product had been consumed and could not be tested.

Plaintiffs bear the burden of proving their allegations, and when a product is not available for testing, it is virtually impossible to prove that the product was defective. This case illustrates the potential for pharmacist liability based on an inappropriate response by a pharmacist to a patient's inquiry. Had the patient been able to produce the product for analysis, the result might have been different. Patient concerns about pharmaceutical product quality should never be dismissed without the inspection of the product by a pharmacist.

Types of Pharmaceutical Product Defects

There are four basic ways in which a pharmaceutical product can be legally considered to be defective and subject to product liability. These four types of pharmaceutical product liability are based on manufacturing defect, warning defect, design defect, and marketing defect. Because pharmaceutical products are produced according to exacting standards, with close FDA oversight and frequent facility inspections, it is rare for there to be a successful manufacturing defect case involving pharmaceutical products. It is not impossible, of course, for a defectively manufactured product to cause harm leading to liability, but it is uncommon. Warning defect cases allege that the manufacturer knew of an adverse effect that could occur from the use of its drug but withheld that information from those who used the drug, causing harm to the users. Design defect cases allege that a product was intended to treat a condition for which it was actually more detrimental than beneficial. For example, a medication that treats atrial fibrillation but elevates blood pressure could be subject to a design defect claim because the very patients who use it might be those in whom it would be potentially fatal. Design defect claims like this are rare, but they are not unheard of. Marketing defect claims are also unusual, because they are based on a theory of product overpromotion that is difficult to causally connect with patient harm. By far, the most common type of product liability claim is that of a warning defect.

Warning Defect

In general, the allegations of a warning defect lawsuit are based on the plaintiff's claim that a known adverse effect was not disclosed in the pharmaceutical product's labeling and that if the warning had been included, then the drug either would not have been used or would have been used in a safer manner. Most warning defect cases base their allegations on the contents of the package insert, and they contend that the adverse effect either was not described in the package insert or was described so vaguely as to be ineffective.

The adequacy of the warning is a question that must be addressed through expert testimony and must then be decided by a jury. Experts in communication effectiveness can evaluate whether the warnings provided by the product labeler used words that appropriately reflected the nature of the risk. In warning defect lawsuits, words like "serious," "major," and "unexpected" are examined by experts to determine whether they would be interpreted by a person reading them to sufficiently convey an accurate message about a drug's risks. Labeling is viewed in its entirety. The experts might conclude that an otherwise adequate warning was undermined by additional contradictory language that was associated with the drug.

The package insert is directed to health professionals, and this is the basis of the often-utilized "learned intermediary rule" that protects manufacturers from liability. Under this rule, the manufacturer has a duty to the patient, yet that duty to the patient can be met by providing a warning to the patient's healthcare professionals rather than directly to the patient. Under most circumstances, manufacturers do not have a duty to warn patients directly because they don't have a direct contact with patients. Manufacturers never see patients. In addition, manufacturers do not know the unique physiology or pathology of any specific patient, so warnings by a manufacturer to a patient would not necessarily reflect that patient's individual need for information. The learned intermediary rule allows manufacturers to escape liability to a patient for warning defect, as long as the warning provided in the package insert is sufficient for a health professional to appreciate the significance of the risk.

Defendants in warning defect cases have often asserted what is generally referred to as the "government standards defense." Under this defense, the argument made is that the FDA approves all product labeling word for word, and for this reason, there should be no second-guessing of the FDA by courts of law in product liability cases. Essentially, the argument is that if the FDA says a warning is good enough, then it must be good enough. This argument has succeeded at times and failed at other times. The reality is that the FDA is a reactive agency. It evaluates labeling submitted to the agency by a manufacturer, based on scientific information provided by the manufacturer. If the manufacturer has withheld or mischaracterized the science, then the decision made by the FDA is subject to reevaluation by a court of law. A court may conclude that the manufacturer did not do anything deceptive with the FDA, yet the product warnings are still inadequate, and the manufacturer will be held liable simply for having placed the product on the market in a defective condition.

A Case of Alleged Inadequate Warnings

A patient was prescribed canagliflozin for the treatment of type 2 diabetes.[3] She alleged that, after two weeks of usage of the drug, she began losing weight and suffered nausea and vomiting. She was admitted to the hospital where she was diagnosed with diabetic ketoacidosis (DKA). Her lawsuit against the manufacturer alleged that the product had been accompanied with inadequate warnings, and that if the manufacturer had properly disclosed the risks associated with the product, she would not have used it because safer alternatives were available.

The lawsuit alleged that at the time she used this medication, the package insert did not warn of the risk of DKA and only stated that "a possible side effect was kidney problems." She claimed that the manufacturer "withheld knowledge that Invokana can cause serious complications, including diabetic ketoacidosis, from plaintiff, other consumers, their physicians, the medical community, and the public." The defendant manufacturer filed a motion to dismiss the case.

In considering the motion to dismiss, the court noted that to establish an inadequate warning claim, a plaintiff must show that (1) the defendant knew, or had reason to know, that the product is likely to be dangerous for the intended use; (2) the defendant had no reason to believe that the user would realize the danger; and (3) the defendant failed to exercise reasonable care to inform the user about the danger. The court further noted the plaintiff's allegation that soon after the product entered the market, numerous reports of adverse reactions, including DKA, were reported to the manufacturer. In addition, the package insert warned against using the product to treat patients with DKA, possibly showing that the manufacturer was aware of an adverse relationship between the drug and DKA. The court ruled that the plaintiff had sufficiently alleged that the defendant manufacturer knew that there was a risk of the product causing DKA. The manufacturer's motion to dismiss was denied.

This case demonstrates that when a drug is initially released onto the market, adverse effects that were not identified or were not significantly appreciated during clinical trials may become evident. There is a duty to update product labeling to reflect new information discovered during the initial period of marketing. The defendant in this case may have met that duty. But the allegations in the lawsuit were sufficient to avoid dismissal of the lawsuit and allow the continuation of litigation until the case was ultimately settled out of court.

Unreasonable Marketing

An unreasonable marketing lawsuit was filed by the mother of a patient who used dexfenfluramine for several months and who died from primary pulmonary hypertension caused by the use of the drug.[4] The lawsuit alleged that the manufacturer had introduced into the market a drug that was "unreasonably dangerous for anyone to use" and that the drug "was so unreasonably dangerous and defective in design that it should never have been on the market." The manufacturer defended the case by arguing that the only basis on which a drug product liability case could be litigated was the presence of impurities in the product or deficient warnings. The trial court dismissed the case, and the plaintiff appealed. An intermediate appellate court reversed the dismissal, and the defendant manufacturer appealed this reversal. The state supreme court then reviewed the case.

The court noted that the plaintiff had chosen to characterize the basis of her lawsuit as "unreasonable marketing," and the defense argued that this was not a recognized category of drug product liability. The court replied that "A company that is responsible for tendering into the market a drug which it knows or should know is so dangerous that it should not be taken by anyone can be said to have violated its duty of care either in design or in marketing. A manufacturer's negligent conduct can occur at any stage of the marketing process: in the initial design of the drug, in the failure to investigate information about the risks the drug poses, and in its decision to continue to sell the drug despite those unreasonable risks. The defendant's unreasonable behavior at any point in this process should be sufficient to give rise to liability when that conduct results in injury. In other words, the substantive allegations are more important than the labels."

The plaintiff explained that the reason she did not present her lawsuit as a traditional "failure to warn" claim was that, in her view, no warning concerning the product would be sufficient. She contended that the law establishes a duty, on the part of manufacturers, which can be viewed as a continuum from the initial warning of dangers, through a stronger warning if justified by emerging knowledge of previously unforeseen risks, through nonmarketing or discontinuance of marketing when it becomes or should become known that a product simply should not be used in the light of its relative risks. The court agreed that this continuum is within the scope of the general framework of a manufacturer's legal responsibility. And the court noted that if the plaintiff chose to characterize her lawsuit as being for unreasonable marketing, then "this is consistent with her prerogative as master of her own claim."

The court concluded that the "primary responsibility for drug safety rests with the manufacturer, which has superior access to information about its drugs, especially in the post-marketing phase as new risks emerge." The court ruled that pharmaceutical manufacturers violate their duty of care if they introduce a drug into the market, or continue to market a previously introduced drug, with actual or constructive knowledge that the drug is too harmful to be used by anyone. The court allowed the case to proceed to trial, although it was then settled out of court.

This case teaches that courts understand the special position of pharmaceutical manufacturers as the best experts regarding the risks and benefits of the drugs that they have developed and have newly introduced into the marketplace. Health professionals have little or no experience with newly released drugs, and they rely on manufacturers to provide them with products that are not so dangerous that they will harm any patient who uses them. This is particularly the case when drugs are potentially fatal, and they are intended for a purpose such as weight loss for which there are nonpharmaceutical options that can be used.

Product Defect and Medication Errors

A hospital in California made an error, using 10,000 unit/mL of heparin to clear a heparin-lock, rather than the standard 10 unit/mL strength.[5] The pediatric patients with whom this error occurred were twins who appear to have made a full recovery. The parents sued the manufacturer of the heparin products, alleging that the products were "unreasonably dangerous because the labels of both vials had a blue background that made them difficult to distinguish." They further alleged "that the background colors should have been different and that the vials should have been completely distinguishable in size and shape." They contended that the defendant manufacturer was negligent because they (1) failed to recall or repackage the 10,000 units/mL vial of heparin or issue an urgent warning to healthcare professionals, when it had actual knowledge of infant deaths that occurred as a result of medication errors, (2) sold different strengths with the same blue background, (3) failed to issue an urgent warning about the fatal medication errors to all healthcare professionals who purchased the product or failed to initiate mandatory education and implement safety measures so that a fatal medication error would not occur, and (4) failed to provide an adequate after-market solution to the existing vials and to assure that none of the existing vials were used until the after-market solution was implemented.

Even though the harm had occurred in California, the plaintiffs filed their lawsuit in Illinois because the defendant manufacturer was headquartered in Illinois and many of the witnesses to actions taken, or not taken, by the manufacturer would be located in or near corporate headquarters. The defendant manufacturer speculated that the plaintiffs were actually forum shopping, looking for a favorable place to file the lawsuit in the belief that their chances of winning were greater in Illinois than in California. The manufacturer filed a motion to dismiss the case in Illinois based on the doctrine of "forum non conveniens" (loosely translated as "not the appropriate place for this lawsuit"). The argument made by the defendant was that the allegations of product defect were so closely tied to the medication error in the hospital that the lawsuit should be heard in California to provide complete context for consideration of the liability of the hospital and of the manufacturer. An Illinois court cannot subpoena witnesses from California, so a lawsuit in Illinois might not be able to provide the full factual story for a jury. The lower court granted this motion to dismiss, and the plaintiffs appealed.

The appellate court evaluated the contentions of both parties. The court noted that the injury occurred in California and "the fact that the injury occurred in California is not fortuitous, since this is where the plaintiffs live and where the twins were born." While the plaintiffs alleged that "the culpable acts occurred in Illinois, the hospital staff's medication error occurred in California," and the court concluded that these two factors were a "wash." Acknowledging that courts often defer to a plaintiff's choice of where to file a lawsuit, the court nevertheless concluded that the plaintiff's choice of Illinois in this case was "entitled to less deference because Illinois is neither their residence nor the site of the injury." The court also acknowledged the inability of the defendant manufacturer to "secure unwilling witnesses" from the hospital in California if the case were to proceed in Illinois. The court affirmed the dismissal of the case in Illinois. Whether the case was ever refiled in California is unclear.

This case explains that the question of whether a pharmaceutical product is defective and unreasonably dangerous may depend on the context within which the product was used. It is possible that the drug was defective. It is also possible that the manner of drug use by hospital personnel was blameworthy. Perhaps both the drug and the manner of its use were to blame. Separating out the issues of medication error and product defect may not provide the depth of analysis that is necessary to resolve a lawsuit after harm has occurred from drug use. These two issues must be considered together by a court that has access to all parties who were involved in the incident.

Alleged Labeling Deficiencies

A lawsuit resulted after a nurse in a hospital mistakenly retrieved and administered 14.6% NaCl when the order was for normal saline.[6] This error resulted in massive, permanent disability for a newborn patient. The patient's conservator settled with the hospital and then sued the manufacturer for failure to provide adequate warnings with its concentrated NaCl product. The manufacturer moved to dismiss the lawsuit, claiming that (1) it had provided adequate warnings to the hospital, (2) it had a right to assume that hospital employees would follow warnings on the product, (3) the action was legally barred since the product was administered by a sophisticated user, and (4) any absence of warning was not the cause of the patient's injury. The plaintiff opposed dismissal, arguing that "the defendant manufacturer failed to provide any warning to the hospital of the particular form of risk here: that concentrated saline could be mistaken for diluted saline." The plaintiff argued that the manufacturer's product warning was inadequate because the manufacturer ignored an FDA letter, and it failed to specifically notify its customers of the risk of mistaken injection of concentrated saline, as well as the fact that such injections were a "foreseeable misuse," which the manufacturer's warnings did not prevent.

The court described the facts of the case, which warrant a lengthy narrative.

When he was born, the patient had good color and respiratory effort. Shortly afterward, he went limp and required resuscitation. Because of his low blood sugar, he was started on intravenous (IV) fluids and transferred to the Neonatal Special Care Unit (NSCU). A nurse in the NSCU detected a low blood pressure reading, and she contacted the patient's attending physician. The physician ordered "Piggyback normal saline, 20 cc over 30 minutes." At this time, the patient was not hyponatremic and he did not have an electrolyte imbalance.

A second nurse overheard the first nurse repeat the physician's order on the telephone, and the second nurse asked if she could help. The first nurse said, "Yes, if you could draw it up." The second nurse did not read the order that was transcribed by the first nurse. Instead, relying on what she had overheard, she understood that the physician had ordered normal saline.

The second nurse removed a vial from the NSCU medication cart. The medication cart contained, in drawers on different levels, both normal saline and 14.6% NaCl. The nurse did not read the label on the vial she retrieved. The nurse later testified that she knew the order was for normal saline, "because you would never add 20 mL of sodium chloride to an IV solution, it would be too large an amount to add to an IV." Nevertheless, the second nurse drew up 20 mL of 14.6% NaCl and gave the syringe to the first nurse. Less than an hour later, the physician again ordered 20 mL of normal saline to be injected into a port in the patient's IV tubing, and the second nurse again drew up 20 mL of 14.6% NaCl in a syringe that she handed to the first nurse.

The second nurse testified that "as soon as I retrieved the empty vials from the trash, I knew it was the wrong concentration," because "it's on the label." She testified, "I made a mistake," and "my thought process did not continue where it should have."

The court stated that the package insert for the 14.6% NaCl said:

> CONCENTRATE
>
> CAUTION: MUST BE DILUTED FOR IV USE
>
> 14.6% SODIUM CHLORIDE Injection
>
> ADDITIVE SOLUTION
>
> CONCENTRATED SOLUTION
>
> FOR USE ONLY AFTER DILUTION WITH COMPATIBLE IV FLUIDS

The external packaging of the vial read:

> CONCENTRATE
>
> CAUTION: MUST BE DILUTED FOR IV USE

14.6%

SODIUM CHLORIDE

The court then described the level of knowledge at the hospital at the time of the medication error. The hospital's director of pharmacy testified that "He knew dispensing medications from floor stock could increase the risk of medication errors. He also knew that nurses could make mistakes when they were using sodium chloride. For instance, he knew that nurses could select the wrong concentration, draw up too much or too little of the right concentration, and not dilute it properly before administration. They could administer it in improper ways, by improper routes, and to the wrong patients." The director of pharmacy knew at the time of the error that one approach to reducing the risk of medication errors was to reduce floor stock items. It was standard hospital practice for the pharmacy to control the dispensing and administration of drugs in order to minimize error, and the director of pharmacy stated he had read literature on the subject. The director of pharmacy testified that he was well aware "that there was a risk of serious adverse reaction if an excessive dose of concentrated sodium chloride was administered to a newborn by IV, and if a doctor had prescribed normal saline but 14.6% NaCl was inadvertently administered instead."

Members of the hospital's nursing and medical staff provided similar testimony regarding their knowledge of the potential for harm from the IV use of 14.6% NaCl.

The plaintiff alleged that, two years prior to the incident, the FDA had sent a letter to manufacturers of 23.4% NaCl, recommending that they add to the product labeling a warning that inadvertent direct injection of concentrated NaCl may give rise to hypernatremia and produce very serious medical results. There was no evidence that the manufacturer defendant in this case ever received that letter. Yet as soon as the defendant manufacturer became aware of it, eighteen months later, the labeling of the 14.6% NaCl was changed in consultation with the FDA.

In light of this evidence, the court said: "In the present case, the facts surrounding the inadvertent injection of concentrated saline are not disputed. The external product label warns—in red ink—that the product is 14.6% sodium chloride, and that it is 'CONCENTRATE,' requiring 'CAUTION: MUST BE DILUTED FOR IV USE.' The package insert further warns of the specific mechanism of injury in the present case: that 'inadvertent direct injection or absorption of concentrated sodium chloride solution may give rise to sudden hypernatremia.' The insert states that sodium overload can occur with intravenous infusion of excessive amounts of sodium-containing solutions." The insert also stated that the product "must be diluted before infusion to avoid a sudden increase in the level of plasma sodium."

Applying the law to the facts of the case, the court made several observations. First, "there is no duty to warn of dangers actually known to the user of a product." Second, "a product is not unreasonably dangerous when its degree of danger is obvious, generally known, or recognized. If a danger is obvious, then its obviousness constitutes a warning, and the product seller's failure to provide a separate warning should not constitute a defect." Third, "there is no duty imposed on a manufacturer to warn or protect against dangers, hazards, or risks which are patent, open, or obvious, and which should have been realized by a reasonable user of the product."

The court concluded that "the plaintiff's injuries were caused when the nurse, although certainly aware that an infant should not be directly injected with 14.6% concentrated sodium chloride, and by her own admission simply stopped thinking, failed to read the label clearly identifying the product as 14.6% concentrated sodium chloride. Hospital pharmacy personnel knew that dispensing medications from floor stock could create additional risks of medication errors. The decision to floor-stock concentrated sodium chloride was made after weighing the risk of medication error against its patients' medical needs."

The defendant manufacturer's motion to dismiss the case was granted.

This case demonstrates that there are limits to the effectiveness of warnings placed on product labeling. The plaintiff in this case claimed that the manufacturer should have provided some sort of warning that would require the user of the concentrated NaCl product to read the labeling of the vial prior to its use and appreciate the meaning of the labeling. This is sometimes referred to as a "forcing function" that makes errors virtually impossible. The court held that there is no legal duty to warn a product user of something that the user already knows. Better warnings cannot prevent all human errors.

Product Adulteration

There are relatively few reports of pharmaceutical products that have been intentionally adulterated by healthcare professionals for nefarious purposes. As few as they may be, these reports warrant significant attention. They may represent rare outliers of healthcare criminality, or they may be the tip of an unseen iceberg that would expose extensive pharmaceutical homicide on closer inspection.

The federal Food, Drug and Cosmetic Act defines adulteration.[7] Here is an abridged version of the statutory language.

A drug or device shall be deemed to be adulterated—

(a) Poisonous, insanitary, etc., ingredients; adequate controls in manufacture

(1) If it consists in whole or in part of any filthy, putrid, or decomposed substance; or (2)(A) if it has been prepared, packed, or held under insanitary conditions whereby it may have been contaminated with filth, or whereby it may have been rendered injurious to health; or (B) if it is a drug and the methods used in, or the facilities or controls used for, its manufacture, processing, packing, or holding do not conform to or are not operated or administered in conformity with current good manufacturing practice to assure that such drug meets the requirements of this chapter as to safety and has the identity and strength, and meets the quality and purity characteristics, which it purports or is represented to possess.

(b) Strength, quality, or purity differing from official compendium

If it purports to be or is represented as a drug the name of which is recognized in an official compendium, and its strength differs from, or its quality or purity falls below, the standard set forth in such compendium. Such determination as to strength, quality, or purity shall be made in accordance with the tests or methods of assay set forth in such compendium.

(c) Misrepresentation of strength, etc., where drug is unrecognized in compendium

If it is not subject to the provisions of paragraph (b) of this section and its strength differs from, or its purity or quality falls below, that which it purports or is represented to possess.

(d) Mixture with or substitution of another substance

If it is a drug and any substance has been (1) mixed or packed therewith so as to reduce its quality or strength or (2) substituted wholly or in part, therefore.

Any action taken by a pharmacist that results in a drug being contaminated with a foreign substance, as well as any action that results in a drug being held under insanitary conditions that may result in contamination, will cause the drug to be legally deemed adulterated. In addition, any action by a pharmacist that results in a drug being dispensed in a strength other than the strength that it purports to represent will cause the drug to be deemed adulterated.

Intentional Chemotherapy Dilution

A Kansas City, Missouri pharmacist, Robert Courtney, was accused of diluting chemotherapy drugs that were intended for patients with cancer who died but would have recovered had the full-strength medication been administered to them.[8] Evidence showed that Courtney diluted the chemotherapy drugs before distributing the drugs for administration to patients with cancer. Courtney billed for the full strength of the diluted products. His profit-making scheme was detected when one of the physicians who ordered the medications from the pharmacist was questioned by a pharmaceutical sales representative about why the physician was not using more of the drug. The physician realized that he was ordering more of the drug from the pharmacist than the manufacturer's records indicated, which was being purchased by the pharmacist from the manufacturer. The difference between the amount of drug that was supposedly being provided by Courtney for patient care and the amount of drug that Courtney was purchasing from the manufacturer suggested that the medication being provided by Courtney was being diluted contrary to the physician's order.

The physician took a sample of the pharmacist's chemotherapy product to a laboratory, and the lab reported that the sample contained only 32% of the drug that it was supposed to contain. The physician then met with the FDA and the Federal Bureau of Investigation agents. The federal agents tested seven additional samples of Gemzar and Taxol that Courtney had supplied for the doctor's patients. They found that the doses contained from 17% to 50% of the chemotherapy drugs they were supposed to contain. The federal agents then had the doctor order doses of Platinol, Zofran, Gemzar, Taxol, and Paraplatin from Courtney using fictitious patient names. Lab testing revealed that these samples contained from 0% to 65% of the dosages that the doctor had ordered and that Courtney had represented they contained by processing them and labeling them as being full-strength medications.

Authorities executed a search warrant at Courtney's pharmacy, and he was arrested and indicted. He pleaded guilty to eight counts of product tampering causing serious bodily injury and twelve counts of adulterating or misbranding a drug. Courtney was sentenced to thirty years in prison.

New England Compounding Center (NECC)

NECC was a pharmaceutical manufacturing facility that pretended to be a compounding pharmacy in hopes that it could escape the FDA regulatory oversight as a manufacturer. NECC compounded sterile products from nonsterile ingredients, in large quantities, for as yet unknown patients who would use the drugs under the care of as yet unknown physicians, by sending these products across state lines where they were to be used in patient care at some future time. Unfortunately, in the fall of 2012, dozens of patients died, and hundreds were injured when three batches of injectable methylprednisolone acetate were contaminated with fungus caused a national outbreak of spinal meningitis.

Two NECC pharmacists, Barry Cadden[9] and Glenn Chin,[10] were charged with second-degree murder and with numerous other regulatory violations. The government alleged that the unlawful activities of the pharmacists included, among other things, the pharmacists' failure to properly sterilize drugs, failure to properly test drugs for sterility, and failure to wait for test results before sending the drugs to customers. Both of these now-former pharmacists (licenses revoked) were convicted in federal court of racketeering, fraud, and conspiracy. They were found not guilty of second-degree murder in their federal trial. States in which patients died from the use of contaminated NECC products have filed their own charges against these two former pharmacists, and those charges include murder. The only clear lesson from the NECC cases is that a pharmacy practice business plan that pushes the envelope in the direction of unlawful activity runs the risk of crossing the line into illegality and exposing the involved pharmacists to criminal liability for patient deaths.

Other cases in the NECC aftermath provide more useful examples of what ought not to be done when one finds oneself working at a questionable pharmacy practice site where the lives of patients are placed at risk. The two principal pharmacists at NECC were not the only people against whom criminal charges were brought. When a pharmacy's unlawful actions result in patient deaths, every member of the pharmacy team at that practice site will be subjected to government scrutiny and to possible criminal prosecution.

Criminal Liability of Pharmacists in Packing Area

In one of the many other NECC cases, three pharmacists who worked in the NECC "packing area" faced criminal charges for aiding and abetting the misbranding of drugs.[11] The defendant pharmacists allegedly "checked drug orders before shipment to NECC customers."

A lower court dismissed criminal charges against the pharmacists because their activities in the packing area did not fit the definition of "dispensing." Under federal law, a drug is deemed misbranded if it has been dispensed without a legitimate prescription. The lower court judge relied on the dictionary definition of the term "dispensing" because it is undefined under federal law. The court ruled that one cannot be guilty of misbranding if one's activities did not constitute dispensing, and the case against the pharmacists was dismissed because packing and shipping dispensed drugs is not dispensing. The government appealed the dismissal.

In support of its appeal, the government alleged that shipments checked by the pharmacists were based on prescriptions for "fake patients" with names such as "Wonder Woman," "Flash Gordon," "L. L. Bean," "Coco Puff," and "Filet O'fish." Therefore, the government alleged that the drugs were misbranded, and the pharmacists had violated the misbranding provisions of federal law, because the pharmacists knew from these fake names that there was no legitimate prescription for the drugs they packed and shipped.

The appellate court considered the pharmacists' argument that they had "acted not as NECC pharmacists but as shipping clerks, performing clerical tasks, like checking addresses on packages." The pharmacists insisted they did not understand from the language of federal law "that they could be criminally liable for helping fill prescriptions they never signed off on, let alone caught sight of."

The court disagreed with the pharmacists' assertion that their role "was limited to confirming that the correct drugs were being sent to the correct facility and did not include checking the prescriptions or patient names or any other aspect of the dispensing process." The court concluded that the language "viewed in context and with common sense connotes the kind of checking that pharmacists regularly do when filling prescriptions, i.e., confirming that legit prescriptions triggered the drug shipments."

The court rejected the argument by the pharmacists that "a nonpharmacist could easily have performed the tasks" assigned to them in the packing area and that they should not be held to the standard of a pharmacist. The court ruled that a pharmacist is held to pharmacy standards regardless of the tasks being performed.

The general lesson of this case is that pharmacists may have legal responsibility for the aspects of the practice system in which they do not actively participate, if the pharmacists are aware of suspicious activities in those other parts of the system. Simply because tasks assigned to a pharmacist and performed by a pharmacist may legally be undertaken by a nonpharmacist, it does not relieve the pharmacist of professional responsibilities associated with the performance of those tasks.

Criminal Liability of a Clean Room Pharmacist

The pharmacist defendant in another NECC case was described as the "Clean Room Pharmacist" at NECC.[12] He was not associated with any of the contaminated injectable methylprednisolone that led to the NECC tragedy.

However, investigations following the tragedy disclosed that the pharmacist had allegedly been involved with other fraudulent activities.

The government asserted that the pharmacist had supervised a pharmacy technician whose license had been revoked. The pharmacist knew of the revocation and advised the technician to conceal the fact that he was working in the clean room by falsely certifying his lab work through the use of the NECC chief pharmacist's initials. The jury also learned that the pharmacist "frequently used expired ingredients in filling customer orders, did not properly test drugs before they were shipped, and that he instructed the technician to do the same." The pharmacist allegedly instructed the technician to leave the clean room whenever state inspectors or NECC customers visited and instead to pretend to be working as a stockman in the warehouse.

The pharmacist was convicted of fraud, and he appealed. The appellate court acknowledged that the pharmacist "did not directly interact with any of NECC's customers." However, "the question is not whether the pharmacist made direct misrepresentations to customers but whether he was a knowing participant in a scheme or artifice to defraud, or for obtaining money or property by means of false or fraudulent pretenses."

The court said, "The government need not prove that the defendant devised the fraudulent scheme; but it must prove willful participation in the scheme with knowledge of its fraudulent nature and with intent that these illicit objectives be achieved."

The pharmacist's alleged deception regarding the pharmacy technician's license revocation was a key factor. Several pharmacy directors who were customers of NECC testified that the credentialing of NECC personnel was "vital" to their decision to purchase NECC products. They had repeatedly been told by NECC salespersons that all NECC pharmacy staff were "licensed or registered or certified, whatever the requirements were by the state, prior to making the product." The pharmacist's fraud conviction was affirmed.

The hard lesson of this case is that those who associate with people who are committing illegal acts may be found guilty by association. Investigators will cast their net wide in search of any wrongdoing. While looking for improprieties on the periphery of a notorious illegal act, investigators will focus on unrelated suspicious activities that could otherwise go undetected, and they will initiate criminal prosecution of those involved with illegal activities.

Lethal Adulteration of Intravenous Solution

In September 2022, Raynaldo Riviera Ortiz Jr., a Texas anesthesiologist, was charged with injecting nerve blocking and bronchodilation drugs into IV bags at a surgical center where he worked, resulting in at least one death and multiple cardiac emergencies.[13] According to court documents, a physician coworker of the defendant experienced a medical emergency and died immediately after treating herself for dehydration using an IV bag of saline taken from the surgical center.

An autopsy report revealed that she died from a lethal dose of bupivacaine. According to the criminal complaint, surgical center personnel identified ten additional unexpected cardiac emergencies that occurred during otherwise unremarkable surgeries between May and August 2022, which the complaint alleged to be an exceptionally high rate of complications over such a short period of time.

In each of those cases, medical personnel were able to stabilize the patient only through the use of emergency measures. Most of the incidents occurred during longer surgeries that used more than one IV bag, including one or more bags retrieved mid-surgery from a stainless steel bag warmer.

The complaint alleged that, in one instance captured in the surveillance video, Ortiz was observed walking quickly from an operating room to the bag warmer, placing a single IV bag inside, visually scanning the empty hallway, and quickly walking away. Just over an hour later, according to the complaint, a 56-year-old woman suffered a cardiac emergency during a scheduled cosmetic surgery after a bag from the warmer was used during her procedure. The complaint alleged that, in another instance, agents observed Ortiz exit his operating room carrying an IV bag concealed in what appeared to be a paper folder, swap the bag with another bag from the warmer, and walk away. Roughly half an hour later, a 54-year-old woman suffered a cardiac emergency during a scheduled cosmetic surgery after a bag from the warmer was used during her procedure.

Ortiz was found guilty on four counts of tampering with consumer products resulting in serious bodily injury, one count of tampering with a consumer product, and five counts of intentional adulteration of a drug.

Conclusion

Pharmaceutical manufacturers can be held liable if they place defective and unreasonably dangerous products on the market. Under some circumstances, a defect in a pharmaceutical product may be determined to be the cause of a patient's death. Under other circumstances, it may be a healthcare professional's error in using the product that caused harm to a patient. It is also possible that a combination of product defect and professional error or an intentional criminal act caused harm to a patient. The likelihood of deliberate adulteration by a criminal healthcare professional should be considered.

Key Takeaways

- Accept responsibility for product quality. Your stock of pharmaceutical products is within your control. Be sure to store products under conditions that will preserve the quality of the products. Be alert for product recalls and remove from stock any product that is subject to a recall. Regularly check your stock for outdated products and remove outdated products from any area in which they may be retrieved for use in filling an order. Identify a secure area where recalled or outdated products can be sequestered prior to their being returned to the distributor or the manufacturer. Always note the lot number of the stock container from which an order is filled for a patient. The failure by a pharmacy to identify the lot number may lead to allegations of liability even when nothing wrong was done at the pharmacy.
- Be alert to the possibility of product defects. If a solid dosage form in your pharmaceutical stock seems to be deteriorating, or if a precipitate appears in a liquid dosage form, then remove the product from your active stock area and investigate what may have happened. If a patient indicates to you that a medication does not smell/taste/look like this medication usually does, then this is another reason for follow-up. If a patient reveals that a medication is not producing the usual therapeutic benefit, or that the medication is causing unexpected adverse effects, then report this to the manufacturer. Also file a MedWatch report with the FDA. Although this type of report may be the result of a misimpression by the patient, if many similar reports are filed, then it suggests a trend based on reality. The trend will become obvious only when a large number of anecdotal observations have been submitted.
- Be vigilant to the possibility of pharmaceutical product adulteration due to criminal motives, but reject conspiracy theories about the intentional poisoning of America by heartless pharmaceutical manufacturers and merciless healthcare professionals. Some people extrapolate from rare, but widely publicized incidents of pharmaceutical product defect, to insist that there is collusion among pharmaceutical manufacturers, the FDA, prescribers, pharmacists, and hospitals, to deliberately provide harmful medications to trusting and unsuspecting people who become ill or die from the pharmaceuticals, thus expanding opportunities for profit from the treatment of

pharmaceutically created illnesses. While there is evidence that people who distribute pharmaceutical products, and who regulate pharmaceutical products, do make occasional mistakes, and on rare occasions there are criminal acts, there is no evidence of a malicious conspiracy to poison America. There are outlier incidents in which people involved with pharmaceutical product distribution commit crimes that put profits over public safety. No industry or profession is immune to criminality by a small number of selfish sociopaths. Be sure to explain to anyone who has concerns about the quality of pharmaceutical products that there are standards to effectively provide these products with the fewest risks possible. Bogus conspiracy theories can lead patients, and even some healthcare professionals, to distrust the system of drug production and distribution. Effective pharmaceutical care is based on trust in the quality of pharmaceutical products. As you protect your patients from preventable adverse drug events, do your best to restore that trust in the mind of your patients, so that they will accept therapies that can cure their diseases and improve their quality of life.

References

1. Miller v. Bernard, 957 N.E.2d 685 (Ind.App. 2011).

2. Maida v. Rite Aid Corporation, 619 N.Y.S.2d 812 (N.Y.App. 1994).

3. Brazil v. Janssen Research & Development, 196 F.Supp.3d 1351 (N.D. Ga. 2016).

4. Lance v. Wyeth, 85 A.3d 434 (Pa. 2014).

5. Quaid v. Baxter Healthcare Corporation, 910 N.E.2d 1236 (Ill.App. 2009).

6. Wright v. Abbott Laboratories, 62 F.Supp.2d 1186 (D.Kan. 1999).

7. 21 U.S. Code § 351—Adulterated drugs and devices.

8. United States v. Courtney, 362 F.3d 497 (8th Cir. 2004).

9. United States v. Cadden, 51 F.4th 32 (1st Cir. 2022).

10. United States v. Chin, 41 F.4th 16 (1st Cir. 2022).

11. United States v. Stepanets, 879 F.3d 367 (1st Cir. 2018).

12. United States v. Leary, 2019 WL 1584508 (D.Mass. 2019).

13. Limehouse J. Texas doctor who tampered with patients IV bags faces 190 years after guilty verdict. *USA Today* (April 17, 2024). https://www.usatoday.com/story/news/nation/2024/04/17/doctor-poisoning-iv-bags-texas-prison-sentence/73357779007/

Chapter 12

Fatalities from Unapproved Drugs

Many pharmacists and other healthcare professionals are surprised to discover that some marketed medications have not been approved by the FDA. An unapproved drug is not necessarily dangerous. In theory, a drug that lacks FDA approval may be generally recognized as safe and effective, and thus may be legally distributed, following decades of use by healthcare professionals in the care of their patients. Approval of a new drug by the FDA does not guarantee that the new drug is safer or more effective than an unapproved drug that has been used safely for many years. It is theoretically possible that an unapproved drug is safe while an approved drug is unsafe. Safety and effectiveness depend on a patient's response to a drug. There are no guarantees of safety or effectiveness in drug therapy, even if a drug has been approved by the FDA.

Availability of Unapproved Drugs

Although pharmacists and patients may consider FDA-approved drugs to be safer than unapproved drugs, new drugs that have been approved by the FDA are not considered harmless. Patients who use FDA-approved pharmaceuticals should not be lulled into thinking that their medications are innocuous, simply because the medications have been approved by the FDA for therapeutic use. Prescription drugs are approved as safe and effective for use under the conditions that are prescribed, suggested, or recommended in the product labeling. They must be prescribed by practitioners based on accepted professional standards, and they must be used by patients as directed for use by medical personnel. The approval of drugs by the FDA does not address safety issues when the drug has been prescribed contrary to professional standards or has been used by a patient contrary to medical directions. Even if used as directed, drugs can cause fatalities. However, the use of unapproved drugs increases the risk of harm from medication use.

Unapproved drug use is different from off-label use of an approved drug. The FDA has consistently stated that approved drugs may be used for a condition that is not described in the product labeling, as long as professional standards for patient care have been met. This is one type of off-label use. Other types of off-label use would include prescribing an approved drug for a patient population that is not referenced in the product labeling or prescribing a dose that is not listed in the product labeling. Off-label drug use does not violate federal law. Pharmacies may fill prescriptions for off-label uses without violating the laws enforced by the FDA. In fact, there are many standard approaches to drug therapy that are technically off-label. On the other hand, distributing a drug that has not been approved by the FDA risks violation of federal law.

The FDA estimates that thousands of currently marketed drugs have not been approved by the agency. Many of these unapproved products have been available from pharmacies for decades and have been used safely (for the most part) during that time, although the clinical trials required by the agency for formal approval have never been conducted. On the other hand, some marketed unapproved drugs have been newly released into the market by unscrupulous businesspeople whose plan is to make a quick profit before their product is forced off the market by regulators. In times of drug shortages, when approved drugs may not be readily available through standard distribution channels, dishonest suppliers may take advantage of an opportunity to market nonstandard and unapproved pharmaceutical products. The prescriber, pharmacist, and patient may not be aware that the products are unapproved.

Pharmacists find themselves in a quandary as to how they can protect patients from approved drugs with identified risks and also from unapproved drugs with unidentified risks. There is a risk of fatality from drug use with both categories of drugs. The risk of fatality from the use of an unapproved drug is likely to be greater than from the use of an approved drug, due to the lack of FDA review. Understanding the new drug approval process and recognizing the risks of fatality from unapproved drug use are a challenge that pharmacists must meet. Pharmacists are ground-zero protectors of patients from unnecessary risks posed by unapproved drugs.

FDA's Online Reference on Drug Approval Status

The FDA provides a means to determine whether a marketed pharmaceutical product has been approved by the agency. In the FDA's online reference book titled, *Approved Drug Products with Therapeutic Equivalence Evaluations* (its short title is *The Orange Book*), all approved products are listed.[1] The primary utility of this book is that it serves as a reference to look up therapeutic equivalence evaluations for generic drug products. More fundamentally, it also serves as a way to verify the approval status of a marketed product. *The Orange Book* lists the name of each approved product, as well as the "sponsor" of a product that submitted a new drug application (NDA) or abbreviated new drug application (ANDA) to the agency and obtained approval through the FDA approval process. Sometimes, the marketer of a product may not be the sponsor. There may be a business arrangement through which the sponsor licenses a marketer to distribute an approved product.

Some people may ask, "Why doesn't the FDA publish a comprehensive list of drugs that are marketed but are unapproved?" That list would be a great thing to have. But it would be difficult, if not impossible, for the agency to do this. The agency simply does not know, and cannot know, all the drugs that are marketed and are unapproved. They discover these drugs based on reports submitted to them from the field. They know some of them, but they can't know all of them. Pharmacists, physicians, and others involved with drug therapy inform the agency if there are harmful drugs on the market, and the agency can then determine whether the drugs are approved. It is a tautology that one can't report a comprehensive list of what one does not know, because one has no way to know what it is that one does not know. This would be considered a "known unknown" in the sense that the FDA knows unapproved drugs are being marketed, but the agency does not know what those drugs are or where those drugs are entering the drug distribution system. The FDA relies heavily on pharmacists to be their "eyes and ears" for suspicious circumstances regarding day-to-day drug distribution.

There are far fewer marketed and unapproved biologics, as opposed to drugs, if there are any at all. However, the need for pharmacists to detect and report harmful biologics is the same as that for harmful drugs. The reference that can be used in determining biologic approval status is a book titled *Lists of Licensed Biological Products with Reference Product Exclusivity and Biosimilarity or Interchangeability Evaluations*. This online FDA reference, which is known as *The Purple Book*, serves the same purpose as the *Orange Book*, but for a different type of product.[2]

Catalysts for Drug Safety Concerns

Just as individual people often act in ways that reflect their history and experience, government agencies have institutional memories that guide agency policy.

Two similar stories, with distinct differences, describe how frustration and success at the FDA serve as guideposts for agency activities in the area of unapproved drugs. The story of frustration is the Elixir Sulfanilamide disaster that could not be prevented by the agency because the agency lacked new drug approval authority prior to passage of the 1938 Food, Drug, and Cosmetic Act. The story of success is the nonapproval of thalidomide, which literally saved both life and limb due to a firm commitment by the agency to public health protection. These two stories are often cited to support the policy of requiring agency approval for all marketed drugs.

In 1937, the drug sulfanilamide had been used in tablet and powder form to successfully treat streptococcal infections. A salesman for S.E. Massengill Co.

reported to headquarters that there was a demand for a liquid formulation of the drug in southern states, where liquid medications were culturally more popular than solid dosage forms. The challenge for the development of a liquid formulation was the insolubility of the drug in water, or in alcohol, or any of the other standard diluents. The company's chief chemist and chief pharmacist worked together, and they discovered that sulfanilamide powder would dissolve in diethylene glycol. The company formulated sulfanilamide in diethylene glycol, then tested the product for taste, appearance, and fragrance, and found it to be acceptable based on those criteria. The new liquid formulation was not tested for toxicity, which was not legally required at that time.

The formulation was labeled as "Elixir Sulfanilamide," and it was distributed throughout the country. Unfortunately, the product was found to be lethal due to toxicity of the diethylene glycol diluent, and it caused hundreds of patient deaths.

The FDA learned of the deaths and immediately seized the products. Because the label used the word "elixir," which could only be used for products containing alcohol, the product was deemed misbranded. The word "elixir" made the labeling untruthful since there was no alcohol in the product. Had the word "solution" been used instead, the FDA would have been powerless to prevent distribution of the product, and many more people would likely have died.

The Elixir Sulfanilamide tragedy was a catalyst for enactment of the FDCA in 1938. Although the agency succeeded in removing the toxic product from the market, the agency had used a technicality as the basis of its action. This experience provided support for the requirement of safety studies prior to the marketing of any new drug. The passage of the FDCA (still the foundational law for federal drug regulation) gave the federal government clear legal authority over the safety of pharmaceutical product distribution.

Thalidomide, the subject of an FDA success story, was developed in West Germany after World War II to treat morning sickness during pregnancy. The company that developed it was Chemie Grünenthal. Without conducting thorough tests on the drug, the company marketed it in 1957 as an over-the-counter product and labeled it as being "completely safe." But the drug was not safe at all. It caused peripheral neuropathy in adults. It also caused limb reductions in children born to women who had used the drug to prevent nausea during pregnancy. Over 13,000 babies suffered phocomelia from the drug, most of them in Germany and the United Kingdom.

What protected Americans from thalidomide was not a lack of desire to market the drug here. Instead, it was the commitment of a new FDA reviewer, Dr. Frances Kelsey, who refused to approve the drug for sale in the United States without additional evidence of safety. Dr. Kelsey felt that the clinical evidence supporting the drug "was more on the nature of testimonials rather than the results of well-designed, well-executed studies." Furthermore, since the drug was not indicated for life-threatening conditions, she believed additional time should be taken to verify the product's safety. As a result of this caution by Dr. Kelsey, American pharmacies never stocked the drug. By 1961, the truth about the drug's toxicity was known.

These two stories, taken together, help explain the perspective of the FDA toward unapproved drugs. Everyone at the agency wants to prevent the occurrence of another Elixir Sulfanilamide. Everyone at the agency wants to produce another success story like thalidomide.

Drug or Food?

The FDCA premarketing approval requirement extends to drugs but not to foods. The definition of "food" and of "drug" can determine whether an unapproved product is legal or illegal.

In the case of *Nutrilab v. Schweiker*,[3] a manufacturer marketed a "Starch Blocker" product without FDA approval. When challenged by the FDA, the manufacturer claimed that approval was not necessary, because the product was a food and not a drug. The product was formulated as a tablet, and it consisted of a protein derived from raw kidney beans. The manufacturer's theory was that the protein in the product would inhibit the alpha-amylase enzyme in the user's GI tract, thus allowing undigested starch to pass through the GI tract, avoiding the consumption of calories and promoting weight loss. The manufacturer contended that the product should be classified as food because it had been sourced from a food product. The FDA contended that the product was a drug because its intended use was as a drug.

In evaluating the opposing arguments, the court reasoned that a food is an article that is "used by people in the ordinary way most people use food—primarily for taste, aroma, or nutritive value." The court concluded that the "tablets at issue are not consumed primarily for taste, aroma, or nutritive value; in fact, they are taken for their ability to block the digestion of food and aid in weight loss." Thus, the product was intended to affect the structure or function of the body but was not a food. The court concluded, "Starch Blockers indisputably satisfy this requirement for they are intended to affect digestion in the people who take them. Therefore, starch blockers are drugs under the Food, Drug and Cosmetic Act."

While the FDA may exercise enforcement discretion regarding foods that are marketed as drugs, the FDCA requires all products marketed as drugs to be approved prior to marketing.

Safety and Efficacy

Technically, under the FDCA, a drug will be considered not new, and therefore it does not require approval, if the drug is generally recognized as safe and effective (GRASE). This classification of safe and effective drugs is sometimes flippantly referred to as a "state of GRASE."

The case of *United States v. Article of Drug Mykocert*[4] sheds light on how much disagreement there must be as to a drug's GRASE status for there not to be "general recognition" of the drug's safety and efficacy.

In this case, the drug in question was intended for use as a gynecological therapy. In opposing the unapproved marketing of the product, the FDA produced affidavits from five academic obstetrician-gynecologists, all of whom swore that in their opinion the drug was not generally recognized as safe and effective. The court said: "While we do not express an opinion as to whether a mere conflict in expert opinion constitutes lack of general recognition, it cannot be denied that the affidavits of five of the leading doctors in the field which deny general recognition creates more than a mere conflict. It is inconceivable that a drug such as this could be considered generally recognized in the face of such learned non-recognition."

The FDA has consistently been successful in showing lack of general recognition by providing the testimony of several qualified scientific experts who do not recognize the safety or efficacy of a product.

Drugs That Are Subject to the Approval Requirement

Under the FDCA, a "new drug" is defined as any drug that is not generally recognized as safe and effective, under conditions prescribed, recommended, or suggested in the drug's labeling, among experts qualified by scientific training and experience to evaluate the safety and efficacy of drugs.

All new drugs must be approved by the FDA prior to their introduction into interstate commerce. Note that the definition of "new drug" is determined by the drug's labeling. Any change in the drug's labeling can cause a drug that is not new to become new and will require an additional approval by the FDA. This approach is consistent with the agency focus on the content of labeling as a trigger for regulatory violations.

The FDCA definition of "new drug" clearly leaves open the possibility that a drug may not be considered new if the drug is generally recognized as safe and effective. This general recognition standard is one factor that has led to some drugs being marketed without approval in the past. However, the FDA has initiated a formal process to require approval of all marketed drugs that have not been approved. This initiative is based on the agency's interpretation that all unapproved drugs are "new drugs."

The FDCA does not specify that all drugs are new drugs. In fact, the existence of separate definitions in the FDCA for "drug" and for "new drug" supports the position that all drugs are not new drugs and that "new drugs" are a subset of "drugs" with the possibility that there could be lawfully marketed "not new" drugs. Otherwise, there would be no need for two separate categories of regulated articles. This literal interpretation of the FDCA is not how the FDA interprets the FDCA. The FDA interprets the FDCA to say that all drugs are new drugs and that therefore all drugs require FDA approval. It is an interpretation that has been upheld by the courts. The "our drug is not new" option is unavailable for all practical purposes to manufacturers who want to avoid going through the NDA (new drug approval) process.

Importance of Labeling

According to the FDCA, a drug "label" is a display of written, printed, or graphic matter placed directly upon the immediate container of any drug. The broader term "labeling" means all labels placed on the immediate container, and other written, printed, or graphic matter either placed upon a drug container or accompanying the drug. The concept of labeling does not include the spoken word. Written, printed, or graphic matter need not accompany a drug product closely for the material to be regulated as labeling. The material may be available at the same location and at the time of drug distribution. If so, it can be considered labeling.

Drug labeling may be directed toward either healthcare professionals or patients. The purpose of drug labeling is to provide accurate information that can be used to promote the safe and effective use of a safe and effective drug.

The foundational document for official drug labeling is the drug package insert (PI). This leaflet is distributed with the drug product from the manufacturer through intermediaries to the drug dispenser.

The PI is approved word-for-word by the FDA. Changes to the PI must be approved by the FDA. All other drug labeling is based on the content of the approved PI. If PI labeling language is not approved, then the drug is considered an unapproved "new drug."

Pre-1938 Drugs

One way in which unapproved drugs have been marketed is through what is often referred to as the "grandfather clause" within the FDCA. Although several different types of "grandfather clause" still exist, the interpretation of them by the FDA renders them essentially irrelevant. The approach taken by the FDA is to allow distribution under a "grandfather clause" only if a drug is marketed today exactly as it was marketed in 1938 or at another time when a grandfather clause was legally implemented. This approach reduces to zero the number of drugs that can qualify for marketing without approval under a "grandfather clause."

The FDA position has not always been so limited. The Original Federal Food and Drug Act of 1906 prohibited the sale of adulterated or misbranded drugs, but it did not require premarket approval. In 1938, when the FDCA was passed, all new drugs were required to be approved for safety. This was the result of the Elixir Sulfanilamide tragedy.

The active ingredients for many drugs were first introduced, at least in some form, prior to 1938. Under the 1938 law, the "grandfather clause" exempted from the definition of "new drug" any drug product that was on the market prior to the passage of the FDCA and which contained in its labeling the same representations concerning the conditions of use as it did in 1938, prior to passage of the FDCA. The 1938 grandfather clause is the most frequently cited of several such grandfather clauses. Grandfathered drugs were not required to be approved by the FDA under the 1938 law and could be legally marketed without approval of the agency.

Between 1938 and 1962, if a drug had been approved by the FDA, the agency approach was to regulate the so-called copycat products that were identical, related, or similar to the approved drug as if they were approved based on the original drug's approval. These products were "deemed" to be approved, even though they had not been approved. Many manufacturers also introduced drugs into the market between 1938 and 1962, based on their assessment that the products were generally recognized as safe, and the FDA issued opinions agreeing with this assessment. All such opinions have now been revoked. Grandfather status is now effectively extinct.

The 1962 FDCA Efficacy Amendments

When the Kefauver–Harris Amendment to the FDCA was passed in 1962, the FDA was faced with an enormous task. The agency was not only required to evaluate all post-1962 drugs for efficacy as well as safety, there was also a retrospective requirement to evaluate the efficacy of drugs approved as safe between 1938 and 1962.

Rather than undertake this job with existing limited agency resources, the FDA contracted with the National Academy of Sciences/National Research Council to evaluate over 3,400 products that were approved for safety only between 1938 and 1962 and had not been reviewed for efficacy. This was called the Drug Efficacy Study Implementation (DESI) process. Initial determinations of efficacy were made by NAS/NRC, and drugs determined to be less than fully effective were allowed to remain on the market subject to the ongoing DESI process that would require years of hearings, appeals, and litigation.

A very few currently marketed yet unapproved products continue to be the subject of DESI review, and they are in a state of regulatory limbo. Other products have completed DESI review and have been subject to withdrawal due to lack of efficacy, yet they remain on the market despite this determination. The FDA considers all such products to be unapproved new drugs that are being marketed illegally.

Criminal Acts

When there is an opportunity for economic gain from illegal activity, there will be illegal activity by criminals who seek that economic gain. The field of pharmaceutical manufacturing and distribution is no more immune to criminal activity than is any other area of commerce.

Some unapproved drugs currently being marketed were introduced to the market after 1962 when the FDA had clear authority to require evidence of safety and efficacy for these products. The illegal marketers of the products have simply ignored the legal requirement of FDA approval.

Limited resources for enforcement within the FDA have allowed these criminals to continue their illegal activities, and the quasi-legal status of many similar products has allowed the clearly illegal products to appear to be legitimate. These products may have a National Drug Code (NDC) number, and they may appear in the Physician's Desk Reference. This does not mean they are approved. When confronted by regulators, the distributors of these drugs may claim that they were confused by the complexity of the FDCA and its amendments and that such confusions and ambiguities misled them into thinking they were complying with the law. The old adage that "ignorance of the law is no excuse" applies as a response to this claim.

A Classic Legal Case of Criminal Unapproved Drug Marketing

Regulatory agencies rely heavily on voluntary compliance. It has often been said that regulations are unnecessary for the vast majority of individuals and businesses who would comply with applicable standards in the absence of legal coercion. On the other hand, regulations are necessary for the small number of individuals and businesses that choose to violate the law to enhance profitability for themselves at the expense of public safety. The marketing of the intravenous vitamin E product known as E-Ferol IV illustrates the reality of this perspective. The facts of this case are hard to believe, but they are true.[5]

A pharmaceutical executive was convicted of misbranding violations and introducing into interstate commerce an unapproved new drug. The product that led to the conviction was E-Ferol IV, which was first marketed in the fall of 1983. It consisted of vitamin E and two polysorbates that were used as emulsifying agents. Approximately 26,000 vials of E-Ferol IV were distributed until a recall was ordered by the FDA and the product was permanently removed from the market in April 1984. The product had been identified as causing the death of approximately 40 premature infants. There were likely many more deaths that were not identified as having been caused by E-Ferol IV.

The development of E-Ferol IV was prompted by the need for an intravenous form of vitamin E to prevent retrolental fibroplasia (RLF) that causes impaired vision or permanent blindness in premature infants. The two principal forms of vitamin E that were available in the early 1980s were an oral formulation and an intramuscular (IM) formulation. Both products were sold as nutritional supplements and not as drugs. The company that developed E-Ferol IV already was distributing an intramuscular injection product known as E-Ferol IM, with labeling that made no reference to RLF or to any other medical condition.

In 1982, a neonatologist wrote to the manufacturer suggesting that there could be a large market for an IV formulation because the IM formulation was difficult to administer to neonates. An executive at the company responded that "the amount of polysorbates needed may be detrimental," and he pointed out that "fat emulsions for IV use are very tricky products and fraught with particulate size problems." The executive was aware that another manufacturer was attempting to obtain FDA approval of an IV vitamin E product. He expressed caution to a colleague noting that "if we make some attempt to solubilize the vitamin E and use the wrong proportions and kill a few infants, we'd have some serious problems."

Notwithstanding these concerns, the manufacturer went ahead and developed E-Ferol IV. The manufacturer never did any testing to determine whether E-Ferol IV would be safe and effective for use in premature infants. The product was introduced onto the market. In the "Clinical Pharmacology" section of the package insert, the manufacturer included this language: "Reports in the literature indicate that substantial doses of vitamin E will reduce the severity of retrolental fibroplasia in neonates, which are administered oxygen because of their low weight, under 1500 grams." A regulatory consultant sent a memorandum to the company stating, "I do not believe that legally we can make a claim that vitamin E is effective against RLF if given to infants. This will require an NDA for the use of vitamin E as a drug." The pharmaceutical executive claimed that he never saw the memorandum.

The E-Ferol IV product was marketed to approximately 1,000 directors of neonatal intensive care units. Nothing in the promotional materials indicated that the product had not been tested for safety and efficacy. Physicians and pharmacists testified at trial that they thought the product had been approved by the FDA based on the manner in which it was being marketed.

Almost immediately concerns about the product were conveyed to the manufacturer. In December 1983, a neonatologist in Honolulu reported that two neonates had developed "unusual symptoms" following the administration of E-Ferol IV. In early January 1984, a pharmacist "expressed concern about the large amount of polysorbate." At about this same time, another pharmacist was critical "of the company representing the product as appropriate for the treatment of RLF without any studies to support this claim."

In late January 1984, a neonatologist in Spokane reported three neonatal deaths resulting from E-Ferol IV use. The company ceased distribution of the product, informing customers that the product was "unavailable because it was on back order," rather than sharing any information about possible toxicities. An attorney for the manufacturer told the company that "the references to RLF in the package insert made the product a drug and that the FDA would probably consider it to be a new drug." The attorney advised the company to stop shipping the drug until experts could evaluate its safety and efficacy.

The manufacturer then revised E-Ferol IV's package insert to omit all references to RLF and with a reduced recommended dosage. However, shipments were resumed before the revised package inserts could be included with the product.

On March 27, 1984, a pharmacist in Tennessee informed the manufacturer that her hospital had stopped administering E-Ferol IV because of neonatal deaths associated with its use. Shipments of E-Ferol IV continued until April 6, 1984, when the FDA contacted the manufacturer resulting in a recall of the product and the permanent removal of the product from the market.

The pharmaceutical executive who was convicted of violating the FDCA by introducing unapproved E-Ferol IV into interstate commerce appealed his conviction. He argued on appeal that (1) FDA policy led him to believe that E-Ferol IV could be marketed lawfully without a new drug approval and (2) that this same policy was so vague and indefinite as to deprive him of fair warning that his conduct was illegal. This argument rests on the notion that ignorance of the law is an excuse for criminality. It is not an effective defense strategy.

The court applied what is known as the "willful blindness theory," under which criminal liability may be imposed on people who recognize the likelihood of wrongdoing but consciously refuse to take basic investigatory steps. The pharmaceutical executive's conviction was affirmed.

The awareness this case brings is that sometimes the profit motive can override safety concerns. Regulatory agencies have been established to prevent this sort of illegal conduct. But regulators can't be in all places at all times. It is the responsibility of health professionals to be knowledgeable of regulatory requirements for new drugs and to protect patients under circumstances where manufacturers or distributors may not be fulfilling this role. The E-Ferol IV case was the impetus for the Unapproved Drug Initiative (UDI) in which the FDA is currently engaged.

Regulatory Priorities

The continued presence of unapproved drugs on the market is in some ways perplexing. These unapproved drugs may be readily available from wholesalers for inclusion in pharmacy inventory, and they are routinely dispensed to patients pursuant to prescriptions issued by physicians. To some people it seems like the FDA is "doing nothing" about a major problem. This is a misperception. The FDA is doing plenty to address the problem of unapproved drugs. What they are doing is methodical and thoughtful. It is an exercise of their enforcement discretion. Just as all regulatory agencies have laws to enforce and the discretion to decide how, when, and where to enforce them, the FDA has authority to determine its own approach to the problem of unapproved drugs.

As a tactical matter, the FDA has decided how to use its limited resources to address a vast problem. It would be irrational and inefficient if the agency did not set priorities for the use of existing resources. One of the limited resources is the resource of knowledge. The agency cannot know immediately when an unapproved new drug enters the pharmaceutical market. It takes time to learn and react.

On a more strategic level, the FDA understands that the regulatory principle of balance is fully applicable to enforcement of laws and rules applicable to unapproved drugs. Some patients are using unapproved drugs successfully in the treatment of disease, with little threat to the public health. It could disrupt the balance between risk and benefit to impulsively interfere with ongoing successful medical care.

Compliance Guidance

The FDCA and the regulations enforced by the FDA are seldom self-explanatory. They address complex issues and are capable of alternate interpretations, even by those who are committed to compliance. For this reason, the FDA publishes compliance policy guides (CPGs) that advise the regulated industry how the agency intends to use its enforcement discretion. Technically, CPGs describe the agency's thinking on a topic and should be viewed as recommendations only. They do not necessarily establish legally enforceable responsibilities. A CPG that is related to the marketing of unapproved new drugs provides FDA guidance on the agency's approach to enforcement, following discovery of a problem during an inspection or after having been alerted by outside sources.

Once an illegally marketed product is identified, taking enforcement action against the product typically involves one or more of the following: requesting voluntary compliance; providing notice of action in the Federal Register; issuing what the agency calls an "untitled letter" to the offender; issuing the far more serious "warning letter" which connotes that enforcement action is imminent; or actually initiating a seizure of the product, injunction against further product distribution, or any other proceedings such as criminal prosecution.

In its 2006 CPG, updated on September 19, 2011, the FDA clarified its approach to the enforcing of laws related to unapproved drugs. The agency indicated that it would continue a risk-based approach to priority setting, giving higher priority to enforcement actions involving relatively high-risk categories of drugs and lower priority to relatively low-risk categories of drugs. These priorities apply only to unapproved drugs that were on the market as of September 9, 2011. The agency drew a line in the sand by taking a zero-tolerance approach to products introduced into interstate commerce without approval following that date. Any product placed on the market after that date without approval will be subject to immediate enforcement action regardless of the stated risk-based priorities described in the CPG. All unapproved drugs after that date are subject to enforcement without notice and without expectation that discretion will be exercised by the agency.

Regulatory Agency Conflict

On November 25, 2020, the U.S. Department of Health and Human Services (HHS) published a notice in the Federal Register terminating the FDA's Unapproved Drugs Initiative. The HHS rationale was that some unapproved drugs need not be approved because they are generally recognized as safe and effective (GRASE) and, therefore, do not require FDA approval since they are not new drugs. The HHS notice also criticized the FDA for changing the law of drug approval through the informal publication of a CPG, when any such change must be done through the more formal notice and comment rulemaking process. The FDA's Marketed Unapproved Drugs Compliance Policy Guide (the CPG previously referred to in this program) was withdrawn by the HHS action.

On May 27, 2021, the FDA published its own notice in the Federal Register. The FDA was highly critical of the previous HHS notice, outlining what the FDA considered to be numerous factual and legal errors in the HHS announcement. Whether this interagency squabble will continue remains to be seen. In the interim, although the original CPG is not necessarily in effect, it reflects the perspective of the agency and must be considered as an effective guide for regulatory compliance in the area of unapproved new drugs.

The FDA has published several explanations of its position regarding unapproved drugs. The agency has clarified the agency position that all drugs are new drugs and that all drugs must be approved before they are placed into interstate commerce.[6] The agency acknowledges that a balance must be struck between public safety concerns that warrant strict enforcement of the Food, Drug, and Cosmetic Act and the correlative concerns related to product access and reasonable cost. A policy of strict enforcement has the potential to reduce access to necessary medications and/or to increase the costs of necessary medications.

Fixing the Biggest Problems First

The FDA has indicated, in its CPG for unapproved drugs (now withdrawn, but likely still a useful statement of policy), that its use of enforcement discretion will focus on six particular areas of concern for unapproved drugs. This approach is likely to continue until a new CPG is issued. Here are the areas in which the agency now focuses its efforts:

- *Drugs with potential safety risks.* Removing potentially unsafe drugs protects the public from direct and indirect health threats.
- *Drugs that lack evidence of effectiveness.* Removing ineffective drugs protects the public from using these products in lieu of available

effective treatments. Depending on the indication, some ineffective products also pose safety risks.

- *Health fraud drugs.* The FDA defines health fraud as "the deceptive promotion, advertisement, distribution, or sale of articles that are represented as being effective to diagnose, prevent, cure, treat, or mitigate disease (or other conditions), or provide a beneficial effect on health, but which have not been scientifically proven safe and effective for such purposes. Such practices may be deliberate or done without adequate knowledge or understanding of the article." Within this category, the FDA places the highest priority on drugs that present a direct risk to health. In setting priorities for enforcement directed toward health fraud drugs, the FDA also considers indirect risks, such as whether the therapeutic claims are significant, whether there are any scientific data to support the safety and effectiveness of the product, and the degree of vulnerability of the prospective user group.
- *Drugs that present direct challenges to the new drug approval and OTC drug monograph systems.* The FDA uses specific, systematic rules to authorize marketing of drugs through the new drug approval system or the OTC monographs. The integrity of these systems is integral to the protection of public health. When a product is placed in interstate commerce with flagrant disregard of the established agency systems, there is a risk that respect for the systems will be diminished. Targeting drugs that explicitly challenge the drug approval or OTC drug monograph systems buttresses the integrity of these systems and makes it more likely that firms will comply with the new drug approval and monograph requirements, which benefits the public health.
- *Unapproved new drugs that also violate the FDCA in other ways.* The agency may choose to use its enforcement authority over unapproved drugs under circumstances where there are other violations of the FDCA, even if there are other versions of the same unapproved drug made by other firms that do not violate the FDCA in other ways. Thus, if a product is in violation of the misbranding or adulteration provisions, for example, the agency may use these violations as the basis for action related to the unapproved status of the product.
- *Drugs that are reformulated to evade an FDA enforcement action.* The FDA has become aware that some companies have anticipated FDA enforcement action directed toward specific types or formulations of an unapproved product and have made product changes specifically to evade that enforcement but have not brought the product into compliance with the new drug provisions. Such a reformulation will not lead the agency to exercise discretion and allow the change.

Regulatory Grace Period

Sometimes, a company will obtain approval of an NDA for a product even though other companies are marketing the drug without approval. The FDA encourages this type of voluntary compliance because it benefits the public health and reduces the expenditure of FDA resources. Since they present a direct challenge to the drug approval system, the FDA is more likely to take enforcement action against remaining unapproved drugs in this situation. However, the agency uses its enforcement discretion, balancing the need to provide incentives for voluntary compliance against the implications of enforcement actions on the marketplace and on medication users who are accustomed to using marketed products.

When a company obtains approval to market a product that other companies are marketing without approval, FDA usually allows a grace period of roughly one year before it will initiate enforcement action against remaining unapproved products. Many companies that have been marketing the unapproved product will then opt to permanently withdraw it from the market. These withdrawals give the company that holds the FDA approval a de facto monopoly over the product's availability. This monopoly status can have significant effects on product price and availability.

Conclusion

There are drugs on the market, and on the shelves of community and institutional pharmacies, that have not been approved by the FDA. These drugs have not necessarily been subjected to rigorous study of their safety and efficacy. The agency is aware of this reality and has undertaken enforcement programs to address it. Through agency action, many unapproved drugs have been removed from the market. Healthcare professionals share with the FDA a responsibility to promote patient safety by protecting patients from the hazards, and potentially fatal hazards, of unapproved drugs.

Key Takeaways

- Be alert to the possibility that the drugs you are dispensing may not be approved by the FDA. Simply because a drug label bears an NDC number does not necessarily mean that the drug has been approved by the FDA. The agency itself recognizes that there are many unapproved drugs on the market. Regardless of any interagency disagreements about how to handle the challenge of marketed unapproved drugs, the reality remains that pharmacists are the last link in a long chain of drug development, production, marketing, and distribution. The FDA can establish standards for drug approval, and the agency can enforce those standards when they are violated by a pharmaceutical manufacturer or distributor, but the FDA can't consistently protect patients from the potential harm of an unapproved drug. The FDA has no direct connection with patients. The FDA's only connection with patients is through the pharmacist. One of your many important responsibilities is to protect patients from harmful drugs, including unapproved drugs. If you have doubts about whether a drug has been approved, look in the *Orange Book* to verify the approval status of a drug that you have been asked to dispense and/or manage.

- Alert the FDA if you see any problems that may be related to an unapproved new drug. It was pharmacists and other committed health professionals who brought to the FDA's attention the deaths that were being caused by E-Ferol IV. The responsibility of pharmacists to provide protection from deadly unapproved drugs goes beyond their own patients to include the general public. Individual reports of fatalities that are submitted to the FDA can be aggregated by the agency into a compelling story of criminal misconduct. What pharmacists scattered across the country see as an anecdote can be collected by the FDA to prompt quick action based on multiple observations. Don't hesitate to report something that seems trivial to you. Let the FDA decide what is trivial and what is significant.
- Although FDA approval is an important step in the use of any medication, resist the temptation to assume that FDA approval means a drug is absolutely safe. Don't get caught in the trap of thinking that all unapproved drugs are unsafe and that all approved drugs are safe. It doesn't necessarily work that way. Patients can die from the use of an approved drug. Patients can be cured by unapproved drugs. The approval status of a drug should not be viewed as a security blanket for a patient who uses the drug.

References

1. Food and Drug Administration. Approved Drug Products with Therapeutic Equivalence Evaluations | Orange Book. https://www.fda.gov/drugs/drug-approvals-and-databases/approved-drug-products-therapeutic-equivalence-evaluations-orange-book

2. Food and Drug Administration. Purple Book: Lists of Licensed Biological Products with Reference Product Exclusivity and Biosimilarity or Interchangeability Evaluations. https://www.fda.gov/drugs/therapeutic-biologics-applications-bla/purple-book-lists-licensed-biological-products-reference-product-exclusivity-and-biosimilarity-or

3. Nutrilab v. Schweiker, 713 F.2d 335 (7th Cir. 1983).

4. United States v. Article of Drug Mykocert, 345 F.Supp. 571 (N.D. Ill. 1972).

5. United States v. Hiland, 909 F.2d 1114 (8th Cir. 1990).

6. United States Food and Drug Administration. Unapproved Drugs. https://www.fda.gov/drugs/enforcement-activities-fda/unapproved-drugs

Chapter 13

Distinguishing Mercy from Murder

Death is inevitable. Taxes are not, of course, as there are many loopholes that a person can find to avoid paying taxes. But there are no loopholes that allow a person to avoid dying.

In 1997, Justice Sandra Day O'Connor of the U.S. Supreme Court had this to say, "Death will be different for each of us. For many, the last days will be spent in physical pain and perhaps the despair that accompanies physical deterioration and a loss of control of basic bodily and mental functions. Some will seek medication to alleviate that pain and other symptoms." Justice O'Connor's observations beg the question whether those who provide medication to persons at the end of life have committed a crime if the medication causes the patient's death. Is it pharmaceutical homicide? This is not an easy question to answer.

Those who live in the United States have been given a liberty interest that allows each person the freedom to pursue that person's own goals as long as that pursuit does not interfere with the similar pursuits of another person. This is often called "positive freedom." There is also freedom not to be subjected to actions by others, regardless of how benevolent the intentions of others may be if those actions are contrary to the beneficiary's wishes. This is often called "negative freedom."

Controversies may arise when, at the end of a person's life, comfort care procedures that are undertaken to ease the person's pain or to otherwise reduce the trauma of the final days of life may be interpreted as hastening that person's death. This is particularly true if the person is a child, or is frail, or is elderly, or may otherwise not be deemed fully competent to assert personal preferences. The withholding of drug therapy (e.g., antibiotics for a patient with pneumonia) or the administration of a drug (e.g., opioids to manage a patient's pain) may lead to accusations that the person who controlled access to the drug has killed the patient either by withholding the drug or by administering the drug. This accusation can result in criminal charges, including charges of murder.

Principle of Double Effect

Under what is often called the "Principle of Double Effect," it is considered morally permissible to perform a risky medical action or procedure that has both foreseeable good effects and foreseeable bad effects, if (1) the act itself is morally good, (2) the good effect is not a result of the bad effect, (3) the bad effect is not intended (although it may be foreseen), and (4) the good and bad effects are in proportion to each other.

Double Effect has been used to justify the provision of pain medications to terminally ill patients, with the intention to relieve pain, while also knowing that death may be hastened by the drugs. The act of relieving pain is a good act, and the foreseeable consequence of shortening life is excused under the circumstances. There is general agreement on this particular application of the principle of Double Effect. On the other hand, a deliberate act that causes death, with the primary intention of ending the life of a person for the specific purpose of relieving that person's suffering because dead people no longer suffer, generally does not fit within Double Effect.

A Classic Legal Case of Double Effect

One of the most poignant legal cases related to the principle of Double Effect was the case of a small-town Kansas physician who appealed his conviction for the attempted murder of one patient and the intentional and malicious second-degree murder of another patient.[1] The facts of the two incidents are lengthy. A brief summary of each situation provides the basic background for understanding how difficult and risky it can be to care for patients at the end of life.

The first patient was a 78-year-old female. She had suffered from terminal cancer for "a number of years," and, according to her son, she "had gone downhill dramatically" in recent days. The son transported his mother to the hospital emergency room because her pain medication was no longer working. The defendant physician explained to the son that he could provide stronger opioids for the patient but that in her condition "it slows respiration and here is a real danger the patient can die." The son instructed the physician "to give her more pain medication." The physician administered a 100 mcg injection of fentanyl. He told the son that his mother was close to death, and the physician recited the Robert Frost poem "Into the Woods" at the patient's bedside. At this point, the son apparently had a change of heart. He told the physician, "Let me make this perfectly clear: I'd rather my mother lay there and suffer ten more days than you do anything to speed up her death." The physician recommended that the patient be transferred to a larger hospital in a neighboring community. The patient died at this new hospital two days later.

The second patient was an 81-year-old male who was "obese and a severe diabetic with a history of heart disease." He had a pacemaker and was using warfarin. The patient was found "slumped over in a booth at a convenience store." Several days before, he had refused to continue taking his warfarin. He was transported to the hospital emergency room where he was seen by the defendant physician. The physician concluded that the patient had suffered a massive stroke. The physician ordered IV norcuron so that the patient could be intubated. Nurses testified that over the next 3 hours the physician worked tirelessly to save the patient's life. This included a second injection of norcuron to keep the patient from "bucking out" his breathing tube. The defendant physician contacted a medical colleague to request a second opinion. The consultant physician concluded that the patient "had no pulse, respiration, or reflexes," and a nurse testified that the consultant physician said, "He's gone." Shortly thereafter, the patient was pronounced dead.

It was his treatment of these two patients for which the physician was charged with attempted murder and first-degree murder. The evidence presented at the trial was conflicting, with three physicians testifying on behalf of the prosecution and six physicians testifying on behalf of the defense. A jury found the physician guilty of the charges made against him.

The physician appealed. On appeal, the court reviewed the trial transcripts as well as three amicus (friend of the court) briefs that had been filed by medical associations. The language of the Kansas Court of Appeals is striking (the court's language is in italics):

In the instant case, there is nothing close to a medical consensus that the defendant physician's actions were homicidal. In fact, there was extremely strong testimony to the contrary. This evidence included the testimony of two physicians who were involved in the treatment of the two alleged victims, although not in the actions which are the subject of this case. They testified that [the defendant physician's] actions were not only noncriminal, but they were medically appropriate.

There was also the consultant physician's testimony that he confirmed the second patient was actually dead, from a medical standpoint (although not technically "brain dead"), before resuscitation attempts were halted.

The evidence also included the testimony of three other highly qualified physicians who were asked to review the records and render their opinions on the reasonableness of the defendant physician's actions. They all found his actions were not only noncriminal but were within the bounds of good medical practice.

Despite this testimony, the jury apparently found, beyond a reasonable doubt, that the defendant physician's actions were totally outside appropriate medical practice. Having found that, it then apparently found there was no reasonable doubt that the source of his actions was homicidal intent. They apparently arrived at this based on the testimony of the three physicians brought in by the State, who disagreed with the opinions of the other six physicians who testified.

We have made a thorough review of the record, which includes a wealth of undisputed evidence and expert medical testimony. We find that no rational jury could find criminal intent and guilt beyond a reasonable doubt based on the record here. When the issue is whether there is reasonable doubt, a jury is not free to disbelieve undisputed facts. What occurred here is generally known. The jury was not free to disbelieve that there was substantial competent medical opinion in support of the proposition that the defendant physician's actions were not only noncriminal but were medically appropriate.

This is not a situation where the evidence in the defendant's favor is trifling. It is extremely strong. When there is such strong evidence supporting a reasonable, noncriminal explanation for the doctor's actions, it cannot be said that there is no reasonable doubt of criminal guilt. This is particularly true in a situation as we are faced with here, where the only way the defendant's actions may be found to be criminal is through expert testimony, and that testimony is strongly controverted in every detail.

We do not say that a physician can always escape criminal conviction for reckless or purposeful homicidal behavior through friendly medical testimony on his or her behalf. But there is a reason why there has yet to be in Anglo-American law an affirmed conviction of a physician for homicide arising out of medical treatment based on such highly controverted expert evidence as here.

All three amicus briefs acknowledge the appropriateness of criminal responsibility where a physician's actions are clearly reckless or purposefully homicidal. However, they note that if criminal responsibility can be assessed based solely on the opinions of a portion of the medical community which are strongly challenged by an opposing and authoritative medical consensus, we have criminalized malpractice, and even the possibility of malpractice.

The instant case is a very good example of this. With no direct evidence of criminal intent, it is highly disturbing that testimony by such an impressive array of apparently objective medical experts, who found the defendant's actions to be not only noncriminal, but medically appropriate, can be dismissed as "unbelievable" and not even capable of generating reasonable doubt.

The quality and quantity of evidence necessary to establish criminal guilt was not presented in this case. We must therefore reverse the convictions on the grounds of insufficient evidence and order the entry of a verdict of acquittal.

The importance of this case is that it illustrates how emotion and misunderstanding of what has occurred in the care of a critically ill patient can lead to a misinterpretation of motives and causation, when evaluating the actions of healthcare professionals who provide end-of-life care. The law does not allow killing, but the law encourages appropriate treatment of those who are dying.

Defining "Death"

It is simplistic and transparently obvious to say that a person has not been murdered until that person is dead. It is less simple to define what is meant by "dead." This was not always as difficult as it is today. For thousands of years, humans considered a previously living person to be "dead" based on the cessation of all cardiopulmonary function, as well as the cessation of all cognitive activity and the cessation of all responsive activity. These physical changes defined death, and they were noncontroversial. All three functions were so closely tied together that this became known as the "heart-lung" definition of death. This was not a scientific or clinical determination. Although in later years it became necessary to have a trained person (a physician or a mortician) certify death, the certification was simply that the person seemed to be dead based on the obvious evidence. Science and clinical skills were not necessary to determine death.

The process of declaring death changed when mechanical substitutes for heart and lung function became available. The "heart-lung" definition of death no longer sufficed, because technically a body could be made to artificially respire and circulate blood forever. But nobody lives forever. At this point, the law became far more important in determining whether a death had occurred. Rather than accepting that a person had died, based on the rudimentary observations of a physician or mortician, legal precepts were developed to define the time at which a death had occurred, based on specific criteria established under the law. These criteria have undergone modification over time. They are still not without controversy. The determination of whether a person has died and when the death occurred, which used to be so simple, is now quite complex.

A 1968 article from *JAMA* explains the rationale for changing the definition of death:

> There are two reasons why there is need for a new definition: (1) Improvements in resuscitative and supportive measures have led to increased efforts to save those who are desperately injured. Sometimes these efforts have only partial success so that the result is an individual whose heart continues to beat but whose brain is

> irreversibly damaged. The burden is great on patients who suffer permanent loss of intellect, on their families, on the hospitals, and on those in need of hospital beds already occupied by these comatose patients. (2) Obsolete criteria for the definition of death can lead to controversy in obtaining organs for transplantation.[2]

For several years thereafter, the American Medical Association and other groups worked to develop a definition of death that would meet legal needs. The result was the Uniform Determination of Death Act (UDDA) of 1980 [3] This is a model act that is not binding on anyone, but it may be used by any state in the drafting of legislation to define death in that state. The state laws that result from adoption of the UDDA are binding within the state. The UDDA currently says:

> An individual who has sustained either (1) irreversible cessation of circulatory and respiratory function, or (2) irreversible cessation of all function of the entire brain, including the brain stem, is dead. A determination of death must be made in accordance with accepted medical standards.

Soon after this approach was adopted in many states, criminal murderers claimed that physicians had killed their victims. The perpetrators asserted that their victims had been "kept alive" in the hospital by mechanical means until they were declared "brain dead" by a physician who "pulled the plug" and caused the victims' death. This argument did not win any acquittals, but it reinforced the need for laws to define death.

The UDDA definition is called the "whole brain" definition. It begs the question: "What about the person who has no cerebral (higher brain) function yet still respires independently due to continued brain stem function?" The controversy regarding whether "whole brain" or "partial brain" death is the most appropriate legal definition continues to occur, although proposals for updated definitions have been suggested.

Defining "Dying"

Death is an event that occurs at an identifiable point in time. Dying is a process that occurs over time. It is important to distinguish between aging and dying. Everyone is aging; by the year, by the week, by the hour, by the minute, and by the second. Aging is of no special significance, other than the modifications that must be made in lifestyle and circumstances to accommodate the changes that occur with aging. Dying is a different matter altogether. There are activities that may be undertaken with a person who is dying that would not be appropriate if done with a person who is merely aging.

Caring for those why are dying requires taking an approach to death that includes elements of pathology, physiology, and psychology. End-of-life care also requires thorough consideration of the decisions and choices that must be made by and for people who are approaching death.

Just as the definition of death has changed with advances in medicine, the nature of dying has changed, and these changes have led to the need for difficult decisions to be made by patients and their loved ones. Hospice care has developed a specialized expertise in providing support during the dying process. The provision of medication to hospice patients has been a significant development. The practice of "terminal sedation" has evolved, and it has been distinguished from intentional killing.

Suicide

Suicide is the act of voluntarily and intentionally taking one's own life. Suicide usually requires that the actor be a person of mature years and sound mind who understands the result of the act. There are strong feelings about suicide in American society. Some people believe that suicide is morally wrong because it is a selfish act that leaves the victim's family to deal with the distressing consequences. There are some people who think that suicide is a sin because only God has the right to decide when death will occur. Yet others think that autonomous individuals should be free to decide for themselves when to die and that this decision should not be interfered with by others. This latter view is particularly the case when the person who commits suicide has been in severe, chronic pain or has another medical reason to choose not to continue suffering.

Personal beliefs about the act of suicide may carry over to policy perspectives on assisted dying for terminally ill patients. In years past, there were laws that declared suicide to be illegal. As a penalty for this crime, the victim's property could be forfeited and not given to the rightful heirs. Those laws have now been repealed. Suicide is not a crime in any state of the United States.

Attempted suicide is also not a crime. However, those who survive a suicide attempt may be subject to legal protections for their own benefit. In most states, the law permits mandatory institutionalization of a person who has attempted suicide for a 72-hour period of observation following the attempt. This is not punishment; it is treatment.

Assisted Suicide

It may seem odd that a person is not legally allowed to assist another person in the performance of an act that the first person is legally permitted to perform.

But in most states that is the law. It is considered illegal in most jurisdictions to assist suicide even though suicide itself is not illegal. The U.S. Supreme Court has affirmed the right of states to criminalize assisted suicide. It is illegal to help somebody do something that is not illegal for them to do. States can also decide to decriminalize assisted suicide if the democratic process in the state results in a preference for that approach.

The federal approach to assisted suicide was established in a pair of cases from New York. The U.S. Supreme Court reviewed a challenge to the New York law that made it a crime to aid another person to commit or attempt suicide.[2] The question asked of the court was whether the New York law violates the Equal Protection Clause of the Fourteenth Amendment to the U.S. Constitution.

The parties who challenged the law were physicians who practiced medicine in New York; they asserted that it would be consistent with the standards of their profession if they were to prescribe lethal medications for mentally competent, terminally ill patients who are suffering great pain and desire a physician's assistance in taking their own lives. The physicians contended that the Constitution should be interpreted to allow them to provide this medical treatment even though the Attorney General of New York had issued an opinion that any such treatment was unlawfully assisting suicide.

The physicians argued that patients already had a right to die by refusing treatment such as nutrition and hydration at the end of life and that a right to be given lethal medications is "essentially the same thing." They argued that outlawing physician-assisted suicide under these circumstances is unequal treatment of equally situated persons.

The court disagreed, saying, "We think the distinction between assisting suicide and withdrawing life-sustaining treatment, a distinction widely recognized and endorsed in the medical profession and in our legal traditions, is both important and logical; it is certainly rational." The court provided various reasons for distinguishing between "letting a patient die and making that patient die." The court disagreed with the physicians' claim that the distinction is arbitrary and irrational.

The state explained that judicial support for the law was based on several factors: prohibiting intentional killing and preserving life; preventing suicide; maintaining the physician's role as their patients' healers; protecting vulnerable people from indifference and prejudice and the psychological and financial pressure to end their lives; as well as avoiding a possible slippery slope toward euthanasia.

This federal ruling does not outlaw physician-assisted suicide. It allows states to choose whether they wish to legalize or criminalize physician-assisted suicide. At least ten jurisdictions (California, Colorado, District of Columbia, Hawaii, Maine, New Jersey, New Mexico, Oregon, Vermont, and Washington) have adopted laws that permit physician-assisted death when specific criteria have been met. Montana has not passed any such specific law, but the Montana Supreme Court has ruled that physician-assisted suicide cannot be criminalized under existing state laws. Advocacy groups in other states are pushing for expanded recognition of a right to physician-assisted death with dignity.

Is Death a Legitimate Medical Purpose?

The medications most frequently used by physicians to assist terminally ill patients in choosing when to die are ultra-short-acting barbiturates. These medications are regulated by the DEA as controlled substances, and as such they fall within the category of medications that may only be prescribed for a legitimate medical purpose and in the usual course of professional practice under federal law. In the case of *Gonzales v. Oregon*, the Attorney General of the United States (AG) challenged the Oregon Death with Dignity Act (ODWDA), contending that under the federal Controlled Substance Act, the State of Oregon did not have the authority to allow the use of federally scheduled controlled substances for anything other than a legitimate medical purpose in the usual course of professional practice.[5] The AG claimed that that death is not a legitimate medical purpose and that causing the death of a patient is not in the usual course of professional practice. The AG contended that a prescription issued pursuant to the OWDA would constitute "drug abuse" and would therefore be in violation of federal law.

Oregon was the first state to legalize what the Oregon law refers to as "death with dignity," allowing some terminally ill patients to choose when they will end their lives. There are a number of conditions that must be met under Oregon law. These conditions include:

- The patient must be a bona fide resident of the State of Oregon.
- The patient must have a diagnosis of "incurable and irreversible disease that, within reasonable medical judgment, will cause death within 6 months."
- A patient must be referred for mental counseling if there is any evidence of impaired mental capacity.
- A consultant physician must confirm the diagnosis of a terminal illness.
- The process requires the issuance of a prescription to be filled by a pharmacist for a patient who self-administers the prescribed drug.

- Physicians or pharmacists who object to participating are allowed to opt out.

Following enactment of the OWDA, the U.S. AG issued an interpretive rule stating that he would deregister from the DEA's list of authorized controlled substance prescribers any physician who prescribed a medication consistent with Oregon law under the ODWDA. The State of Oregon challenged the position taken by the AG, and the U.S. Supreme Court eventually reviewed that challenge. In their ruling, the court stated:

> By this logic, the AG claims extraordinary authority. If the AG's argument were correct, this power to deregister would include the greater power to criminalize even the actions of registered physicians, whenever they engage in conduct he deems illegitimate. It would be anomalous for Congress to have so painstakingly described the AG's limited authority to deregister a single physician or schedule a single drug, but to have given him, just by implication, authority to declare an entire class of activity outside the usual course of professional practice, and therefore a criminal violation of the CSA.

The Supreme Court noted reasons why ruling in favor of the federal government could have broad and long-lasting negative consequences:

> Under the government's theory, the medical judgments the AG could make are not limited to physician-assisted suicide. Were this argument accepted, he could decide whether any particular drug may be used for any particular purpose, or indeed whether a physician who administers any controversial treatment could be deregistered. To read prescriptions for assisted suicide as constituting "drug abuse" under the CSA is discordant with the phrase's consistent use throughout the statute, not to mention its ordinary meaning.

The court concluded that "The structure of the CSA, conveys unwillingness to cede medical judgments to an executive official who lacks medical expertise." The court further observed, "This presumption works against a conclusion that the AG has authority to make quintessentially medical judgments." Finally, the court said, "This confirms that the authority claimed by the AG is both beyond his expertise and incongruous with the statutory purposes and design."

The State of Oregon's challenge to the U.S. Attorney General was upheld. States, and not the federal government, have the authority to determine standards of practice for healthcare professions, and this state authority extends to the legalization of controlled substance use for the purpose of death with dignity.

Euthanasia

Euthanasia is mercy killing. The word is derived from the Greek words "eu" and "thanatos," which translates as "good death." It is a broad concept with heavy baggage. The term "euthanasia" is seldom used within a human healthcare context, due to its ambiguity and moral implications. Some people who say they oppose euthanasia discover that they actually are not in disagreement with those who say they support euthanasia, because the seeming disagreement is based on an understanding of the terms being used and the circumstances to which they are being applied. Terms and circumstances matter a lot when euthanasia is discussed.

There are three circumstances in which euthanasia will ordinarily be considered: at the beginning of life, at the end of life, and following an incident that results in the diagnosis of a persistent vegetative state.

The question of euthanasia arises at the beginning of life when a child has been born in such a challenging physical and/or mental condition that prospects for what some people would consider to be a happy and enjoyable life are very low or nonexistent. Under these circumstances, the decision about terminating a life usually involves the quality of life the child can expect, as well as the impact on the family, and the resources available to support the child.

At the end of life, the question of euthanasia may reflect the preferences of the dying patient to either continue or forego medical treatment. There is no moral obligation by medical staff to continue futile treatment, particularly if the patient refuses the treatment.

Euthanasia may be discussed after a tragic accident or other event has led to hypoxic brain damage from which it is expected that the patient will never recover. This is not always an easy diagnosis. Questions will arise about whether continued treatment is prolonging life or instead is prolonging the dying process. Euthanasia may be offered to allow the patient to die with dignity.

The terminology of euthanasia requires consideration of both voluntariness and what is referred to as the active/passive distinction. As a preliminary matter, it is important to state that all actions that fall under the umbrella of "euthanasia" are benevolent in nature and are done for the good of the person who dies or to fulfill a public responsibility. Malevolently killing another person merely to benefit oneself is simply considered to be murder and does not even enter into the conversation of euthanasia.

Active euthanasia is commissive. It requires physical effort to mercifully end a person's suffering and meaningless existence. Active euthanasia causes death directly, rather than allowing for a death to occur. The administration of a large dose of a lethal drug is active euthanasia.

Passive euthanasia requires an act of omission, when something could be done to prolong a person's life, but that thing is intentionally not done. Sometimes, this is referred to as "letting die" as opposed to "killing." The failure to quickly initiate life support (sometimes referred to as a "slow code") is passive euthanasia.

Some people object to the passive/active distinction based on the argument that the intent and the result are the same in each case. Other people see a difference between actively interfering with the natural course of things and passively letting nature take its course.

Voluntary euthanasia occurs when the person who dies has expressed a clear desire to die and has consented to the procedures, or to the withholding of procedures, which will lead to the person's death.

Nonvoluntary euthanasia occurs when the person who dies is not able to express a desire to die and cannot consent to procedures that will lead to death. Such persons may be in a persistent vegetative state or they may be too young to consent or may have a mental disability. Proxy decisions must be made by responsible parties who represent the best interests of the person who will die.

Involuntary euthanasia occurs when a person dies against that person's expressed wishes.

The combinations of these concepts yield scenarios of varying complexity.

The least complicated scenario, from a legal perspective, is active, involuntary euthanasia. Aside from government-sanctioned activities such as warfare or the execution of condemned prisoners, this is considered murder. Criminal charges will be filed against anyone who commits active, involuntary euthanasia.

Active, nonvoluntary euthanasia is essentially the same. It is not legal and will likely result in criminal charges, perhaps murder charges. Surrogate decision-makers are generally not allowed to consent to direct acts that lead to death.

Passive, voluntary euthanasia is also relatively easy to deal with legally. Within a healthcare setting, when a competent patient chooses to be left alone and die in peace, this event has no legal consequences. Freedom means the right to be independent of interference by others.

Passive, involuntary euthanasia does present complex legal issues when a patient insists on being treated, but the treatment is withheld, leading to the patient's death. Criminal neglect charges are likely in this situation, although there may be a viable defense based on other relevant facts.

Active, voluntary euthanasia is legal in those jurisdictions that currently permit it, within the parameters that have been established in those jurisdictions.

That leaves passive, nonvoluntary euthanasia, in which surrogate decision-makers decline treatment on behalf of the incapacitated patient. Under the law, many jurisdictions permit this to occur, as long as a specific process is followed, and the best interests of the patient are the paramount concern of the surrogate decision-makers.

Because euthanasia as a concept involves so many different variants, it is often not a useful word or concept as applied to healthcare. For that reason, the alternative language generally used in healthcare is "physician-assisted dying" or "death with dignity." These are phrases that have clear meaning in the places where they are used. Their legality, within specific limits, has been established under the law, and those who meet legal requirements are given a safe harbor from criminal prosecution for euthanasia or for murder or for other crimes.

The Right to Die

The concept sometimes referred to as the "right to die" means that a person has the right to choose when and how death will occur when death is imminent. This choice may be asserted for a person by a legal representative of that person, who legally stands in the shoes of the person.

Two well-known cases, referred to as "Quinlan" and "Cruzan," have established the right to die in the United States.

The Quinlan case was decided by the Supreme Court of New Jersey in 1976.[6] Karen Quinlan became comatose following the ingestion of drugs and alcohol, and she was mechanically ventilated. Her parents initially authorized physicians to use any possible treatment that might lead to Karen's recovery. Nothing worked. When the parents were convinced that Karen would never recover, they authorized the hospital to withdraw ventilation. Karen's physicians refused to follow the parents' directive because they claimed that it would violate medical ethics. The parents then sued the physicians and the hospital.

The Supreme Court of New Jersey ruled that Karen had a constitutional right of privacy that could be safeguarded by her legal guardians and that the private decision of the guardians should be honored. The court also ruled that the hospital would be exempt from criminal charges for discontinuing artificial respiration. Karen lived for 10 more years after artificial respiration was discontinued.

Cases that followed Quinlan resulted in mixed holdings based on differing facts and legal arguments. States continued to assert their interest in preserving life and in protecting the standards of the medical profession.

In 1990, the U.S. Supreme Court issued a landmark decision in the Cruzan case.[7]

Nancy Cruzan was left in a persistent vegetative state following an automobile accident. She had no chance of recovery, although with artificial nutrition and hydration she could likely have lived for several decades. Her parents' efforts to remove life support were initially approved by a lower court but were reversed by the Missouri Supreme Court. Her parents appealed to the U.S. Supreme Court.

The court held that the Fourteenth Amendment to the Constitution contains a liberty interest but that this interest does not prevent a state from insisting that there be "clear and convincing" evidence of an incompetent patient's prior expressed wish to have treatment withdrawn should there be no hope of recovery. The court confirmed that a competent patient has a constitutionally protected right to refuse unwanted medical treatment. But an incompetent person in a persistent vegetative state cannot make an informed choice to exercise that right. In the absence of clear and convincing evidence that Nancy would want life support withdrawn, the court upheld the state's right to prohibit this from happening.

The court left open the possibility that new evidence might be found to comply with the clear and convincing standard. A friend of Nancy's from years before heard of the case on the news and informed Nancy's parents that she had discussed the issue with Nancy and that Nancy had said she would not want to be maintained artificially alive if she had no hope of recovery. With this evidence, the Cruzan family went back to court, and they were permitted to authorize withdrawal of nutrition and hydration. Nancy died 12 days after her feeding tubes were removed.

The lesson of these cases is that the wishes of a competent patient will be honored. To protect the right to die, if one wants to exercise that right should one become incompetent, a living will and/or an advance directive should be made. The method of making these documents, with sufficient protection for involved relatives and health professionals, varies from state to state.

A Duty to Die?

Futility is a difficult situation to manage for people who are committed to the value of technology and who claim the ability to solve any problem through technology. The reality is that many people reach a stage in their lives where the future is bleak, and nothing can be done to change that prognosis. Medical care at that stage of life tends to be very expensive, and the return on investment is low, perhaps even nonexistent. Technology has its limits.

There are some health policy analysts and ethicists who have begun to ask whether, faced with the reality that no reasonable medical options exist, people at the end of life have a duty to forego expensive and futile therapies. The argument is that healthcare resources are finite and that those who would benefit from resources should be given priority over those for whom the resources will provide no benefit.

The idea of a terminally ill patient's duty to decline futile treatment, in favor of others who might be denied useful treatment, has been labeled as a "duty to die" by those who are horrified by the notion.

There is currently no trend in the direction of recognizing a legal duty to die, but the conversation is occurring. It is possible that notions of what can and must be done for dying patients will someday be determined, perhaps to a limited degree, by a morally applied cost–benefit analysis.

Dr. Jack Kevorkian

For obvious reasons, most physicians who assist the death of terminally ill patients maintain a low profile. Michigan physician Jack Kevorkian was an exception to this rule.[8] As a crusader for assisted dying, Dr. Kevorkian publicized his provision of fatal medication doses to dying patients, and he dared prosecutors to file criminal charges against him.

Dr. Kevorkian claimed to have participated in 130 patient suicides before he was convicted in 1999 of second-degree murder. His previous four trials, all on charges of assisted suicide, had resulted in three acquittals and one mistrial.

The incident that led to Dr. Kevorkian's conviction was the videotaped death of a patient who suffered from ALS. The patient consented to physician-assisted dying. Dr. Kevorkian injected the patient with secobarbital, succinylcholine, and KCl. Using an EKG, Dr. Kevorkian established that the patient's heart had stopped. What was different about this incident, as opposed to previous incidents, was the direct injection of the drugs by Dr. Kevorkian, rather than the use of a device through which patients self-injected drugs made available to them by Dr. Kevorkian. In the four previous cases that had not resulted in a criminal conviction, Kevorkian had provided the medication to the patients, and they had self-administered the medications.

After being convicted of murder, Dr. Kevorkian was sentenced to 10 to 25 years in prison. He was paroled after only 8 years. He died in 2011, leaving a legacy of controversy. Some people sympathized with him, and others were horrified. He accomplished his goal of attracting attention.

Dr. James Gallant

Oregon physician Dr. James Gallant was disciplined by the state licensing agency for engaging in the "mercy killing" of a patient. Dr. Gallant was found to have committed "unprofessional conduct." He was reprimanded and his medical license was suspended for 60 days.[9] The state Court of Appeals affirmed the discipline in 1999. There is no record of a criminal case having been filed.

The facts of the case showed that the 76-year-old patient awakened one morning with a severe headache. She collapsed while calling for emergency assistance. In the ER, a neurosurgeon determined that the patient had suffered a massive intracerebral hemorrhage from which she would soon die.

As her primary care physician, Dr. Gallant was called. The patient's daughter arrived and insisted that no artificial methods be used to prolong her mother's dying but that her mother be kept comfortable. Dr. Gallant removed a respirator that had been installed. He prescribed diazepam and morphine for comfort. He expected the patient to die quickly, but she did not. After returning to his clinic to see other patients, Dr. Gallant contacted the ER frequently. The patient was still alive, and the daughter requested that the patient's cardiac pacemaker be deactivated, but Dr. Gallant did not know how to do this.

An ER nurse called Dr. Gallant about an hour later to report that the patient's family members were concerned that the patient was suffering needlessly. The nurse then suggested to Dr. Gallant that succinylcholine is sometimes used "in these situations." Dr. Gallant ordered that the drug be injected, and the patient died. Three weeks later, the hospital reported the incident to the licensing agency.

In the appeal of his discipline by the state agency, Dr. Gallant contended that adequate due process had not been observed in the administrative action taken against his license. He cited the Oregon Death with Dignity Act as legal authority for his conduct. The court disagreed and affirmed the discipline, noting that the case had nothing to do with the Oregon Death with Dignity Act, where patient consent is necessary and the patient self-administers the prescribed lethal medication.

Bonnie Savoy

Desperate situations may lead to drastic actions. The unexplained death of a frail and/or elderly person may implicate the spouse or partner as the culprit in an assisted suicide, if the facts indicate that the victim had expressed a desire to die.[10] Vulnerable people may be physically incapable of taking their own lives, and they may request the assistance of a loved one. Under most circumstances, it is a crime to honor any such request. Even in states that have legalized death with dignity, the process of carrying out a planned death is narrowly regulated. Any killing of another person that is outside that process is murder.

Bonnie Savoy was convicted of first-degree premeditated murder in the death of her husband from an overdose of insulin.[11] The husband suffered from multiple sclerosis and had become a challenge to care for. The evidence showed that the couple were facing financial difficulties that would lead to foreclosure on their home. The husband was not diabetic. Savoy regularly injected her husband with interferon beta-1b. A friend of hers was diabetic, and the friend noticed that insulin was missing from her supply following a visit by Savoy to the friend's home. The investigators alleged that Savoy had used insulin stolen from the friend's home and that she had switched the insulin for the interferon beta-1b when administering the regular injection to her husband. There was no direct evidence that the substitution had been made.

Savoy challenged her conviction based on the insufficiency of the evidence. At trial, Savoy did not dispute that the husband died from a purposeful injection of a lethal dose of insulin. However, she contended that the husband administered the lethal dose of insulin himself. Due to the husband's physical condition, this argument was subject to considerable skepticism, and the jury did not believe it. The court concluded that the prosecution had presented sufficient evidence from which a rational jury could conclude, beyond a reasonable doubt, that Savoy had injected the insulin. The conviction was affirmed.

Regardless of how poignant a seemingly impossible situation may be, people who engage in mercy killing of their partners are murderers. It does not matter that the victim may have requested assistance in dying. Vulnerable people deserve the protection of the law. Circumstantial evidence will support the murder conviction of a person who kills a partner, even if the killing was done benevolently.

Pharmacists and Assisted Dying

The language typically used in state laws with reference to "physician-assisted dying" is in many ways a misnomer. A patient's decision to choose when to die certainly requires the assistance of a physician who must order the medication, but it also requires the assistance of a pharmacist who must dispense or distribute the medication that is used in the procedure, and it may require the assistance of a nurse to administer the medication. Policymakers often overlook the role of the pharmacist and nurse. That is, they overlook those necessary roles until a pharmacist or nurse declines to participate, and then the roles of pharmacists and nurses become very relevant to ongoing policy discussions.

Organized pharmacy does not have a specific rule that allows or requires or prohibits participation by pharmacists in physician-assisted dying. Rather, the pharmacy profession recognizes that individual pharmacists may assert their own personal objections to morally problematic procedures, as long as professional responsibilities are met. In jurisdictions where assisted dying is illegal, the pharmacist's role is clear. No pharmacist should participate in an illegal procedure. When assisted dying is legal, the analysis is one of ethics, and many pharmacists look to ethical standards of the profession. As a general rule, the pharmacy profession allows pharmacists to decline participation in assisted dying by "stepping out of the way" of these activities. The pharmacy profession generally does not support pharmacists who "step in the way" through activities that are intended to sabotage a legal procedure ordered by a patient's physician, to which the patient has consented.

The process of stepping out of the way is generally referred to as "conscientious objection," and the process for exercising it is consistent with a long history of support for conscientious objection to military service in the United States. When a conscientious objector to war wishes to step away and not participate as an active combatant in a war, this wish can be granted after the objector has explained the reason for the objection to the draft board. But the war will nevertheless continue with others participating. The objector is not allowed to stop the war. Stopping a war would be a political action rather than an appeal to individual conscience. A disruption of the war effort (e.g., by causing defective weapons to be manufactured) would be considered an act of treason.

Organized pharmacy respects the right of a pharmacist to step away from assisted dying and not provide medications that are to be used in the process. As is the case with conscientious objection to military service, there may be conditions that would apply to asserting this right in a pharmacy setting.

The first of these conditions is publicity. A pharmacist who works in a healthcare setting where assisted dying takes place must "publicize" their conscientious objection by explaining the objecting to pharmacy management, so that alternative ways of having the legal pharmacy services made available can be found. A pharmacist is not allowed to "surprise" management by unexpectedly asserting a right to conscience at a time when no alternative pharmacists are available and, thus, sabotage a planned procedure.

The second condition is authenticity, and this is far more difficult to apply. An authentic objection based on conscience is founded on personal beliefs that lead a pharmacist to say something like, "I could not live with myself if I were to do that." It is not impermissible for management to ask a pharmacist to explain the nature of the conscientious objection to assure that it is authentic. A pharmacist who says to management, "I just don't want to do it, and I can't give you a reason," will not qualify for conscientious objection.

Some pharmacists will choose to work in a practice setting where assisted dying is unlikely to occur and where the pharmacists will not be called on to participate in procedures that they find to be morally objectionable. Some pharmacists will choose to be politically active in issues related to physician-assisted dying, and these political activities should be pursued outside the work environment. As the population of the United States ages, and as end-of-life care becomes more technologically complex, the legal and ethical issues surrounding end-of-life care will present challenges to pharmacists. It is important for pharmacists to anticipate those challenges so that patient needs can be met.

Law and Ethics at the End of Life

Standards of pharmacy practice do not recognize special circumstances that justify an ethical exemption from pharmacy laws for end-of-life care. A legal case from Louisiana explains this point quite clearly.[12] A patient was enrolled in hospice care, and the hospice physician prescribed a fentanyl patch, with morphine suppositories for breakthrough pain. The morphine prescription was for a total quantity of 40 suppositories, with specific instructions for the pharmacist to initially dispense only 20 suppositories, and additional authority for the pharmacist to dispense the second supply of 20 suppositories 72 hours later. The initial 20 suppositories were dispensed on a Friday.

On Sunday morning, the patient's son requested release of the remaining 20 suppositories. The pharmacist consulted the prescriber, who refused to authorize the early release of the second supply. The physician contacted the patient's son, telling him that a nurse would need to visit the home and assess his father before release of the additional supply of suppositories could be authorized. The son became threatening and abusive and refused to allow the nurse to visit for the assessment. The physician advised the son that the father was dismissed as a hospice patient, and he instructed the son to take the father to the emergency room, which the son did. The father died that night.

The lawsuit filed by the son alleged that the pharmacy and the physician should have allowed release of the remaining 20 suppositories because this was the ethically right thing to do for a dying patient in excruciating pain. The physician defended the lawsuit by citing medical standards that require patient assessment when a dosage of opioids is increased. The pharmacy defended the lawsuit by referencing the requirement that prescription drugs be dispensed only on the order of an authorized prescriber. The pharmacy explained that there was no legal authority to dispense the remaining 20 suppositories, absent notification from the prescribing physician that the additional supply could be dispensed. The court agreed with the pharmacy and dismissed the case. There was no ethical basis for violating the law. Even in a patient's last hours of life, basic legal requirements must be honored.

Conclusion

The aggressive use of palliative medications at the end of a patient's life can hasten a patient's death. The emotion that surrounds the dying process can lead to misinterpretations of what is happening and perhaps can also lead to litigation based on misunderstandings. Healthcare professionals who are involved in the provision of medication that causes the death of a dying patient, or that may have caused the dying patient's death, may be suspected of having committed a crime. It is important that these activities be undertaken with transparency and compassion to avoid misunderstandings that may lead to legal proceedings.

Key Takeaways

- Be aware of the rights of vulnerable patients at the end of life who may be exploited by well-intentioned family members or by healthcare professionals. Also be aware of each patient's right to determine their own destiny. Do your best to put yourself in the circumstances of the patient. Find out what you can about the patient's previously expressed preferences if you feel uncomfortable with any end-of-life care situation that you encounter. If you are in a jurisdiction that has legalized death with dignity, understand that the method through which dying patients are allowed to choose the time of their death is the issuance of a prescription for them by their physician, and the dispensing of medication to them by their pharmacist pursuant to that prescription. Death-with-dignity statutes permit the exercise of conscientious objection by a pharmacist who wishes to step aside and not fill such a prescription. Consider in advance whether you would choose to participate in the filling of a prescription for an intentionally lethal medication. Tell your manager and/or your colleagues of the choice you have made. If you think your participation would be conditional, then let your manager and/or colleagues know the conditions under which you would decline to participate.

- Recognize that the end of a patient's life can be an extremely emotional time for the patient, for the patient's family, and for healthcare professionals who know the patient and have provided care for the patient. In both the institutional and community pharmacy practice settings, it is common for the volume of medications to escalate at the end of a patient's life. When you see from your records that a patient is of a certain age, and when the patient's medication use has changed to indicate a critical illness that may be fatal, prepare yourself to professionally handle questions and concerns by the patient or family members. It is perfectly acceptable for pharmacists to show their emotions in times of sadness. The death of a patient is a sad time. However, during the dying process, it is important to provide the best information possible when questions are asked about a patient's medication. Emotion, natural though it may be, cannot get in the way of quality pharmaceutical care.
- Be alert for questions about lethal medication doses when a patient is in declining health and may be considering a fatal overdose. If a patient asks how much of a medication would constitute a lethal dose, and if you detect that the patient is thinking about committing suicide, then don't disregard the question as frivolous. This is the time to begin a conversation. Try changing the subject by asking, "How is your medication working for you?" Discuss the benefits of the medication and explain the risks as well. Emphasize the importance of taking all medications as they have been prescribed. If you continue to be concerned that the patient may be suicidal, then contact the patient's primary care physician. It is not a HIPAA violation to disclose what you know about a patient to the patient's physician. If the patient does not have a primary care physician, and if the patient's intentions seem

to be serious, then ask, “Is it your intent to take an overdose of this medication?” If the patient says yes, or if the patient seems ambivalent, then call your local suicide prevention line and ask for help. Suicide prevention counselors will be able to suggest solutions that can help the patient and that do not require you to violate patient confidentiality. There are continuing pharmacy educations programs that address suicide prevention. Consider completing one of these programs.

References

1. State v. Naramore, 965 P.2d 211 (Kan.App. 1998).

2. A Definition of Irreversible Coma: Report of the Ad Hoc Committee of the Harvard Medical School to Examine the Definition of Brain Death. *JAMA*. 1968;205(6):337–340.

3. Lewis A. The Uniform Determination of Death Act is Being Revised. *Neurocrit Care*. 2022 Apr;36(2):335–338.

4. Vacco v. Quill, 521 U.S. 702 (1997).

5. Gonzales v. Oregon, 546 U.S. 243 (2006).

6. Matter of Quinlan, 355 A.2d 647 (N.J. 1976).

7. Cruzan v. Director, Missouri Department of Health, 497 U.S. 261 (1990).

8. People v. Kevorkian, 639 N.W.2d 291 (Mich.App. 2002).

9. Gallant v. Board of Medical Examiners, 974 P.2d 814 (Or.App. 1999).

10. Salari S. Patterns of intimate partner homicide suicide in later life: Strategies for prevention. *Clin Interv Aging*. 2007;2(3):441–452.

11. Savoy v. Washington, 2010 Westlaw 5327346 (S.D. Mich. 2010).

12. McGregor v. Hospice Care of Louisiana, 36 So.3d 272 (La.App. 2010).

Chapter 14

Liability for Fatal Healthcare Practices

Pharmacists can be exposed to legal liability for any medication error that leads to the death of a patient. All preventable patient deaths will lead to consequences for an erring pharmacist. While these consequences may not be criminal in nature, they are nevertheless career-altering, if not career-ending. From a patient safety perspective, there is a clear connection between the avoidance of criminal liability and civil liability for a fatal medication error. Making a mistake that kills a patient is a shockingly transformative experience that must be appreciated and understood so that it can be avoided.

The law of "torts" serves as the basis for evaluating a claim made by a patient (or the patient's estate if the patient has died) against a pharmacist who has allegedly practiced below the applicable standard of care. Under the legal principle of "*respondeat superior*" (translated as "let the master answer"), a pharmacy that employs a negligent pharmacist can be sued for harm caused by the malpractice of its pharmacist. It is also possible to sue a pharmacy directly if the nature of the malpractice allegation is that the pharmacy practice site created a substandard and dangerous practice situation that led to a pharmacist's negligent error.

Elements of Medication Malpractice Liability

There are four elements of a pharmacy malpractice case based on allegations of negligent conduct. All four of these elements must be proven by the plaintiff for there to be a successful malpractice case against a pharmacist or pharmacy. These four elements are:

- *Duty Owed.* A pharmacist or pharmacy may be held liable for malpractice only if a duty of care was owed to the person who allegedly was harmed through a pharmacist's negligence. This first element is relatively straightforward. If a pharmacist is alleged to have dispensed a medication in error (wrong drug, wrong directions, wrong strength, etc.), or if a pharmacist provides inaccurate advice (counseling that two drugs can be safely taken together, when in fact there is a major drug–drug interaction), then the duty of the pharmacist is clear. Pharmacists have a duty to accurately process medication orders and provide accurate information to patients. The duty-owed element has been met. On the other hand, if a pharmacist is alleged to have failed to correct a prescriber's misdiagnosis, then the duty owed is far less clear. Pharmacists are generally not required to act as diagnosticians. If a patient has suffered harm due to the failure by a prescriber to appropriately diagnose the patient's ailment, then a malpractice lawsuit against the pharmacist who dispensed the incorrectly prescribed medication that was accurately dispensed will likely fail because there is no duty owed by a pharmacist to correct the inaccuracy of a prescriber's diagnosis.

- *Breach of Duty.* If a pharmacist or pharmacy owes a duty to a patient who was allegedly harmed though negligence, the next step is to show a breach of that duty. The customary way to show a breach of duty is through expert witness testimony. The plaintiff must produce an expert in the profession of pharmacy who is of the opinion that the defendants did not comply with the standard of care when they provided products and/or services to the patient. The plaintiff's expert is required to establish a foundation for the opinions that are expressed in support of the plaintiff's case. The plaintiff's expert must explain the relevant standard of care and must clarify how the actions taken by the defendants were not consistent with the standard of care. The defense is allowed to provide their own expert to rebut the testimony of the plaintiff's expert. Usually, a defense expert will explain that the pharmacy standard of care is different from what the plaintiff's expert identified and that the defendant's conduct met the standard of care. This point–counterpoint disagreement is sometimes referred to as a "battle of the experts." A jury will decide which expert's version to accept as credible.
- *Causation.* A pharmacist who owes a duty and who has breached that duty will nevertheless win a malpractice lawsuit if the harm experienced by the patient was not caused by the erring pharmacist. If the harm was caused by a factor other than the pharmacist's error, then there can be no pharmacist liability for the harm. For example, a patient's underlying disease may have progressed rapidly, and the facts may show that the patient actually died from the disease and not from the pharmacist's error. It may also be possible to defend an erring pharmacist by showing that there was another factor that more proximately caused harm to the patient. For example, a pharmacist may have erred in filling a prescription for an obvious overdose of an opioid. Yet if the facts show that the patient committed suicide by intentionally ingesting a large quantity of the medication, then the proximate cause of the patient's death could be the voluntary ingestion of medication and not the pharmacist's error. An intervening act that is not foreseeable to an erring pharmacist will break the chain of causation and will relieve the pharmacist of liability.
- *Damages.* A plaintiff must have suffered actual damages to support a lawsuit for malpractice against a pharmacist. Theoretical damage will not suffice. For example, a patient may contend that a pharmacist's

error caused no physical harm but did cause the patient to have "fear of medication use" because the patient is devastated by the thought of what might have happened due to the error. This sort of speculative harm will not support a case of malpractice. Only actual damages will support a pharmacy malpractice case. Actual damage is usually not difficult to prove. Experts can explain the extent of the damage suffered by a patient. It is up to the jury to determine the amount of money to award based on the severity of the damages and the economic consequences to the patient of the damages. In the absence of gross negligence, compensatory damages will comprise the entire award for pharmacist malpractice. If the evidence shows that the defendant pharmacist acted with malice or with utter disregard for the patient's welfare, then a jury may award punitive damages. The purpose of punitive damages, as the phrase suggests, is to punish the pharmacist for morally culpable conduct that goes beyond mere inadvertence or inattention.

Corrective justice is the theoretical basis of malpractice law. Corrective justice links a victim with a wrongdoer, and it requires the wrongdoer to repair the wrongful losses caused to the victim. For a loss by the victim to be wrongful, it need not be a loss for which the wrongdoer is morally to blame. It need only be a loss that is incident to the violation of trust that has been placed in the wrongdoer by the victim.

According to corrective justice, any malpractice liability that is based on "ordinary negligence" does not imply condemnation, because a defendant can be liable for malpractice even though no intentional harm was done to a patient. Corrective justice is a form of transactional (or contractual) justice. Pursuant to this contractual relationship, an agreement has been reached through which a healthcare professional will provide competent services to a patient, and the patient will provide payment to the healthcare professional both through monetary exchange (which can be delivered through the patient's health insurance) and through adherence to the care plan established by the healthcare professional. A violation of the terms of this transaction occurs if the healthcare professional makes an error causing harm to the patient, and the healthcare professional must repair the damage done to the patient in the same way that a debt is repaid (this repayment can be delivered through malpractice insurance).

Corrective justice acknowledges a difference between "ordinary negligence" and "gross negligence." The concept of "gross negligence" carries with it an element of moral condemnation. There must be consequences for conduct that rises to the level of intentional indifference, and those consequences are administered through an award of punitive damages. Although punitive damages can be a windfall for the plaintiff because they may exceed actual damages, they may also be viewed as compensation to the plaintiff for having undergone the experience of being the object of deceitful and/or immoral conduct. An award of punitive damages based on gross negligence is primarily focused on the action of the person who caused harm, but the rights of the person who was harmed are also a consideration.

Ordinary Negligence as the Basis of Pharmacist Malpractice Liability

The tort of negligence has not always been a recognized legal principle of Anglo-American law. When the United States became an independent country, communities were relatively small and close-knit. Harm done by one person to another was generally worked out through informal social systems. Crimes were punished by the government, but civil wrongs such as negligent professional practice did not require a government framework for their resolution. Friends worked out their differences in ways that were culturally expected and accepted. Even when one person inadvertently caused the death of another person, and when no crime had occurred, disagreements between the perpetrator and the survivors of the victim were resolved without the need for government intervention.

As communities became more complex and as close connections among residents became less common, differences in cultural perspectives about how to identify wrongdoing and how to "right a wrong" required the development of a governmental forum at which individual disagreements could be fairly and objectively heard and resolved. In the mid-1800s, when the tort of negligence began to develop in the United States, pharmacy cases were among the first lawsuits to recognize a civil remedy for harm caused to a person through the carelessness of another person. The potentially lethal nature of the medications provided by pharmacists led to pharmacists being the subject of early malpractice litigation.

In a case from 1852, a patient filed a malpractice lawsuit against a pharmacist for negligently dispensing extract of belladonna when the patient's physician had prescribed extract of dandelion.[1] The court described extract of belladonna as a "deadly poison." The patient recovered, although for a short time it was thought that she would die. The court based a determination of pharmacist liability on the general principle that "every man is bound under the law to avoid that which endangers another." The court concluded:

> The defendant's duty arose out of the nature of his business and the danger to others incident to its mismanagement. Nothing but mischief like that which actually happened could have been expected from sending the poison falsely labeled into the market; and the defendant is justly responsible for the probable consequences of the act.

The plaintiff was awarded money damages to compensate her for the harm caused by the pharmacist's error.

A similar case, also from 1852, arose from harm caused by a pharmacist's compounding of a medication using a mill that had not been adequately cleaned following its previous use.[2] The residue of a poisonous substance was unintentionally included in a patient's medication. The patient survived but suffered severe adverse effects. The patient sued the pharmacist for malpractice. The court said:

> The purchasers of wines and provisions, by sight, smell, and taste, may be able, without incurring any material injury, to detect their bad and unwholesome qualities, but many are wholly unable, by the taste or appearance of many drugs, to distinguish those which are poisonous from others which are innoxious, so close is their resemblance to each other; purchasers have, therefore, to trust their druggist. It is upon his skill and prudence they must rely. It is, therefore, incumbent upon him that he understands his business. It is his duty to know the properties of his drugs, and to be able to distinguish them from each other. It is his duty so to qualify himself, or to employ those who are so qualified, to attend to the business of compounding and vending medicines and drugs, as that one drug may not be sold for another, and so that, when a prescription is presented to be made up, the proper medicines, and none other, be used in mixing and compounding it. As applicable to the owners of drug stores, or persons engaged in vending drugs and medicines at retail, the legal maxim should be reversed. Instead of *caveat emptor*, it should be *caveat vendor*.

Although there had been no intent to cause harm to the patient, the lawsuit against the pharmacist succeeded and the patient was awarded money damages. Perhaps more importantly, the tradition of *caveat emptor* ("let the buyer beware") was firmly replaced with *caveat vendor* ("let the seller beware") as applied to pharmacy practice transactions.

Modern-day pharmacists are held to a similarly exact standard. The law requires absolute accuracy in order processing. The fact of error speaks so loudly that, when a patient has received a medication in error, a presumption of ordinary negligence arises, and the pharmacist is virtually powerless to rebut the presumption. The pharmacist may have been careful and attentive when the order was being processed, but what matters is that an error occurred and not how careful the pharmacist was in processing the order. Careful practice does not absolve a pharmacist of liability following the commission of an error under tort law. The resulting exposure to liability is similar in pharmacist malpractice cases alleging the failure to warn of adverse drug effects or the failure to screen prescription orders for potential problems. An error is an error. Pharmacists cannot successfully defend cases of malpractice by showing the application of skill and caring at the time an error occurs.

Ordinary Negligence: Pharmacy Perspectives and Legal Perspectives

From a pharmacy perspective, the phrase "ordinary negligence" is perplexing. In a profession that prides itself on accuracy, the notion that any sort of negligence could be considered as "ordinary" boggles the pharmacist mind. Those who practice the profession of pharmacy see nothing ordinary about negligence in pharmacy. A pharmacist who is alleged to have been negligent is likely to be offended by the allegation. It is countercultural in pharmacy to accept that negligence is ordinary.

From a legal perspective, the phrase "ordinary negligence" makes perfect sense. Malpractice law is based on the tort of negligence. If an error is made by a healthcare professional, resulting in harm to a patient, and if an award of damages is legally justified, then the only basis on which that award can be made is negligence. If there is no negligence, then there can be no malpractice award. No offense is intended toward a pharmacist when a lawyer alleges ordinary negligence by the pharmacist. It is simply a means to obtain corrective justice for the lawyer's client.

Reconciliation of the differing pharmacy and legal perspectives on ordinary negligence may be facilitated if the nature of pharmacy errors is considered within a legal context. There are two fundamental types of pharmacy errors that lead to malpractice liability based on negligence. The first type of error is often referred to as the "execution failure," while the second type of error is often referred to as a "planning failure." Execution failure can be subdivided into "slips" that result from attentional or perceptual inaccuracies, and "lapses" that generally involve errors of memory. Planning failure is different. It usually occurs when a person accurately carries out an action, but the goal is not achieved.

An example of an execution failure in pharmacy practice would be the delivery of a correctly processed prescription to the wrong patient. An example of a planning failure in pharmacy would be the attachment of a note to a bagged prescription waiting in will-call, indicating that a pharmacist must consult with the patient about a possible drug–drug interaction, but the note falls off the bag and the consultation does not take place. What these errors have in common is that they are inadvertent. They are the types of errors that can occur at any pharmacy. They are human errors. In this sense, they are "ordinary" because they can be anticipated to occur from time to time in any pharmacy. The effects of these errors can be tragic for the patient. Yet the errors themselves do not represent catastrophic failures of the pharmacy practice system. The erring pharmacist, and the pharmacy where the error occurred, can be held liable for compensatory damages based on ordinary negligence, but there will likely be no award of punitive damages because there is no intent to do harm and there is no willful disregard for the patient's best interests.

Gross Negligence as the Basis of Pharmacist Malpractice Liability

The law of professional malpractice is primarily intended to compensate a person who was harmed as the consequence of an error in professional practice. Secondary to compensation, there is also a punitive side of professional malpractice law that can result from the commission of "gross negligence" by a professional person. The word "gross" refers to the scale of the negligence (large rather than small) as well as to the accepted slang meaning (disgusting and offensive). A legal determination of gross negligence is hugely significant because it can lead to an award of punitive damages in addition to compensatory damages. Pharmacists and other health professionals who have made an obvious error will often feel vindicated if they can avoid punitive damages, even when compensatory damages have been awarded against them.

Jurisdictions vary in the language they use to describe the sort of conduct that qualifies under the category of "gross negligence." Phrases like "morally culpable" or "wanton and willful" or "so reckless as to be in utter disregard of the consequences" are often used to define gross negligence. The key factor in distinguishing between ordinary negligence and gross negligence is that the latter is seen as being the result of intentional misconduct, while the former is seen to be an error of mere inadvertence. Acts of gross negligence are committed purposefully rather than involuntarily.

Continuing to engage in dangerous pharmacy practices that have caused harm in the past can be interpreted as intentional misconduct. The cover-up of a pharmacy error that could have been remediated to avoid or to lessen harm requires intentionality by the person who engages in the cover-up. The deliberate violation of well-established rules is an intentional act. Each of these actions demonstrates malice on the part of the actor. In this sense, malice refers to selfishness and lack of concern for the welfare of others. It does not connote hatred or spite or ill will.

Some states do not allow insurance coverage of punitive damages. The public policy justification for this approach is that debts incurred through malice should not be repaid by third parties. Just as a person convicted of a crime cannot hire another person to serve the convict's prison sentence, a healthcare professional who commits gross negligence may not be allowed to use malpractice insurance to pay an award and, through this insurance coverage, be allowed to purchase the right to behave immorally.

Many state legislatures have passed laws labeled as "tort reform" that attempt to reduce the incidence of frivolous malpractice lawsuits while allowing the pursuit of valid malpractice claims, subject to some limitations. One common limitation on a valid malpractice claim is the placement of a "cap" on the dollar value of a compensatory award for a plaintiff. The "cap" may provide that only a certain amount of money may be paid to the victim of a medical error, even if the harm to the plaintiff vastly exceeds that amount. When this happens, the plaintiff may have no recourse other than to argue for punitive damages based on gross negligence. There will likely be a separate cap on punitive damages, and a claim for punitive damages provides one additional pool of money from which to obtain an award if the cap on compensatory damages is too restrictive.

Punitive damages are the means through which malpractice liability litigation rewards those who have been harmed through egregious pharmacy errors. The law of punitive damages is best illustrated through several legal case studies.

Legal Case Study: Lack of Institutional Controls

One of the classic cases in pharmacy law is from the State of Alabama, and it is based on an ordinary error that led to an extraordinary judicial ruling.[3] The defendant pharmacy received from the patient a handwritten prescription that was intended to order Tamoxifen, but the pharmacist misread the prescription and the pharmacy erroneously dispensed Tambocor. The pharmacy in this case did not dispute that the error had occurred or that it should be held liable for compensatory damages based on the actions of its employees. What was remarkable about the case was the patient's contention that the pharmacy should also be held liable for punitive damages based on wantonness on the part of the pharmacy corporation.

The trial court allowed the jury to award the plaintiff punitive damages based on a finding of corporate "wantonness." The pharmacy appealed this ruling. The appellate court noted that in Alabama, as in most states, "wantonness" is defined as "conduct which is carried on with a reckless or conscious disregard of the rights or safety of others." The court then posed the question of whether the plaintiff had presented sufficient evidence that the pharmacy had acted with reckless disregard for the safety of others. The court summarized the evidence that the pharmacy had acted with reckless disregard (this language is quoted from the court's own summary):

- "The prescription was illegible."
- "The pharmacist knew that the prescribing physician was an oncologist."
- "The pharmacist gave the plaintiff Tambocor, and antiarrhythmic drug used by cardiologists to treat arrhythmias, although the prescription actually called for an oncology drug."
- "The pharmacist did not attempt to call the physician to verify the accuracy of her reading of it and did not even try to question the patient about why her oncologist would prescribe a heart medication for her."
- "The pharmacist did not re-read the prescription to verify the accuracy of her reading of it."
- "The prescription was refilled incorrectly on two other occasions over a 5 ½ month period."
- "After the patient heard a news report about cancer and the newest treatment for cancer, which included Tamoxifen, which was not what she had been taking for 5 ½ months, she inquired of the pharmacy whether Tambocor was another name for Tamoxifen, and only then was it determined that the pharmacy had made an error with her prescription."

Based on this set of facts, the court considered whether the jury had appropriately reached the conclusion that punitive damages were warranted based on a claim of wantonness. The court concluded:

> Although the pharmacy argues that specialists regularly prescribe medicines for ailments outside their specialty, we believe that a prescription from an oncologist that a pharmacist believes to call for Tambocor, a heart medication used by cardiologists to treat arrhythmias or serious heart ailments, should cause her grave concern and necessarily prompt further inquiry. The extreme unusualness of a prescription from a cancer specialist supposedly calling for a dangerous heart medication, combined with the alleged illegibility of

> the prescription, is sufficient evidence of a reckless disregard of the safety of others to create a jury question as to whether the pharmacy acted wantonly. A jury could infer that the pharmacy's actions under these circumstances rose to the level of a conscious or reckless disregard for the safety of the patient. We note that the jury was informed of 233 incident reports that had been prepared by pharmacy employees during the three years preceding the incident. Those reports dealt in some way or another with patient complaints of errors on the part of pharmacy employees in filling the prescriptions, and the vast majority of them indicated that pharmacy employees had committed errors. This evidence, in addition to evidence filed with the State Board of Pharmacy and the evidence of lawsuits filed alleging that pharmacy employees had mis-filled prescriptions, was relevant to show the pharmacy's knowledge of problems within its pharmacies and, thus, was admissible in connection with the wantonness claim, predicated on the pharmacy having failed to initiate sufficient institutional controls over the manner in which prescriptions were filled.

Based on this rationale, the jury verdict that awarded punitive damages against the pharmacy was affirmed on appeal. This was the first legal case recognizing primary liability of a pharmacy corporation for the failure to initiate sufficient institutional controls over order processing at the pharmacy. It is interesting to note that the pharmacist was considered to be part of the pharmacy system, but the pharmacist was not considered to be the entirety of the system. The pharmacy management's knowledge of prior incidents of error, and an apparent lack of effort to modify the system to prevent errors, was a critical factor that supported a conclusion of system failure and that justified punitive damages.

The significance of this case is recognition that to avoid punishment through an award of punitive damages, pharmacies must organize and maintain effective systems that are designed to capture errors made by pharmacy team members and repair those errors before patients suffer preventable harm. Pharmacists, pharmacy technicians, and other pharmacy personnel have a significant role to play in the development and implementation of those error reduction systems.

Legal Case Study: Ignoring Device Manufacture Instructions and Warnings

High-tech medical devices are commonly used in contemporary hospital pharmacy. These specialized technologies are accompanied by manufacturer's instructions that explain potential precautions for their use, and pharmacists are aware that any technology can occasionally fail. A particularly relevant case reviewed a lower court's award of punitive damages based on a hospital pharmacist's failure to follow the manufacturer's directions while compounding a cardioplegia solution.[4] A jury awarded the plaintiff $92,000 in compensatory damages and $400,000 in punitive damages, and the hospital appealed the punitive damages award.

The cardioplegia was used during an arterial grafting procedure to protect the patient's heart from damage while it was stopped. When the physician attempted to restart the patient's heart, he was unable to do so. Laboratory results showed that the solution did not contain a sufficient amount of dextrose and that this deficiency caused the patient's death.

The appellate court noted that the cardioplegia compounder used by the pharmacist was accompanied by a manual that said, "Compounding should be monitored at the start of a cycle and at intervals thereafter to assure solutions are being transferred within acceptable limits." The pharmacist testified that she had prepared this physician's specific solution over 150 times before the fatal incident. She said that she heard the compounder start when she pushed the start button. She then turned away from the compounder to do other work. It took about 10 minutes for the compounder to mix the solution and during that time the pharmacist was nearby. She testified that she heard the compounder running the whole time it was operating. She said she would have heard an alarm if one had sounded.

The pharmacist testified:

> I could either stand there for 10 minutes and watch it, or I could watch it to see that the wheels were turning, do something else, turn around and work, turn back and see that the wheels were turning and that the fluid levels were changing. I could do that. I did it through part of the run. I turned my back to do my calculations. By the time I was able to finish my calculations and turn back, the dextrose run had already been completed. It was on its water cycle at that time.
>
> I did not look at the machine while the dextrose cycle was being operated. I do not remember that I ever saw the dextrose wheel turning. At the end of the dextrose cycle, I did not look at the dextrose bottle to see if the level had changed. If I had needed to, I would have been able to check the difference in fluid levels in the bottles.
>
> Just periodically watching does not guarantee that you know what went in the bag. If I had looked at the level on the dextrose bottle and seen that it had not changed, it never would have left the pharmacy.

> If I had looked at the machine for just an instant during the dextrose cycle and seen that the machine was not turning, I would have known something was wrong, but the machine should have sounded an alarm if that wheel was not turning.

An expert witness retained on behalf of the hospital testified that biomedical equipment is similar to all types of computer equipment and that "they can and do malfunction quite regularly." He further testified that computers are susceptible to spontaneous failure from voltage irregularities. In his opinion, the compounder was capable of malfunctioning even if it had been properly programmed and the malfunction would cause it not to transfer the correct amount of solution. In his opinion, the compounder malfunctioned when the pharmacist used it to compound the patient's solution. He testified that "the very first thing" that's pumped into the container for the cardioplegia solution is the dextrose" and that the compounder would pump the dextrose "in approximately 20 seconds." He said, "All the operator has got to do to see if dextrose is going in there is to stand there for 20 seconds and watch it."

After reviewing this evidence and testimony, the court recited the standard for an award of punitive damages: "The acts of a defendant which justify the imposition of punitive damages are those which are willful, wanton, malicious or so reckless as to be in utter disregard of the consequences. Such acts are clearly distinguished from negligence. While they need not always include an intent to do harm, they must show such a conscious disregard for another's rights as to amount to willful and intentional wrongdoing."

With this standard in mind, the court summarized the evidence:

> The cause of death was the insufficiency of the dextrose as a component of the cardioplegia solution; according to the manufacturer's manual, compounding should be monitored at the start of a cycle and at intervals thereafter to assure solutions are being transferred within acceptable limits; although the compounder contained an alarm system, that fact did not, according to the manual, dispense with the need for monitoring; the solution was not end tested after it was compounded, and this was a factor which emphasized the need for proper compounding; water and D-50 dextrose solution are both clear solutions, making it impossible for a visual inspection to disclose the deficiency; by watching the compounder, the pharmacist can see the pump wheels turn as the fluid is going through the machine; the pharmacist did not see the wheels turning for the dextrose bottle, nor did she watch to see whether the fluid levels changed in the bottles; she did not look at any time to see whether the dextrose wheel was turning; the hospital had

> no policy requiring her to do other than what she did in operating the compounder; she had not read the manufacturer's manual, nor did hospital policy require her to read it; the dextrose in the cardioplegia solution was less than 10 milligrams per deciliter, and the proper amount was 5,000 milligrams per deciliter; it was good standard practice for the operator of a compounder to observe the wheels of the compounder operating; biomedical equipment of this type malfunctions regularly and is susceptible to spontaneous failure from voltage irregularities; the dextrose cycle, if the solution is compounded properly, requires about 20 seconds; the fact that this solution contained so little dextrose permits the inference that the wheel on the dextrose pump operated, if at all, for a period substantially less than 20 seconds.

The hospital's primary defense was that the compounder had malfunctioned and that this malfunction was the manufacturer's fault and not the pharmacist's fault. The hospital also argued that no expert witness had characterized the incident as anything other than an unfortunate and tragic mistake. There was no expert testimony to the effect that the pharmacist or anyone at the hospital had engaged in conduct that rose to the level of willful and intentional wrongdoing.

The court concluded: "This solution was compounded for the specific purpose of using it to protect a human heart from damage while it was stopped. The potential harm arising from mis-compounding could not have been greater. This court holds that the evidence was sufficient to support an award of punitive damages."

The most important learning point from this case is that mechanical failures are predictable. People who operate mechanical devices must protect patients from harm due to mechanical failures. Operating manuals for mechanical devices should be read by those who operate the devices, and instructions for use contained within the manuals should be followed.

Pharmacy department policies should reflect the content of the operating manuals, with an understanding that mechanical devices cannot be expected to be fail-safe. Overreliance on mechanical devices may constitute willful disregard for the well-being of patients. The failure to read a device manufacturer's operation manual and to follow the directions in the manual may justify an award of punitive damages.

The preventable death of a patient may not result in criminal charges, but it will result in serious consequences for the pharmacist whose negligence caused the fatality. All medications have the potential to cause lethal effects, but some medications have greater lethal potential than others. Killing a patient due to negligence in the preparation of a high-risk medication is likely the worst outcome a pharmacist can imagine.

Legal Case Study: A Cascade of Preventable Errors

A lawsuit was initiated by the survivors of a patient who died as the result of a pharmacy error. During the trial of the case, the court granted a verdict for compensatory damages in favor of the plaintiff and against the defendant pharmacy.[5] However, the trial court denied the plaintiff's request for punitive damages. This ruling by the court meant that the jury was not allowed to even consider the possibility of punitive damages. From the trial court's denial of punitive damages in this case, the plaintiff appealed.

The facts of the case, as recited by the appellate court, showed that the deceased patient had been discharged from the hospital, and a nurse had telephoned the defendant pharmacy with several prescriptions for the patient, including daily metolazone to treat fluid buildup in the patient's lungs. A pharmacy technician at the defendant pharmacy took the telephone order. According to the court, this technician "had no formal pharmacy training or education before becoming a pharmacy technician." The technician "made numerous errors transcribing the prescriptions. She made spelling errors on several of the medication orders. She misspelled the nurse's name and recorded an incorrect birth date for the patient." She also made a mistake on the dosage for an albuterol inhaler. The dosage "was ten times the correct dosage, and potentially could have caused heart arrhythmias and palpitations along with other complications."

Most significantly, the technician entered an order for a daily dose of methotrexate rather than metolazone. A pharmacy expert testifying on behalf of the plaintiff explained that if a pharmacy technician were to take an order over the telephone without knowing what the drug is, the technician would look at a drop-down menu on the computer and select a drug after typing in the first few letters. The expert explained that "if a person is looking for something that starts with the three letters M-e-t and has a 2.5 mg strength, it's a very common mistake to pick the first one that meets those two criteria and pick methotrexate rather than metolazone."

The supervising pharmacist testified that he reviewed the patient's prescription prior to its being processed but that "for some reason [he] didn't recognize the weekly versus daily. It didn't click in [his] mind." The pharmacist testified that the pharmacy used a computer system that provided alerts to pharmacists when prescriptions presented potential problems for patients but that the alert system did not flag this methotrexate prescription.

The pharmacy expert testified that methotrexate is a "high-alert" medication based on classifications provided by the Institute for Safe Medication Practices. He further testified that a pharmacy computer system should be programmed with a "hard stop" to alert a pharmacist if an order for methotrexate were entered with directions to take one tablet daily.

The patient's husband picked up the patient's prescriptions at the pharmacy. An employee at the pharmacy counter asked the husband if he had any questions for the pharmacist. When the husband said that he did not, the employee provided no counseling or warnings about any of the medications. The court explained that a policy and procedures manual at the pharmacy "strongly recommends that all patients with new prescriptions receive patient counseling, even if not required under the law." The pharmacy expert explained that patient counseling should be provided when a patient receives a "high-alert" drug for the first time.

The patient took the methotrexate as instructed on the pharmacy label, and she died less than a month later as a result of methotrexate toxicity.

In considering the plaintiff's appeal of the trial court's dismissal of the claim for punitive damages, the appellate court ruled that the evidence in this case was sufficient to permit a jury to determine that the pharmacy "acted with complete indifference to, and conscious disregard for, the safety of others, in circumstances which presented a high probability of injury." The appellate court ruled that the trial court had erred when the punitive damages evidence was kept from the jury's consideration. The court then explained the basis of its conclusion.

First, the court explained that an award of punitive damages was warranted due to the supervising pharmacist's failure to review the prescription prior to dispensing it to the patient. Despite the pharmacist's insistence that he had performed the review but that the dosage had not "clicked in his mind," the court concluded that an error of this magnitude would have been noticed by any pharmacist who reviewed the prescription. A corporate representative from the defendant pharmacy testified that "the pharmacist really did not perform a medication review of this drug and of this patient." The corporate representative further explained that the pharmacist's failure was "a breakdown in the system."

Second, the court faulted the pharmacy for its failure to perform a heightened review of the prescription because it had been received by a technician through telephone communication. The law of the state in which this occurred does not forbid the technician from taking telephone orders for new prescriptions, but it does require an extra layer of direct pharmacist supervision when this practice is undertaken. The court said, "even if pharmacy technicians were not prohibited from taking telephone orders for new prescriptions, the evidence indicated that technicians should only take telephone orders under the direct supervision of a pharmacist. The court also noted, "evidence concerning the technician's lack of pre-employment education and training, and of the number of errors she made in transcribing the prescriptions, which would have permitted the jury to conclude that the pharmacy's pharmacists should have been aware of a substantial risk of errors if the technician's work was not subject to meaningful pharmacist review."

Third, the court said, "the fact that the pharmacy failed to have a pharmacist personally counsel the husband when he picked up the prescription for a 'high alert' medication would also support an award of punitive damages." The court pointed to testimony by the corporate representative who "testified that her personal practice was to always place a note with a prescription for methotrexate, requiring that a pharmacist have a direct consultation with the patient, because methotrexate is potentially dangerous on the issue of daily versus weekly administration." The supervising pharmacist testified that "he knew how to require that a patient speak with a pharmacist before receiving a medication, but he did not use that mechanism in this case."

The court noted that the pharmacy could have required all pharmacists to follow the practice of the corporate representative and personally speak with patients before dispensing new prescriptions for high-alert medications like methotrexate. Had the jury been allowed to consider punitive damages, the jury could have concluded that the pharmacy's policy of leaving the "decision whether to counsel patient to the discretion of individual pharmacists exhibited conscious indifference to patient safety, when the consequences of prescription errors were potentially lethal."

Finally, the court faulted the pharmacy defendant for having "made no meaningful changes to its procedures as a result of the patient's death." The court said: "In particular, no changes were made to the practice of permitting pharmacy technicians to take telephone orders for new prescriptions; patients were still merely offered counseling when they picked up new prescriptions despite the strong recommendation in the policy manual; and high alert medications like methotrexate were still not treated any differently than other drugs."

The corporate representative "could not identify any specific change to the pharmacy's practices which had resulted from the patient's death." In particular, the representative "agreed that as long as the state allows it, the pharmacy was going to continue to let pharmacy techs, even the ones that might make multiple errors on prescription slips, continue to take new prescriptions over the phone." Although the representative acknowledged that the pharmacist's failure to review the patient's prescriptions was "a breakdown in the system," she also testified that she was unaware of any way in which the pharmacy "could have prevented the outcome in this case." The court reasoned that a jury would be entitled to conclude that the pharmacy's "failure to institute remedial measures suggested by the evidence exhibited its indifference to, and disregard for, the serious risk of injury to patients."

The appellate court ruled that the trial court had erred in dismissing the punitive damages claim against the pharmacy, and the case was remanded back to the trial court for a new trial on the issue of punitive damages.

There are multiple layers to the errors that occurred in this case. Cumulatively, these errors led to a ruling that the pharmacy must be punished for having caused the patient's death. The lack of technician training and poor technician supervision, the absence of a computer alert to potentially fatal overdose, the failure to counsel the patient's husband on the need for care in using a high-alert drug, and the continued use of practices that had been identified as potentially lethal to patients justified an award of punitive damages.

The bad news of this case is that there are multiple ways in which lethal medications can be mistakenly provided to patients, resulting in fatality. The good news is that these challenges can be met through the development and utilization of effective patient safety systems.

Legal Case Study: The Pharmacist's Duty to Warn

Pharmacists have killed patients not only through acts of commission, but they have also failed to act in ways that would have saved patients' lives. Under some circumstances, pharmacists have a legal duty not only to avoid order processing errors but also to provide consultation when necessary to prevent a patient's death. In a relevant "duty to warn" case against a pharmacy, the court considered the duty of care that a pharmacist owes to patients.[6] The issue presented to the court was whether a pharmacist's only duty is to fill a patient's prescription with the correct medication and directions or if, under certain circumstances, a pharmacist may have a duty to do more than accurately process a patient's prescription. The court concluded that when a pharmacist has knowledge of a patient-specific risk with respect to a prescribed medication, the pharmacist has a duty to exercise reasonable care in warning the patient or notifying the prescribing doctor of this risk.

The facts of the case showed that a patient visited a physician for the first time, and while filling out paperwork concerning her medical history, the patient indicated that she might have a sulfa allergy. After discussion with the physician's medical assistant, this possible sulfa allergy was recorded on the patient's medical chart with a question mark ("Sulfa?").

Six months later, the patient returned to the physician's office, complaining of "abdominal fullness." After performing routine tests, the physician diagnosed the patient with a **urinary tract infection**. The physician told the patient that under normal circumstances, her infection could be treated most effectively with trimethoprim/sulfamethoxazole. Given the notation in her chart, however, the physician asked the patient to clarify how certain she was of her sulfa allergy. After further discussion, the patient downplayed the previous notation and asked the physician to write her a prescription for trimethoprim/sulfamethoxazole. The physician complied, and the patient dropped off the prescription at her pharmacy on her way home from the physician's office.

Later that same day, the patient's caretaker returned to the pharmacy to pick up the prescription. Upon asking a pharmacy technician to release the prescription, the technician told the caretaker that the patient's prescription had been "flagged" by the pharmacy's computer system while it was being filled. The technician told the patient's caretaker that the prescription had alerted the pharmacist to the patient's profile that indicated the patient was allergic to sulfa-based drugs. The caretaker then asked the employee to call the patient and to speak with her directly.

A pharmacist called the patient and conveyed the information that her prescription had been flagged because of her sulfa allergy. In response, the patient reportedly indicated that she had taken trimethoprim/sulfamethoxazole in the past and that she had not experienced any adverse reaction to it. Satisfied with this clarification, the pharmacist then manually overrode the computer system's alert, and the prescription was released to the patient's caretaker.

Later that day, after taking the medication, the patient complained that she felt "itchy." The following day, the patient called the physician's office and left a voice mail in which she stated that she was wrong about not having a sulfa allergy. The patient's condition continued to worsen, and she was taken to the emergency room. After being diagnosed with SJS/TEN, the patient was transferred to a burn center, where she eventually lapsed into a coma and died. At the time the patient was removed from life support, she had burns covering 40% to 50% of her body.

The patient's two children (the plaintiffs) filed a wrongful-death action against the pharmacy, alleging that its pharmacist breached the duty of care owed to their mother. Specifically, the plaintiffs contended that the pharmacist breached her duty of care by failing to adequately warn their mother of the prescribed medication's risks in light of her allergy to it or, alternatively, by failing to call the physician to clarify whether he really meant to prescribe a medication to which the patient was allergic.

The court ruled that a narrow duty to warn exists where, as in this case, a pharmacy has patient-specific information about drug allergies and knows that the drug being prescribed is contraindicated for the individual patient. Under such circumstances, a pharmacist has a duty to warn either the prescribing physician or the patient of the potential danger. It is unclear whether the conversation between the pharmacist and the patient was sufficient to meet the recognized duty. The court refused to dismiss the case due to insufficient evidence that the duty had been met. When a patient's life is at significant risk, maximal effort is required to protect the patient from lethal drug effects. A single casual conversation will likely be considered as insufficient.

What a pharmacist sometimes knows, without investigation, and even a treating physician may not know, is susceptibilities of particular patients of the pharmacy to the side effects of a drug that it provides to them. These susceptibilities are significant because of other drugs that the pharmacist knows the patient is taking or a preexisting physical or mental condition again known to the pharmacist that makes the drug contraindicated for the patient. When a pharmacist has such knowledge, the pharmacist must warn either the patient or their physician. The warning must include a description of the risk to the patient and a recommendation for alternate therapy that lessens the risk.

Conclusion

Malpractice law provides a means through which patients who have been harmed by an inadvertent pharmacy error can be compensated for the suffering they have experienced. Malpractice law can also punish pharmacists and pharmacies that caused harm to a patient through willful neglect of their professional duties. The punitive aspect of malpractice law provides for an additional financial award to the harmed patient or to the patient's family if the pharmacy error resulted in the patient's death. An award of punitive damages recognizes that some errors in pharmacy are so egregious that mere compensation is inadequate to reflect the disgraceful violation of pharmacy's commitment to protect the public from harm.

Key Takeaways

- *Manage the risk of harm to your patients.* The role of a risk management department is to protect corporate financial assets from claims of negligence that are asserted by a patient who has been harmed by a pharmacy error. Practicing pharmacists can support this business objective by meeting practice goals that have been established to protect patients from harm. The intentions of those who provide patient care and of those who conduct risk management coincide. Adherence to the pharmacy standard of care in clinical practice will promote patient well-being and will protect the institution from legal liability. Be mindful that the goal is risk management and not risk elimination. There are always risks in the provision of pharmaceutical products and services. Eliminating the risk of harm to patients can also eliminate the possibility of benefit. The standard of care in pharmacy is to measure the risks of drug therapy for each patient and to take only those risks that are necessary to provide safe and effective patient care.

- *Avoid taking unnecessary risks that could harm your patients.* Shortcuts may be tempting, particularly during busy times when demands on personnel are great. Nevertheless, shortcuts must be rejected as being unnecessarily risky to patients. One particularly risky shortcut is the assumption that since many other healthcare professionals are involved with a patient's care, errors that occur by any one person will be discovered by someone else before they cause problems for a patient. Assuming that an experienced technician has performed a task correctly is an unnecessary risk. Allowing a patient to decide whether consultation with a pharmacist is needed is an unnecessary risk. Presuming that the directions for using a medical device are clear, operating a device routinely and perfunctorily without reading and remembering the manufacturer's directions, especially any precautions about what can possibly go wrong and how to prevent them, is an unnecessary risk. When you are faced with a challenging situation, consider what your answer would be if an error were to occur and if you were asked to explain the error. Any answer that begins with the words, "Well, I assumed that...." is a wrong answer. Professional people don't assume. They find out. They make sure. Punitive damages can result from making incorrect assumptions.
- Give yourself a periodic professional checkup. Can you explain the standard of care for the professional activities in which you engage? What flexibility is there within the standards that apply to your area of professional practice? How do you apply your knowledge and skills for the benefit of patients within your practice setting? If there are any uncertainties in your answers to these questions, then conduct a due diligence introspective inquiry to find out what changes you must make (if any) to your professional practices. The inquiry may require discussions with trusted colleagues, internet-based research, and attendance at continuing pharmacy education programs. Don't allow yourself to be lulled into a complacent approach to practice within a

dynamic and expanding period of increasing professional responsibilities. Complacency may be interpreted as dangerous and reckless practice, and it may support an award of punitive damages. It may result in the preventable death of your patient.

References

1. Thomas v. Winchester, 6 N.Y. 397 (N.Y. 1852).

2. Fleet & Semple v. Hollenkemp, 52 Ky. (1 B Mon.) 219 (1852).

3. Harco Drugs, Inc. v. Holloway, 669 So.2d 878 (Ala. 1995).

4. Schroeder v. Lester E. Cox Medical Center, 833 S.W.2d 411 (Mo.App. 1992).

5. Oyler v. Hy-Vee, Inc., 539 S.W.3d 742 (Mo.App. 2017).

6. Klasch v. Walgreen Co., 264 P.3d 1155 (Nev. 2011).

Chapter 15

Criminalization of Medication Errors

A basic principle of criminal law is that intentionality is a precursor to culpability. A person who intentionally causes harm to another person has committed a crime under most circumstances. A person who inadvertently causes harm to another person is generally not guilty of criminal conduct. This foundational principle of law extends to healthcare generally and to pharmacy practice specifically. If a pharmacist's unintentional error harms a patient, then the erring pharmacist may be held civilly liable for money damages under malpractice law or may be administratively liable through disciplinary action by an agency such as the board of pharmacy. Yet criminality is usually not considered as an effective or appropriate response to an inadvertent pharmacy error.

Crime of Imperfection

When a patient dies due to an error committed by a healthcare professional, exposure to criminal prosecution is always possible, although it rarely occurs. If a criminal investigation does occur, it is inevitable that an evaluation of actions taken by the suspect healthcare professional will disclose seemingly simple error avoidance steps that could have been implemented to avoid the patient's death but were not taken. The challenges to success that existed at the time the healthcare professional made the error tend to disappear when law enforcement personnel examine the facts with the benefit of hindsight. The response made by the healthcare institution where the error occurred can be the difference between prosecutors allowing the institution to manage the situation internally and, instead, filing criminal charges against an alleged murderer.

Two contrasting cases from university teaching hospitals in the Southeast illustrate how a response to human error can either cause or prevent the filing of criminal charges.

RaDonda Vaught was a nurse at Vanderbilt University Medical Center who provided care for a 75-year-old female patient with a subdural hematoma.[1] The patient's attending physician ordered Versed to be administered to the patient in preparation for a scan. Vaught retrieved the drug from an automated dispensing unit, but she erroneously removed vecuronium when she overrode an alert from the dispensing unit. Although Versed was available in the dispensing unit, it was listed under the generic name midazolam. Apparently, the similarity of the two drugs' names starting with the same two letters caused the inadvertent error to occur. Vaught had chosen the wrong drug from a menu of drug names.

The patient died due to the error. Vaught immediately admitted what she had done. The patient's death was listed as having resulted from natural causes. The death was not reported to the Centers for Medicare and Medicaid Services (CMS) as is required. Vanderbilt quickly and quietly settled a malpractice lawsuit but did not report the incident to the state.

Just under a year later, an anonymous caller reported the incident to CMS. This report led to an investigation that ultimately resulted in Vaught losing her nurse license and to a conviction for criminally negligent homicide. The criminal conviction was widely criticized in the public media and in professional journals for having singled out Vaught as the responsible party when a faulty system and unsafe culture at the medical center set her up for error. On the other hand, Vaught was criticized for failing to take steps necessary to avoid errors, regardless of the system or culture that existed at the medical center when the error occurred. Nobody has ever suggested that RaDonda Vaught intended to kill anyone. This case serves as a rare example of how an inadvertent error can lead to criminal liability.

Pharmacist Edna Irizarry committed a similar inadvertent error, but the result was very different. Irizarry was a pharmacist at Shands Hospital at the University of Florida. She received an order for a 3-year-old patient prescribing 5.75 grams of the amino acid arginine. Instead of the prescribed dosage, 60 grams of arginine was dispensed.[2] A nurse did not recognize the error, and the overdosage was administered to the patient, resulting in the patient's death.

The error was immediately documented and reported to the state as a serious incident. The medical examiner was told of the error, and the error was documented as the cause of death. The hospital conducted a thorough evaluation of all system factors that could have contributed to the error, and multiple system upgrades were implemented to avoid similar errors in the future. A settlement was reached with the patient's parents who established a foundation at the hospital to create a full-service pediatric wing.

Irizarry was fined $1,000 by the state board of pharmacy. The licensing agency recognized that the pharmacist's error was inadvertent and that she was a secondary victim of several institutional system failures. None of the involved healthcare professionals lost their licenses, and nobody was charged with a crime.

To Err Is Human

Humans make mistakes. Fallibility is a condition of human existence. Pharmacists and other healthcare professionals generally accept responsibility for the consequences of the human errors that they make. If a pharmacist's error causes harm to a patient, then the erring pharmacist is expected to step up and admit the error. It is a moral imperative for individual pharmacists to participate in error analysis to prevent future errors. Denial of error interferes with the prevention of future errors. It is considered unethical for a pharmacist to cover up an error, and a cover-up may increase the likelihood of criminal charges against the pharmacist.

The same is true of an error that is caused by a poorly functioning pharmacy system. The system designer or administrator should concede that the system error has occurred. To deny an error that has been discovered and that warrants evaluation to support system improvement is unethical.

The legal challenge is to determine what is a fair response when a pharmacy team member or pharmacy system designer or an administrator accepts responsibility for an error that caused harm to a patient. It is a moral imperative for the legal system to react productively and proactively to an incident of human error. Focusing on what happened in the past, as opposed to looking toward a better future, does not necessarily rectify the problem and does not necessarily prevent similar events in the weeks or months ahead.

Dr. Lucien Leape and colleagues have stressed the importance of a "Just Culture" in healthcare.[3] In making this point, Dr. Leape means that a culture of blame and punishment must be replaced by a culture of forgiveness and improvement. Here is a quote from Dr. Leape:

"The single greatest impediment to error prevention in the medical industry is that we punish people for making mistakes."

The context within which Dr. Leape conveys this important message is the legal response to inadvertent errors made by health professionals who are trying hard to be safe but who commit an unsafe slip or lapse that leads to error. True justice, according to Dr. Leape, would lead to forgiveness of the inadvertent error and to mandatory implementation of steps that will prevent future errors of the same type. Dr. Leape suggests that punishment of the error stands in the way of individual or system improvements and that punishment does not prevent future errors.

This "forgive and remember" approach to errors in healthcare would not be applicable under all circumstances. For example, when a pharmacist intentionally decides not to check a technician's work to speed up order processing to meet a financial quota, forgiveness might be less likely. It might also be inapplicable when a pharmacist ignores obvious indicators that a controlled substance prescription is invalid and fills the questionable prescription, because taking the time to verify prescription legitimacy is too burdensome. In these situations, punishment of the error may be the appropriate response. What Dr. Leape refers to as being forgivable are the normal errors that result from the human condition. Nobody is perfect. Everybody makes mistakes.

"Retributive justice" is the conceptual category of justice through which prosecutorial approaches to criminal punishment have evolved under the law. Based on the idea that a person who causes harm to another must receive their "just deserts," retributive justice results in punitive action taken toward a person who has deliberately harmed another person. In this context, a "just deserts" refers to a deserved punishment. Intentionality by the perpetrator is often used as justification for punitive action. Gross carelessness or glaring disregard for the interests of others may also justify the application of retributive justice.

The concept of retributive justice rests on three basic assumptions:

- *Proportionality.* It is a valid exercise of government authority to punish those who commit certain wrongful acts, in proportion to the harm caused by the wrongful act.
- *Morality.* It is intrinsically good for a representative of the people (a government prosecutor) to punish those who commit acts that are harmful to the public.
- *Verification.* The evidence on which punishment rests must be weighed by a nonbiased evaluator and must have been found to be true.

Many people who support retributive justice believe that those who commit crimes should be punished even if there is no practical value to be gained from the punishment. For example, punishment may be considered justifiable if a pharmacist commits a fatal error while practicing pharmacy, even if the pharmacist's license is permanently revoked. The former pharmacist can no longer endanger patients. Criminal punishment will not deter future crimes by the former pharmacist in a professional role; nor will the former pharmacist need to be incapacitated. That problem has been solved through licensure revocation. A person whose pharmacy license has been revoked is no longer a pharmacist and cannot commit crimes as a pharmacist. There is no practical value in punishing this person because the crime cannot be repeated. Nevertheless, those who criticize regulatory policies that are "soft on crime" may support criminalization of the pharmacist's fatal error out of revenge rather than for an achievable purpose.

Even if the justifications for retributive justice have already been achieved through license revocation, many people will support criminal punishment of the pharmacist through incarceration as a matter of setting things right and restoring balance to the pharmacist–patient relationship pursuant to the view that incarceration of the pharmacist is a reasonable equivalent to the death of the patient. It is considered fair to take away the freedom of a person who has taken away the freedom of another person.

Consequences of Risk Avoidance

Drug therapy is an inherently risky enterprise. It cannot be made risk free. Even when drugs are approved as safe and effective, are appropriately prescribed and dispensed, and the patient uses them as prescribed, they may still cause severe harm or death. Pharmaceutical risks can be managed, but they cannot be eliminated. Patients are always exposed to the risk that a drug will be ineffective or that the drug will cause adverse effects. Pharmacists are exposed to the risk of liability for failing to meet the standard of care in providing products and services to patients. Prescribers and manufacturers face similar risks in their prospective roles. It is a risky business.

As a general rule, pharmacists must be willing to accept the risk that they will be held liable for malpractice when they commit inadvertent human errors. They have no choice in the matter if they wish to continue practicing pharmacy. But the risk of criminal liability for inadvertent error changes the risk calculation unfavorably for pharmacists. The cost of criminal liability for a pharmacist is too high. Incarceration and/or a criminal record are risks that are not worth taking in pharmacy. To avoid this risk, the prospect of criminal liability may cause pharmacists to adopt overly conservative practices that reduce their own risk of criminal liability but deny patients beneficial yet risky therapies. If this approach to risk avoidance becomes widespread in the pharmacy profession, then criminalization of pharmacy error is detrimental to the public good because patients will not receive medications that they need.

Arguments Justifying the Criminalization of Medication Error

There is no rule that says pharmacists or other health professionals cannot be criminally punished for the inadvertent errors they make.[4] A pharmacist whose error kills a patient can be charged with murder due to the error. That this rarely happens is of little consolation to pharmacists. There are a number of reasons that prosecutors use to justify filing criminal charges based on pharmacy error.

The first justification often used to support criminal charges filed against a pharmacist is vengeance. When a person is harmed from something as seemingly simple as transferring a medication from one container to another, and placing the prescriber's instructions on a label, there may be emotions of surprise, anger, and even outrage. People might say, "How could such an easy task be done in error unless the pharmacist was careless and recklessly inattentive?" We live in a vengeful society, where "an eye for an eye and a tooth for a tooth" is sometimes seen as an appropriate, or even necessary, response to harm caused by one person to another.

A related justification is penance. While vengeance often is seen as a way to meet the emotional needs of the victim, punishment is often seen as a way to show the perpetrator that society will not stand for this sort of behavior. The perpetrator must be made to repent for the error.

Perhaps the most frequently offered justification for criminal prosecution of pharmacy error is deterrence. The basic idea of deterrence is that the threat of criminal punishment, and pharmacists' knowledge that criminal punishment has occurred and does occur, will lead to more careful decisions and actions by pharmacists to avoid criminal prosecution. There is some initial appeal attached to this justification because people frequently change their behaviors based on knowledge of the consequences of those behaviors. Insofar as deterrence is directed toward truly careless actions by pharmacists, it may make some sense. Pharmacists who are intoxicated should ask a partner to take a shift for them. Pharmacists who consistently mistake drug A for drug B, because the two drugs are placed on the storage shelf next to each other, should move one or the other of the drugs to a different location and prevent that error from happening again. To do otherwise might be considered criminally careless and recklessly indifferent.

A fourth justification used by prosecutors who file criminal charges against erring pharmacists is to instill public confidence. In many jurisdictions, prosecutors are elected by popular vote. In virtually every jurisdiction, prosecutors have some level of political connection or ambition. It is no surprise that prosecutors feel the need to show that public confidence in them is well placed. When a death occurs due to pharmacist error, prosecutors may want to publicly demonstrate that they, as the person who is obligated to provide legal protection for the public, are doing a competent job. Criminal prosecution of a pharmacist is a method for achieving that goal.

Last, a justification for criminalizing pharmacy error is that filing criminal charges is a relatively simple approach to solving one aspect of the problem of pharmacy error. Even if punishing an erring pharmacist doesn't solve any underlying system problem, it gives the outward appearance of a solution. It is a "play to the crowd" move by a prosecutor. While the problem of error in pharmacy is complex, and the solutions are difficult, at least punishment of the pharmacist allows the prosecutor to act as if some steps are being taken toward a solution, even if that step is pointless.

Arguments Criticizing the Criminalization of Medication Error

The filing of criminal charges against a pharmacist or other health professional, following a fatal error, is not without significant criticism.[5] Prosecutors who file criminal charges following a medication error are sometimes quite surprised to discover that the filing of these charges is controversial. Public support for pharmacists can be significant, even when a pharmacist has made a serious mistake. The public understands that everyone makes mistakes.

One key criticism of criminalizing pharmacy error is that the deterrent effect of criminal charges is minimal. The threat of criminal prosecution does not deter inadvertent errors, because pharmacists are not mindful of an inadvertent error when it occurs. A prosecutor could threaten to execute any pharmacist who makes an error, but inadvertent errors would continue to occur, because they are nonvolitional. The deterrent effect applies only to obviously careless and reckless situations, and these situations are quite rare in pharmacy.

A related criticism of criminal charges against erring pharmacists is over-deterrence. The threat of criminal charges may lead to very conservative pharmacy practices with highly toxic drugs because a mistake with these drugs can be fatal. Over-deterrence can result in patients being denied necessary medications or in delays that inconvenience patients.

A major concern related to criminal prosecution of pharmacists is that it addresses only part of the problem. If one accepts the idea that systems set up pharmacists for errors, then focusing on only the erring pharmacist is unfair. The culprit may be the system and not the pharmacist. Although the pharmacist is part of the system, there are many other components of a drug delivery process. What about the manufacturer that chose almost identical packaging and labeling for two drugs that are quite different? What about the prescriber whose order was unclear or nonstandard? How about the physical design of the pharmacy that distracted the pharmacist? It is considered unjust to only blame the pharmacist for an error when the system contributed to the error.

A final criticism of criminalization is that it will lead to the cover-up of errors. An erring pharmacist who knows they will be punished for an error is less likely to document or report the error, and remediation is less likely to occur.

A brief summary of several well-known pharmacy cases places the issue of criminalizing pharmacy error in the context of busy pharmacy practice and a system that challenges pharmacists to avoid errors.

Case Law: Medication Errors and Prosecutorial Power

Ohio Pharmacist Eric Cropp did not adequately check a technician's work and did not discover that the technician had prepared a chemotherapy order with 23.4% NaCl rather than with 0.9% NaCl. This error proved fatal to the one-and-a-half-year-old patient.[6] The evidence showed that when Cropp came to work that day, the hospital's computer system had been down and there was a backlog of orders to fill. There was only one technician who was focused on planning her wedding, rather than on order processing accuracy. A nurse placed a stat order for the chemotherapy, although there was no urgent need for the medication. Because the pharmacy was short-staffed, Cropp had no time for work breaks. Despite this evidence, the prosecutor referred to the overwhelmed pharmacist's failure to detect the technician's error as "outrageously negligent." Cropp was originally charged with negligent homicide. He entered a plea of no-contest to involuntary manslaughter, and he spent six months in jail.

Since his release from incarceration, Eric Cropp has spent considerable time speaking to pharmacy groups about the need to avoid errors due to dysfunctional pharmacy systems that set pharmacists up to commit fatal errors. Ohio state law has been amended to increase qualifications and standards of practice for pharmacy technicians.

Case Law: Standard of Care Not Relevant to Criminal Charges

Iowa Nurse Michael Buman worked the night shift in a long-term care facility (LTCF).[7] A resident complained to the nurse that he had not received his clozapine for several days. A colleague had twice noted "NA" on the medication administration record (MAR) next to the resident's clozapine, signifying that it was not available. Buman discovered that the clozapine had not been included in the most recent two-week supply of medication delivered by the pharmacy. The clozapine "could not be located anywhere in the nurses' station."

Based on this information, Buman concluded that the clozapine "had been discontinued or otherwise changed to something else and that someone had failed to make that notation in the MAR." To correct what he believed was a clerical error, Buman noted "DC'ed" beside the entry for clozapine in the MAR. In fact, the clozapine had not been discontinued by the resident's physician. Due to Buman's error, the resident did not receive his medication for a total of 10 days. The resident was hospitalized for "worsening psychotic illness because his clozapine was inadvertently stopped."

The state filed felony criminal charges against Buman for "wanton neglect of a resident in a health care facility." The state contended that Buman had "on his own and without doctor authorization discontinued the resident's antipsychotic medication." A jury convicted Buman, and he appealed the conviction.

The appellate court noted that the state had the burden of proving that Buman "knowingly acted in a manner likely to be injurious to the physical or mental welfare of a resident." The trial judge had instructed the jury on the minimum standard of care as set out in Board of Nursing regulations, which require that a nurse either carry out the orders of a prescribing physician or notify the prescribing physician that the orders cannot be carried out. Buman contended that reference to the Board of Nursing regulations was misleading because "although a violation of the minimum standard of care may be relevant in a license revocation hearing, it does not require that a nurse intentionally act in a way that would probably cause injury."

The court agreed with Buman, ruling that the reference to the regulations was "ill advised" because the language used in the regulations "could confuse the jury or lead it to misapply the law on whether the nurse knowingly acted in a manner likely to injure the resident." The criminal conviction was reversed. Failure to meet the relevant standard of care does not suffice as evidence that a crime has been committed.

Normality of Error

Dr. James Reason has helped draw a distinction between what could informally be referred to as "honest mistakes" and "careless indifference."[8] It is the latter that prosecutors seek to punish, and the former that critics of prosecutorial overstepping seek to prevent from being punished. But how can prosecutors tell the difference? The two can oftentimes look the same when in fact they are very different. As the cases above show, sometimes prosecutors see what they expect to see rather than what is really there.

Dr. Reason begins with the position that human error is "normal." By that he means that human beings are imperfect. They make mistakes. This is a natural part of the human condition.

Normal error occurs when a person unintentionally does something other than what ought to have been done. This may happen, for example, when a pharmacist selects the wrong "sig code" from a drop-down computer menu, resulting in a patient being instructed to take a drug once daily rather than once weekly. Or it may happen when a pharmacist fails to appreciate the significance of a serious drug–drug interaction alert.

Dr. Reason suggests that errors of a different sort (not normal) result from recognized "at-risk" behaviors. An at-risk behavior increases risk when risk is not recognized or is mistakenly believed to be justified. A community pharmacist who has little experience with intravenous admixtures would engage in an "at-risk" behavior when supervising a technician in an IV room. The participation in "at-risk" behaviors increases the likelihood that a pharmacist will be criminally blamed for an error.

An institutional pharmacist might engage in an "at-risk" behavior when counseling an ambulatory patient about a serious drug–drug interaction. These risky behaviors are permitted for all pharmacists. They are required for all pharmacists. Yet they are "at-risk" behaviors for some pharmacists, but not for all pharmacists. Pharmacists who recognize what is for them an "at-risk" behavior, because it is new and unusual for them, are expected to take special care under James Reason's typology.

The most problematic activity under Dr. Reason's typology of error is what he calls "reckless" behavior. This behavior is characterized by a conscious choice to disregard a substantial and unjustifiable risk. It is hard to imagine this happening in a pharmacy, but it has occurred. For example, the failure to end-test a cardioplegia solution after having identified recurrent problems with a compounding device would fit into this category. Telling a patient not to worry about a drug allergy that previously led to a hospital admission for this patient is another example. This level of recklessness might warrant criminal charges against a pharmacist.

Moral Luck

Even within the category of reckless behavior, there is the possibility for the law to react differently to two similarly reckless persons based on what is known as "moral luck." Here is what a highly respected judge had to say about moral luck, in a pharmacy case:

> The concept has infiltrated the law. If two drivers are equally careless, and one driver has had an accident in which another person is killed and the other driver has no accident, the first gets charged with homicide and the second gets a ticket (maybe). Yet they'd made identical choices and performed identical acts, and the difference in consequences was a matter purely of chance. But consequences, even when fortuitous have an effect on the goodness or badness of an act.[9]

Under this rationale, if two careless pharmacists make the same order processing error, and one patient dies (perhaps this patient is particularly susceptible to adverse drug effects) while the other patient is unaffected by the mistake (perhaps this patient discovers the pharmacist's mistake and never uses the drug), the reality of the first patient's death speaks loudly and may lead to punishment. It is a matter of moral luck. The carelessness of the two pharmacists is equal. The consequences for the two pharmacists are unequal. Most judges and juries will recognize that luck should not be used as the basis for filing criminal charges against a pharmacist due to a fatal outcome caused by an inadvertent human error.

When Criminalization Makes Sense (Maybe)

Concerns about the fallibility of the human condition, and the reality of moral luck, have led some healthcare policy analysts to develop a formula for determining which erroneous acts in healthcare are worthy of criminal punishment.

Dr. Paul Monks contends that there is a difference between those who err despite trying hard not to err and those who haven't even made any attempt to avoid their errors.[10]

Monks is particularly critical of several situations leading to error in healthcare:

- Disregarding known past experience in failing to avoid a present dangerous situation.
- Failing to speak up when circumstances threaten a patient's care.
- Placing profits ahead of public service.
- Covering up a small problem leads to a much larger problem.

These are the factors, perhaps still difficult to identify and document, that distinguish between an "honest mistake" and "reckless disregard," according to Monks. While the former should not be characterized as criminal conduct, the latter may be so characterized.

Characteristics of Medication Error Criminal Cases

The types of cases that result in criminal charges can also be helpful in developing pharmacy practices that avoid criminal prosecution. A search for criminal cases brought against pharmacists between 1966 and 2023 based on errors made by the pharmacists produced 15 cases for analysis. The cases break down in this way:

- All cases located were "wrong drug" cases. In 5 of the 15 cases, the order was for cancer chemotherapy drugs; the other 10 cases involved an assortment of unrelated drugs.

- In 12 of the 15 cases, the patient who was harmed was a child of 6 years in age or under.
- In the 8 cases based on incidents that occurred in 2000 or before, only one case resulted from a technician error that went undetected by the pharmacist.
- In the 7 cases based on incidents that occurred after 2000, all 7 resulted from technician errors that went undetected by the pharmacist.
- In 12 cases out of 15, the erring pharmacist did not regularly work at the pharmacy where the error occurred.

While it is difficult to generalize based on such small numbers, one might conclude from this information that particular care should be taken in reviewing work by a technician, when the patient is a child, when the drug is for chemotherapy, and when the pharmacist does not regularly work at the pharmacy where this activity is being done.

The Alternative of Professional Discipline

The pharmacy profession can police itself. It need not rely on law enforcement to file criminal charges as a means to protect the public. Pharmacists are subject to disciplinary action by their licensing agency if they make a mistake that harms a patient and if they commit an intentional act that leads to patient harm. One of the primary responsibilities of a licensing agency such as the state board of pharmacy is to review practices of licensees that may have caused the death of a patient. Professions regulate themselves for the benefit of the public being served. If professions engage in effective self-regulation, the need for criminal investigation and prosecution following a fatal error can be mitigated.

State Boards of Pharmacy

A state board of pharmacy is authorized to discipline a pharmacist, or a pharmacy, based on violations that are outlined in the state's pharmacy act or in the board of pharmacy's administrative regulations. Some states exhaustively list virtually every specific violation that might be committed. Other states list only a very few specific violations that can be broadly applied to many situations. The board of pharmacy is charged with the responsibility of determining whether disciplinary action is appropriate and, if so, how severe the discipline should be.

The most challenging situations faced by boards of pharmacy are those in which the board must decide what to do when a pharmacist has inadvertently made an error that has resulted in the death of a patient. Since imperfection is a quality of the human condition, and since pharmacists are all humans, it is foreseeable that imperfect pharmacists will make unintentional mistakes. This reality begs the question: "If a pharmacist makes a human error that kills a patient, should be pharmacist be punished for being a fallible human?" And one further question: "If there is to be punishment by a board of pharmacy for human fallibility, then is license revocation a reasonable punishment for an inadvertent fatal error?"

Boards of pharmacy will usually conduct a very intensive investigation of any complaint that alleges the commission of an error that has caused the death of a patient. By examining the circumstances of the incident, boards of pharmacy will be able to learn whether the error was committed despite the best efforts to prevent it or whether the error instead resulted due to no efforts having been made to prevent the error. In other words, was the pharmacist trying hard to avoid errors, or was the pharmacist hardly trying to prevent errors? For boards of pharmacy, the answer to this question can be critical.

Boards of pharmacy will be inclined to severely discipline the "hardly trying" pharmacist or pharmacy, and they will be disinclined to severely discipline the "trying hard" pharmacist or pharmacy. It is usually the effort that matters most to a board of pharmacy and not the result. For the public, this approach of emphasizing effort over result may be difficult to accept. Since the role of the board of pharmacy is to protect the public, members of the public may not make see any distinction between the "hardly trying" pharmacist and the "trying hard" pharmacist. This is a disconnect that is important to appreciate. State boards of pharmacy will need to provide an acceptable explanation to the family of a person who was victimized by the error of a "trying hard" pharmacist, if the decision is to impose a relatively light disciplinary action.

If a board of pharmacy does not revoke the license of a pharmacist whose error results in the death of a patient but instead imposes a fine and a period of probation, the public will likely interpret this penalty as "doing nothing." It would not necessarily matter to the public that the erring pharmacist was following all standard policies and procedures of the profession and that the patient's death was a tragic result of an unavoidable human error.

It can be challenging for a board of pharmacy to persuade the survivors of deceased patients that the public is best served through mandatory improvements in the practices of pharmacists who have erred and through compulsory pharmacy system upgrades that promote the detection and rectification of pharmacist errors before harm occurs to patients. Yet the purpose of the board of pharmacy is not to provide vindication to the friends and family of patients who are the victims of an inadvertent pharmacist error.

The purpose of the board of pharmacy is to assure that pharmacy practitioners and pharmacy practice sites provide safe pharmaceutical products and services as a matter of public health protection.

Discipline of Pharmacy Based on Pharmacist Errors Is Upheld

An important legal case illustrates the context within which pharmacists and pharmacies work together to meet patient needs and perhaps are subject to discipline together when patient harm occurs.[11]

A state board of pharmacy received information indicating that an error in dispensing phenytoin had occurred at a pharmacy. The board's investigation revealed that the pharmacy had received a prescription that called for "Dilantin 100 mg capsules bid" as well as a second prescription for the same patient that called for "Dilantin 50 mg capsules bid." The pharmacy did not stock 50 mg Dilantin, so the pharmacist on duty dispensed liquid Dilantin calling for 150 mg bid, indicating that "10 cc = 50 mg." In fact, this was an error by the pharmacist. The label should have read that "2 cc = 50 mg." The error led to a five-fold overdose. The patient died as a result of the overdose. The pharmacy board's investigation revealed that "the pharmacist had committed four other dispensing errors during a two-month period, including dispensing the wrong drug, dispensing the wrong strength of the right drug, and using the wrong patient's name on a prepared drug order."

The board of pharmacy sent a notice of hearing to the pharmacist and to the pharmacy. The evidence presented at the hearing indicated that all of the cited errors had been initially committed by pharmacy technicians who worked under the pharmacist's supervision. The evidence also showed that the pharmacist had been terminated from employment.

The board of pharmacy suspended the pharmacist's license for seven days, with the suspension delayed for two years on the condition that the pharmacist complied with several board requirements. The board also suspended the pharmacy's permit for seven days, with the suspension also stayed for two years upon the pharmacy complying with restrictions on the number of prescriptions it could fill, more stringent requirements for reporting dispensing errors to the board, and other conditions.

The pharmacist accepted the discipline, recognizing that a fatal error had occurred and that the pharmacist was responsible for the error.

The pharmacy appealed the discipline, contending that the board had exceeded its statutory authority and that it had improperly imputed to the pharmacy the findings of negligence made against another subject of its investigation. Essentially, the pharmacy was arguing that the threat to patient safety was due to the pharmacist, and not due to the pharmacy, and that firing the pharmacist had remedied the threat to public safety. The pharmacy contended that "vicarious liability," under which an employer can be held to account for the conduct of an employee, could not be the basis of board of pharmacy disciplinary action against a pharmacy that had merely employed a pharmacist who had made a mistake.

The trial court agreed with the pharmacy, ruling: "The board does not have the authority to discipline a pharmacy permittee for the negligence of a pharmacist employee who is also licensed by the board." The trial court reasoned that the pharmacy technicians who were negligent were being supervised by the pharmacist licensee and that the pharmacist was responsible for the negligence of the technicians that he was supervising. The court concluded that the board had no authority to discipline the pharmacy on the theory of vicarious liability: "If the legislature intended this, then it must expressly say so and the law does not."

The board of pharmacy appealed this lower court ruling to an appellate court. The appellate court admitted that the statutory language was unclear: "The statute does not make it clear whether it is limited in its application to conduct actually committed by a permit holder, or whether a permit holder can be disciplined for conduct that is committed by a licensed pharmacist employed by the permit holder." To address this ambiguity, the appellate court analyzed the purpose of the state pharmacy practice act that served as the enabling statute for the board of pharmacy.

The appellate court then ruled: "In light of the purpose of the act to ensure minimum standards of competency and to protect the public health, safety, and welfare, we conclude, contrary to the decision of the trial court, that the legislature did intend for the board to have authority to discipline a permit holder for the conduct of one of its licensed pharmacists."

The appellate court clarified its ruling, explaining that: "One permitted to maintain and conduct a pharmacy may be disciplined by the pharmacy board for the unlawful acts of his employees while engaged in the conduct and operation of the pharmacy, although the permittee does not authorize the unlawful acts and did not have actual knowledge of the activities. This would be particularly true of a corporate permittee which could act only through its officers, agents, or employees."

The important message of this case is that licensed pharmacists and permitted pharmacies are closely connected in the responsibility to provide safe pharmaceutical products and services. They are equally connected in the acceptance of consequences when safety expectations have not been met. Boards of pharmacy have authority over both pharmacists and pharmacies.

Pharmacist-in-Charge License Revocation Reversed

Boards of pharmacy must not only address substantive violations by licensees, but in doing so they must adhere to procedural requirements that have been established under the law to assure fairness in the professional disciplinary process. The constitutional requirement of procedural due process was the basis for reversal of a pharmacist-in-charge (PIC) license revocation by a state board of pharmacy.[12] The PIC had worked at a pharmacy where he was the only pharmacist. There were several pharmacy technicians who had begun working at the pharmacy prior to the arrival of the PIC. A patient died from an overdose of opioids, and the PIC's pharmacist license was revoked based on "clearly excessive furnishing of controlled substances."

The facts showed that the pharmacy owner (not a pharmacist), and a physician whose office was nearby, as well as the patient who died, were all three close friends. The physician had issued opioid prescriptions for the patient, and these prescriptions were filled by the nonpharmacist owner who used a key that he had retained himself to allow him unsupervised access to the dispensing area. A computer-generated patient profile for the patient indicated that the PIC had dispensed the medications, although the PIC had not done so. The medications had been dispensed by the nonpharmacist owner using the PIC's login information. Even though the PIC had a responsibility to review and sign daily dispensing reports, he did not do this because he "was too busy to review the daily reports and because he assumed that he knew everything that was dispensed, he saw no need to review the reports." The PIC was eventually tipped off by a technician that the illegal activity was occurring, but the patient had died by that time and the board of pharmacy was already investigating the case. Revocation proceedings were begun against the PIC.

After a hearing before an administrative law judge, the judge commented regarding the PIC's explanation of what had occurred:

> His demeanor and attitude while testifying, his often-inconsistent testimony, and his non-responsive answers weaken his credibility. His sole interest is in producing a record number of prescriptions per day. He has no insight into the fact that his focus on volume and speed caused him to neglect duties which are meant to safeguard against the wrongful or excessive dispensing of controlled substances. He does not accept any responsibility for the excessive dispensing which was allowed to occur on his watch. He chooses to place blame on

> everyone but himself. He shows no concern or interest in revising his negligent ways. He gives every indication that if allowed to continue the practice of pharmacy he will continue to ignore his statutory and common-sense responsibilities.

Based on these findings, the administrative law judge recommended licensure revocation, and the board adopted an order revoking the PIC's pharmacist license. From this order of revocation, the pharmacist appealed.

The PIC's argument on appeal was that the board had formally charged him with personally dispensing excessive controlled substances, yet at the hearing the board had argued that the PIC negligently allowed another person to dispense excessive controlled substances. In the legal notice provided to the PIC, the board had used the active voice, alleging that the PIC had "dispensed" and "furnished" opioids to the deceased patient. The pharmacist argued that he had unfairly been surprised by this change in board of pharmacy tactics, from alleging a personal failing to allegations of a failure in the supervision of another person, and that he had not been able to prepare a defense to the new charges.

The reviewing court agreed with the PIC:

> On this record, it is clear that the accusation did not afford the PIC the basic, appropriate elements of procedural due process, in that he was misled by the accusation into believing that he needed to prepare a defense to the personal dispensing charges. During the hearing, it became apparent to the board that the personal dispensing charges could not be sustained, and so without notice to the PIC the board shifted its theory to one of negligence as the pharmacist-in-charge.

The court concluded that the failure of the board's accusation to inform the PIC that the board was going to rely upon a negligent supervision theory, rather than a personal negligence theory, constituted a procedural due process violation. The revocation of the PIC's license was reversed.

The important message of this case is that licensees can't be "sandbagged" into thinking that they are being charged with a particular offense and then be subjected to license revocation based on a different offense. Every licensee who faces the possibility of license revocation has the right to provide a defense to the charges being made. Unless the charges against a licensee are known by the licensee, a defense cannot be developed and effectively presented to a hearing officer. In this case, the PIC was prepared to explain that he had not filled the prescriptions himself. He was not prepared to defend allegations of negligence in the oversight of actions taken by a nonpharmacist owner, because he had no way to anticipate that change in prosecutorial tactics. The board of pharmacy overstepped its authority in revoking the PIC's license.

Value of Professional Self-regulation

The purpose of a state board of pharmacy is to protect the public from unsafe pharmacy practices, including potentially lethal pharmacy practices. This purpose is achieved by enforcing regulatory standards of practice through disciplinary action when the established standards have not been met. Government action must serve a public purpose.

Basic principles of justice guide the conduct of disciplinary action taken by administrative agencies against pharmacists, pharmacies, and other licensed or permitted healthcare entities. Disciplinary action taken by a board of pharmacy is based on the principles of both corrective justice and retributive justice.

The primary goal of both corrective justice and retributive justice is to look back at a potentially harmful incident, or a series of potentially harmful incidents, and to make right the wrong(s) that occurred. A licensing agency need not wait for a tragedy to occur before taking action to prevent a tragedy from occurring. A secondary goal of both corrective justice and retributive justice is the deterrence of future wrongdoing. The concept is that if an actor understands that corrective justice and/or retributive justice will be meted out for the commission of a harmful act, then the actor will refrain from behaviors that are likely to result in harmful acts.

The discipline undertaken by boards of pharmacy toward pharmacist licenses and pharmacy permits combines both corrective justice and retributive justice. If the continuation of a license or permit would be harmful to the public health, then that license or permit can justly be revoked. It is, in effect, the correction of an incorrectly issued license or permit. The licensee or permittee who is the object of disciplinary action is also the subject of retributive justice due to the penal nature of the board's action. In all cases, the board of pharmacy's primary goal is deterrence of future harmful conduct. A board of pharmacy's recognized purpose is to protect the public from harmful outcomes that have not yet happened. Whereas criminal prosecution must be reactive, disciplinary action by a licensing agency can be proactive. Strong disciplinary action by the self-regulating profession of pharmacy, through its state board of pharmacy, has the potential to avoid the need for criminal prosecution.

Conclusion

Criminal prosecution is an action taken by the public against an individual who the prosecutor believes has violated social expectations and has caused harm to all the people through unnecessarily risky actions that perhaps have harmed only one person but could have harmed anyone. Prosecutors are elected or appointed to represent the people through the charging of crimes against the people. Although it is rare for a pharmacist to be charged with a crime for an error in practice, it is not out of the question. When a pharmacist's error appears to have been the result of recklessness and disregard of the best interest of patients, the pharmacist may be exposed to criminal prosecution. The avoidance of criminal prosecution requires that errors be reduced in frequency and magnitude and that steps be taken to demonstrate that when an error does occur, it happened despite the best efforts to prevent it.

Key Takeaways

- *Establish and follow pharmacy practice policies and procedures that are designed to prevent the harmful effects of pharmaceutical products and pharmaceutical services.* Criminal prosecutors will look for aberrations from the norm to determine whether a pharmacist who committed a fatal error was careful or reckless. A pharmacy's policies and procedures can serve as the basis on which that determination is made by a prosecutor. Compliance with P&Ps (policies and procedures) can be interpreted as being standard and expected practice. Violation of P&Ps can be interpreted as reckless practice. Pharmacists cannot guarantee good outcomes from drug therapy, and prosecutors recognize this reality. Pharmacists can guarantee that they will consistently take care in the provision of products and services to their patients. To protect themselves from criminal charges following an error that has caused harm to a patient, pharmacists must show prosecutors evidence that competent care was provided, even though an adverse outcome may have occurred.
- *Show that you care.* In everything you do, make sure that your care for patients shows. This includes the language you speak and the documentation you write. Abruptness and distraction can be misinterpreted as recklessness, even when the reality is that much more pressing matters require your attention and you simply are not able to devote the time to an additional concern. Take the time to explain that you care for the patient and that you care about the outcomes of the services that you provide. Let people see that you care. Whether it is a professional colleague or a patient who requests your attention, avoid any action or language that may result in that person later saying, "she/he didn't seem to care about the problem,

and look what happened." This assessment, wrong though it may be, can be misunderstood by a prosecutor as evidence of recklessness.

- *Don't let the system drag you down.* The healthcare system, of which the pharmacy system is a component, is far from perfect. These imperfections can set up individuals within the system to fail, potentially leading to criminal prosecution for the commission of a fatal error. Participate actively in institutional system enhancements. Resist the temptation to see yourself as the sole solution to systemic problems. You can't fix the system by yourself. Also resist the temptation to see yourself as the victim of the system's problems. That approach doesn't help anyone. When you see a problem with the system that poses immediate threats to patient safety, including lethal threats, then involve management in discussions of how to implement immediate solutions. Do not invite criminal prosecution by attempting to practice pharmacy in a system where significant harm to patients is inevitable.

References

1. Townley JN, Pogue CA, McHugh MD. Criminal prosecution of clinician errors: A setback to the progress toward safe hospital work environments. *J Hosp Med.* 2022 Oct;17(10):850–853.

2. Cohen J. The path between Sebastian's hospitals: Fostering reconciliation after a tragedy. *Barry L. Rev.* 2011 Fall;17(1):89–131.

3. Leape LL, Shore MF, Dienstag JL, Mayer RJ, Edgman-Levitan S, Meyer GS, Healy GB. Perspective: A culture of respect, part 2: Creating a culture of respect. *Acad Med.* 2012 Jul;87(7):853–858.

4. Ferner RE. Medication errors that have led to manslaughter charges. *BMJ.* 2000 Nov 11;321(7270):1212–1216.

5. Booth KN. Medical malpractice as murder? Using root cause analysis as a guiding framework for criminal medical malpractice. *West. Virg. Law Rev.* 2023 Fall;126(1):265–298.

6. Kaufman MB. New York State Council of Health-system Pharmacists: 2013 52nd Annual Assembly: Medication Safety. *P T.* 2013 Jul;38(7):425–426.

7. State v. Buman, 955 N.W.2d 215 (Iowa 2021).

8. Reason J. Human error: models and management. *BMJ.* 2000 Mar 18;320(7237):768–770.

9. United States v. Muoghalu, 662 F.3d 908 (7th Cir. 2011).

10. Monks P. Frankly my dear, I don't give a damn. *Med Sci Law.* 1996 Jul;36(3):185–187.

11. Sunscript Pharmacy Corporation v. North Carolina Board of Pharmacy, 555 S.E.2d 629 (N.C.App. 2001).

12. Smith v. California State Board of Pharmacy, 43 Cal.Rptr.2d 532 (Cal.App. 1995).

Afterword

Medications are similar to many other commercial goods because they can be both beneficial and detrimental. Lawn equipment, kitchen appliances, and power tools come to mind as the types of commercial products that can lead to both good and bad outcomes from their use. These are valuable and necessary products, yet they can be harmful products as well. What makes these other beneficial but potentially harmful products different from pharmaceutical products is the obviousness of the harm that they can cause. The possibility that a chain saw, or a hedge clipper will cut off a finger, or cause even worse damage to its user, is easy to see. Likewise, kitchen knives and pots of boiling water on a stove pose easily identified risks of harm. The potential hazards of automobiles and motorcycles are also quite clear. People continue to use these products despite the potential harm they represent, because the risks of using them can be understood and minimized through caution and attentiveness.

Medications are different. Their risks are not obvious. A solid or liquid drug dosage form may appear to be innocuous yet may contain a chemical entity that would be lethal if misused for a purpose other than legitimate pharmacotherapy. It is often a matter of a person's susceptibility to the effects of a chemical entity, when administered in a specific dose, and at a specific time, that determines whether the chemical entity will save a life or take a life. The role of the pharmacist is to promote the safe use of medications and to prevent the unsafe use of medications. This is an easy sentence to write and recite, but it is a difficult goal to meet.

Pharmacists are required to place patients at risk of harm, because there can be no benefit from medication use unless some level of risk is accepted. However, the risks to which patients are exposed must be measured risks. The use of a risky medication must be considered "worth the risk" in order to achieve therapeutic objectives. The knowledge and skill of a pharmacist can prevent harm from medication use, just as the knowledge and skill of an ordinary user can prevent harm from lawn equipment, kitchen paraphernalia, and transport vehicles. The pharmacist's knowledge is specific to one type of commercial product, and the pharmacist is responsible for anticipating and preventing harm that may be caused by that product.

In distributing medications, and in monitoring the effects of medications, pharmacists have a professional responsibility to anticipate and prevent criminal conduct with those medications. Pharmacists can't protect everyone from everything that may happen due to criminal conduct with a medication. But pharmacists can protect some people from being victimized by some criminals who consider some medications to be the "perfect weapon."

Pharmacists can make the “perfect crime” “less perfect” through their awareness of how medications have been used in the past by causing harm to innocent victims of a murderer’s criminality.

Patterns of criminality tend to repeat themselves. Copycat criminals learn from others. Pharmacists can identify circumstances that suggest an ill motive by a potential criminal or that demonstrate the vulnerability of a potential victim. As the health professionals who control access to the beneficial, yet risky, pharmaceutical product that is potentially lethal, pharmacists are not mere bystanders in either therapeutics or forensics. Pharmacists have a key role to play in the prevention of crimes with medications.